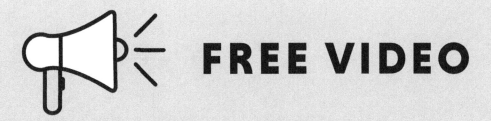

Essential Test Tips Video from Trivium Test Prep!

Thank you for purchasing from Trivium Test Prep!
We're honored to help you prepare for your exam.
To show our appreciation, we're offering a

FREE *Essential Test Tips* Video

Our video includes 35 test preparation strategies that will make you successful
on your big exam. All we ask is that you email us your feedback and describe
your experience with our product. Amazing, awful, or just so-so:
we want to hear what you have to say!

> To receive your **FREE** *Essential Test Tips* Video, please email us at
> **5star@triviumtestprep.com.**

Include "Free 5 Star" in the subject line and the following information in your email:

1. The title of the product you purchased.
2. Your rating from 1 – 5 (with 5 being the best).
3. Your feedback about the product, including how our materials helped you meet
   your goals and ways in which we can improve our products.
4. Your full name and shipping address so we can send your
   FREE *Essential Test Tips* Video.

If you have any questions or concerns please feel free to contact us directly at:
5star@triviumtestprep.com.

Thank you!

– Trivium Test Prep Team

CEN Review Book and Study Guide:

Comprehensive Review Manual
with Practice Test Questions
for the Certified Emergency Nurse Exam

E.M. Falgout

TABLE OF CONTENTS

ONLINE RESOURCES

To help you fully prepare for your Certified Emergency Nurse (CEN) Exam, Ascencia includes online resources with the purchase of this study guide.

PRACTICE TEST

In addition to the practice test included in this book, we also offer an online exam. Since many exams today are computer based, getting to practice your test-taking skills on the computer is a great way to prepare.

FLASH CARDS

A convenient supplement to this study guide, Ascencia's flash cards enable you to review important terms easily on your computer or smartphone.

FROM STRESS TO SUCCESS

Watch "From Stress to Success," a brief but insightful YouTube video that offers the tips, tricks, and secrets experts use to score higher on the exam.

REVIEWS

Leave a review, send us helpful feedback, or sign up for Ascencia promotions—including free books!

Access these materials at: www.ascenciatestprep.com/cen-online-resources

INTRODUCTION

Congratulations on choosing to take the Certified Emergency Nurse (CEN) Exam! Passing the CEN is an important step forward in your nursing career.

In the following pages, you will find information about the CEN, what to expect on test day, how to use this book, and the content covered on the exam. We also encourage you to visit the website of the Board of Certification for Emergency Nursing (https://bcen.org) to register for the exam and find the most current information on the CEN.

THE BCEN CERTIFICATION PROCESS

The **Certified Emergency Nurse (CEN) Exam** is developed by the **Board of Certification for Emergency Nursing (BCEN)** as part of its certification program for emergency nurses. The CEN measures the nursing skills necessary to excel as a nurse in an emergency department. To qualify for the exam, you must have a current Registered Nurse license in the United States or its territories. The BCEN also recommends that you have at least two years of nursing experience in an emergency department. There's no level of experience that's *required* for the exam, but many nurses find that the practical knowledge they have acquired while working in the ED is vital to passing the exam.

To register for the exam, you must first apply through the BCEN website (https://bcen.org/cen/apply-schedule). After your application is accepted, you will receive an email with instructions on how to register for the exam. The CEN is administered at PSI testing centers around the nation.

Once you have met the qualifications and passed the exam, you will have your CEN certification, and you may use the credentials as long as your certification is valid. You will need to recertify every four years. You can earn your recertification by taking continuing education courses or by retaking the exam. If you are taking the exam for recertification, you must submit your application 91 days before your certification lapses. You must then pass the exam within the 90-day testing window.

CEN Questions and Timing

The CEN consists of **175 questions**. Only 150 of these questions are scored; 25 are unscored, or *pretest* questions. These questions are included by the BCEN to test their suitability for inclusion in future tests. You'll have no way of knowing which questions are unscored, so treat every question like it counts.

The questions on the CEN are multiple-choice with four answer choices. Some questions will include exhibits such as ECG reading strips or laboratory results. The CEN has **no guess penalty**. That is, if you answer a question incorrectly, no points are deducted from your score; you simply do not get credit for that question. Therefore, you should always guess if you do not know the answer to a question.

You will have **3 hours** to complete the test. During this time you will also need to complete the BCEN Examination Rules and Regulations Agreement. You may take breaks at any point during the exam, but you will not be given extra time, and you cannot access personal items (other than medications).

CEN Content Areas

The BCEN develops its exams based on feedback from emergency nursing professionals about the nursing concepts and skills that are most important to their work. This feedback has been used to develop an exam framework that emphasizes the assessment, diagnosis, and treatment of conditions emergency nurses are likely to encounter in the ED.

The framework is broken down into seven sections loosely based on human body systems and one section devoted to professional issues. The table below gives the breakdown of the scored questions on the exam. The content outline objectives are listed at the beginning of each chapter.

QUICK Summary of CEN Test Sections	
Section	**No. of Scored Questions**
1. Cardiovascular Emergencies	19
2. Respiratory Emergencies	18
3. Neurological Emergencies	18
4. Gastrointestinal, Genitourinary, Gynecology, and Obstetrical Emergencies	18
5. Mental Health Emergencies	11
6. Medical Emergencies	14
7. Musculoskeletal and Wound Emergencies	13
8. Maxillofacial and Ocular Emergencies	11
9. Environment and Toxicology Emergencies, and Communicable Diseases	14
10. Professional Issues	14
Total	150 questions

EXAM RESULTS

Once you have completed your test, the staff at the Pearson VUE testing center will give you a score report; you can also request to receive the report via email. The score report will include your raw score (the number of questions you answered correctly) for the whole test and for each content area.

The report will also include a pass/fail designation. The number of correct answers needed to pass the exam will vary slightly depending on the questions included in your version of the test (i.e., if you took a version of the test with harder questions, the passing score will be lower). For most test takers, **a passing score will be between 105 and 110** questions answered correctly.

If you do not pass the exam, you will be able to reapply and retake the test after 90 days.

USING THIS BOOK

This book is divided into two sections. In the content area review, you will find the pathophysiology, risk factors, signs and symptoms, diagnostic findings, and treatment protocols for the conditions included in the CEN framework. Throughout the chapter you'll also see Quick Review Questions that will help reinforce important concepts and skills.

The book also includes two full-length practice tests (one in the book and one online) with answer rationales. You can use these tests to gauge your readiness for the test and determine which content areas you may need to review more thoroughly.

ASCENCIA TEST PREP

With health care fields such as nursing, pharmacy, emergency care, and physical therapy becoming the fastest-growing industries in the United States, individuals looking to enter the health care industry or rise in their field need high-quality, reliable resources. Ascencia Test Prep's study guides and test preparation materials are developed by credentialed industry professionals with years of experience in their respective fields. Ascencia recognizes that health care professionals nurture bodies and spirits, and save lives. Ascencia Test Prep's mission is to help health care workers grow.

1 CARDIOVASCULAR EMERGENCIES

Cardiovascular Anatomy and Physiology

- The heart has four chambers: the left atrium, right atrium, left ventricle, and right ventricle.
  - The **right atrium** collects blood from the body.
  - The **right ventricle** pumps blood to the lungs.

- The **left atrium** collects blood from the lungs.
- The **left ventricle** pumps blood to the body.
- The atria are separated by the **atrial septum**; the ventricles are separated by the **ventricular septum**.
- The **atrioventricular valves** are located between the atria and ventricles and cause the first heart sounds (S1) when they close.
  - The **tricuspid valve** separates the right atrium and right ventricle.
  - The **mitral valve** separates the left atrium and left ventricle.
- The two **semilunar valves** are located between the ventricles and great vessels and cause the second heart sound (S2) when they close.
  - The **pulmonic valve** separates the right ventricle and pulmonary artery.
  - The **aortic valve** separates the left ventricle and aorta.

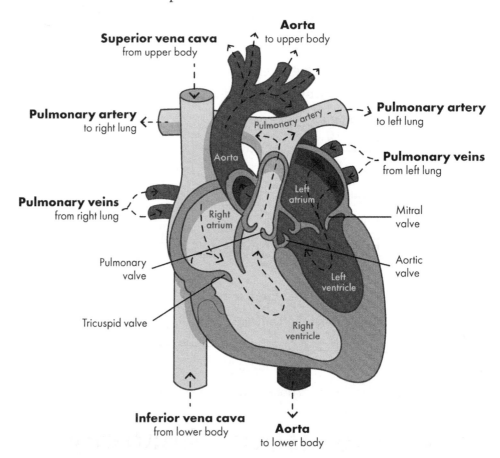

Figure 1.1. Anatomy of the Heart

- The heart is formed by layers of tissue.
  - **pericardium:** the outermost protective layer of the heart, which contains a lubricative liquid
  - **epicardium:** the deepest layer of the pericardium, which envelops the heart muscle

□ **myocardium**: the heart muscle

□ **endocardium**: the innermost, smooth layer of the heart walls

■ The heart's blood supply comes from the aorta, which branches into the **left main coronary artery (LCA)** and **right coronary artery (RCA)**. The LCA further divides into the **left anterior descending (LAD) artery and left circumflex artery**.

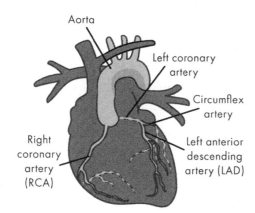

Figure 1.2. Coronary Arteries

■ The heart's pumping action is triggered by the **cardiac conduction system**, which produces and conducts the electrical signals in the heart that cause it to pump.

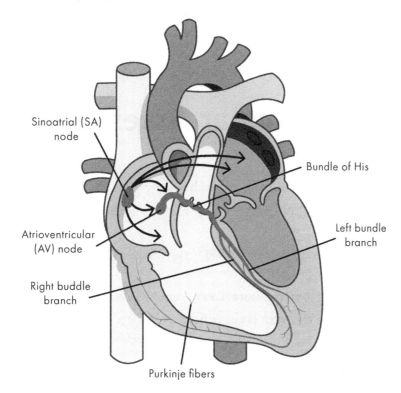

Figure 1.3. The Cardiac Conduction System

- During normal electrical conduction, the **sinoatrial (SA) node** sets the heart's pace by sending out electrical signals that cause the atria to contract. It is located in the anterior wall of the right atrium.
- The **atrioventricular (AV) node** relays the electrical impulse from the sinoatrial node to the ventricles. The impulse is delayed to allow the atria to fully contract and fill the ventricles. The node is located at the base of the right atrial wall.
- The **bundle of His** carries the electrical signal from the AV node to the **right** and **left bundle branches**.
- The end point of the conduction system is the **Purkinje fibers** in the endocardial layer that depolarize muscle cells, causing contraction of the ventricles.

- During the **cardiac cycle**, the heart alternates between **diastole** (relaxation) and **systole** (contraction) to move blood.
  - During atrial systole, the atria force blood into the ventricles.
  - During ventricular systole, the ventricles force blood into the arteries.
  - If the atria are in systole, the ventricles are in diastole; if the ventricles are in systole, the atria are in diastole.

HELPFUL HINT:

Coronary artery perfusion occurs during diastole. An elevated heart rate reduces the amount of time in diastole, thus reducing coronary artery perfusion by decreasing both the volume of blood flow and the time for perfusion to occur.

QUICK REVIEW QUESTION

1. Left-sided heart failure can cause pulmonary edema, while right-sided heart failure is more likely to cause edema in the abdomen and extremities. How does the anatomy of the heart produce this difference?

_____

Cardiovascular Assessment

HEMODYNAMICS

- **Heart rate (HR):** A normal pulse should be 60 – 100 bpm and regular.
- **Blood pressure (BP)** is the pressure exerted by blood on the inside of blood vessels.
  - **Systolic blood pressure (SBP)** is the pressure that occurs while the heart is contracting.
  - **Diastolic blood pressure (DBP)** occurs while the heart is relaxed.
  - The **pulse pressure** is the difference between the systolic and diastolic blood pressure (e.g., BP 120/80 = pulse pressure of 40).

TABLE 1.1. Classifying Blood Pressure

Blood Pressure Category	Systolic mm Hg		Diastolic mmHg
Normal	less than 120	and	less than 80
Elevated	120 – 129	and	less than 80
Hypertension, Stage 1	130 – 139	or	80 – 89
Hypertension, Stage 2	140 or higher	or	higher than 90
Hypertensive Crisis	higher than 180	and/or	higher than 120

- **Stroke volume (SV)** is the volume of blood pumped from the left ventricle during one contraction. Stroke volume is determined by:
  - **preload:** how much the ventricles stretch at the end of diastole (a measure of ventricular end-diastolic volume)
  - **afterload:** resistance the heart must overcome during systole to pump blood into circulation (a measure of aortic pressure and systemic vascular resistance [SVR])
  - **contractility:** the force of the heart independent of preload and afterload

TABLE 1.2. Hemodynamic Parameters

Parameter	Description	Normal Range
Central venous pressure (CVP) or right atrial pressure (RAP)	pressure in the vena cava; used to estimate preload	2 – 6 mm Hg
Pulmonary artery pressure (PAP)	pressure in the pulmonary artery	8 – 20 mm Hg
Stroke volume (SV)	volume of blood forced from the left ventricle with each contraction	60 – 100 mL/beat
Cardiac output (CO)	volume of blood pumped in a unit of time (usually per minute) $CO = SV \times HR$	4 – 8 mL/min
Cardiac index (CI)	CO relative to patient size $CI = CO/BSA$	2.5 – 4 L/min/m²
Mean arterial pressure (MAP)	average BP during a complete cardiac cycle $MAP = SBP + (2 \times DBP)/3$	70 – 100 mm Hg

continued on next page

TABLE 1.2. Hemodynamic Parameters (continued)

Parameter	Description	Normal Range
Systemic vascular resistance (SVR)	total peripheral vascular system resistance to blood flow $SVR = 80 \times (MAP - CVP)/CO$	700 – 1200 dyne · sec/cm^5
Pulmonary artery occlusion pressure (PAOP) or pulmonary capillary wedge pressure (PCWP)	indirect measurement of left atrial pressure; uses Swan-Ganz catheter to "wedge" inflated balloon into a branch of the pulmonary artery	6 – 12 mm Hg
Pulmonary vascular resistance (PVR)	vascular resistance to blood flow in the lungs $PVR = 80 \times (MPAP - PAOP)/CI$	255 – 285 dyne · sec/cm^5
Mixed venous saturation (SvO$_2$)	fraction of oxygen-saturated hemoglobin in veins (taken from pulmonary artery catheter [PAC])	60% – 80%
Central venous oxygen saturation (ScvO$_2$)	fraction of oxygen-saturated hemoglobin in veins; surrogate for SvO$_2$ (taken from central venous catheter)	> 70%
Left ventricular end-diastolic pressure (LVEDP)	pressure in the left ventricle before systole	5 – 12 mm Hg

QUICK REVIEW QUESTION

2. The nurse is reassessing a patient with severe sepsis after a fluid bolus and administration of vasopressors. What hemodynamic value would indicate an improvement?

_____

Cardiac Biomarkers

- **Cardiac biomarkers** measure damage to heart tissue.

TABLE 1.3. Cardiac Biomarkers

Test	Description	Normal Range
Troponin I (cTnI), troponin T (cTnT), and high sensitivity troponin (hs-cTnT)	proteins released when the heart muscle is damaged; high levels can indicate an MI but may also be due to other conditions that stress the heart (e.g., renal failure, HF, pulmonary embolism [PE]); levels peak 24 hours post-MI and can remain elevated for up to 2 weeks	cTnI: < 0.04 ng/mL cTnT: < 0.01 ng/mL hs-cTnT: < 22 ng/L for males and < 14 ng/L for females

Test	Description	Normal Range
Creatine kinase (CK)	responsible for muscle cell function; an increase indicates cardiac or skeletal muscle damage	22 – 198 U/L
Creatine kinase–muscle/brain (CK-MB)	cardiac marker for damaged heart muscle; often used to diagnose a secondary MI or ongoing cardio-vascular conditions; a high ratio of CK-MB to CK (high CK-MB/CK) indicates damage to heart muscle (as opposed to skeletal muscle)	normal CK-MB: 5 – 25 IU/L CK-MB/CK suggesting possible MI: 3 – 5%
B-type natriuretic peptide (BNP) and NT-ProBNP	elevated BNP reflects increased ventricular wall stress; strongly associated with myocardial infarction (MI)/damage and heart failure (HF); often ordered to assess for fluid volume overload as the results are quantitative	BNP: < 100 pg/mL NT-Pro BNP: < 125 pg/mL (under age 74), < 450 pg/ml (age 75 or above)
Lactate dehydrogenase (LDH)	enzyme released in the setting of organ or tissue damage; test is not specific to the heart but is asso-ciated with elevated levels 1 – 3 days after an MI	140-280 U/L

HELPFUL HINT:

The normal ranges given here are general guidelines; reference ranges will vary by facility.

QUICK REVIEW QUESTION

3. What laboratory findings indicate likely heart damage from NSTEMI/STEMI?

Heart Sounds

- **Heart sounds** are produced as blood moves through the heart.
  - The **S1** sound is caused by the closure of the AV valves and indicates the end of diastole and the beginning of systole. It coincides with the R wave on ECG.
  - The **S2** sound is caused by the closure of the semilunar valves and indicates the end of systole and the beginning of diastole.
  - The **S3 (ventricular gallop)** is an extra heart sound heard after S2 and caused by a rush of blood into a ventricle. It is found in patients with decompensated CHF, a normal finding in children and during pregnancy, and sounds like the word "Ken-tuc-ky."
  - The **S4 (atrial gallop)** sound is an extra heart sound heard before S1 and caused by the atrial contraction of blood into a noncompliant

ventricle. It occurs with conditions like MI and left ventricular hypertrophy (LVH) and sounds like the word "Ten-ne-ssee."

- □ A **summation gallop** is when S3 and S4 are heard together. This sound strongly suggests severe myocardial failure.

- **Murmurs** are the sounds made by turbulent blood flow in and around the heart.
  - □ Murmurs can be systolic (occurring during ventricular contraction) or diastolic (occurring during ventricular filling).
  - □ Murmurs are graded by how easily they can be auscultated.

TABLE 1.4. Grades of Murmurs

Grade	Description
Grade I (1)	barely audible
Grade II (2)	audible but faint
Grade III (3)	moderately loud; easily heard
Grade IV (4)	loud; associated with a thrill
Grade V (5)	very loud; heard with one corner of stethoscope off the chest wall
Grade VI (6)	loudest; audible with the stethoscope off the chest

- □ Abnormal murmurs can be caused by septal defects, infections, or structural damage (e.g., stenosis or endocarditis).

- **Pericardial friction rub** is a high-pitched, leathery sound heard characteristically in pericarditis.
  - □ heard loudest at the fourth and fifth intercostal spaces, with patient leaning forward
  - □ will continue even if patient is holding breath

- **Carotid bruits** are abnormal sounds heard over the carotid artery caused by turbulent blood flow. They can be heard with a Doppler or stethoscope and may indicate carotid artery disease.

QUICK REVIEW QUESTION

4. Which abnormal heart sound might a nurse expect to hear in a patient with HF?

_____

ELECTROCARDIOGRAMS (ECG)

- An **electrocardiogram (ECG)** is a noninvasive diagnostic tool that records the heart's electrical activity.

■ **Electrodes** placed on the skin detect the electrical signals sent by cardiac tissue and produce a waveform that can be examined for changes in heart rate or rhythm.

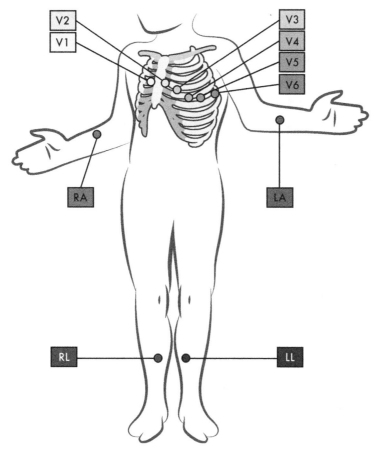

Figure 1.4. Twelve-Lead ECG Electrode Placement

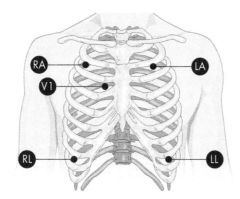

Figure 1.5. 5-Lead ECG Electrode Placement

■ Sets of electrodes form **leads** that show electrical activity in specific parts of the heart.

   □ When current flows toward a lead, it produces a positive deflection (an upright wave).

☐ When current flows away from a lead, it produces a negative deflection (a downward wave).

- A **12-lead ECG** includes three types of leads: **limb leads** (I, II, and III), **augmented limb leads** (aVR, aVL, and aVF), and **precordial leads** (V1 – V6).

- **Posterior leads** (V7, V8, and V9) are placed on the patient's back when a posterior infarction is suspected.

- **Right-side leads** (V3R, V4R, V5R, and V6R) are placed on the patient's right side in a mirror image of V3 – V6 when a right ventricular infarction is suspected.

- A **5-lead ECG** shows leads I, II, and II and one precordial lead. A **3-lead ECG** shows only leads I, II, and III.

- The waveforms and intervals on the ECG strip correspond to the cardiac cycle.

  ☐ **P wave:** represents atrial depolarization and should measure 0.06 – 0.11 seconds

  ☐ **PR interval:** represents the AV conduction time and should measure 0.12 – 0.20 seconds

  ☐ **QRS complex:** represents ventricular depolarization and should measure 0.08 – 0.10 seconds

  ☐ **T wave:** represents the repolarization of the ventricles

  ☐ **U wave:** theorized to represent late repolarization of the His-Purkinje system

  ☐ **QT interval:** represents the total time of ventricular activity (depolarization and repolarization) and should measure 0.36 – 0.44 seconds

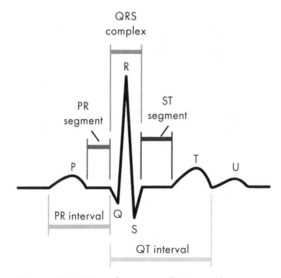

Figure 1.6. Waveforms and Intervals on an ECG

- ☐ **ST segment:** shows the early part of ventricular repolarization
- ☐ **RR interval:** the distance between QRS complexes
- **Normal sinus rhythm** reflects the normal pathway of electrical impulses through the cardiac conduction system.

QUICK REVIEW QUESTIONS

5. Which waveform or interval is highlighted in the figure below?

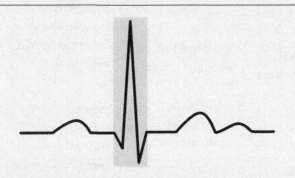

6. If a rhythm is missing P waves, which area of the heart is having difficulty conducting?

Cardiovascular Pharmacology

TABLE 1.5. Cardiovascular Medications			
Category	**Action**	**Indications**	**Common Side Effects**
ACE inhibitors (ACE-Is) lisinopril, ramipril, enalapril, benazepril	lower SVR, resulting in decreased BP	• hypertension (first line) • CHF • medical management post-MI	dry cough contraindicated in hyperkalemia
Alpha1-adrenergic agonists methoxamine, midodrine, phenylephrine	increase SVR, resulting in increased BP	• hypotension • shock	hypertension pounding in the ears

continued on next page

TABLE 1.5. Cardiovascular Medications (continued)

Category	Action	Indications	Common Side Effects
Arterial vasodilators hydralazine, minoxidil	relaxes vascular smooth muscle leading to arterial vasodilation	• hypertension (as adjunct therapy)	reflex tachycardia
Angiotensin II receptor blockers (ARBs) valsartan, losartan, irbesartan	use a mechanism of action similar to that of ACE inhibitors but cause fewer adverse effects	• hypertension (second line if intolerant to ACE inhibitors) • HF • medical management post-MI (second line if intolerant to ACE inhibitors)	hyperkalemia renal impairment
Anticoagulants warfarin, apixaban, rivaroxaban, enoxaparin, heparin	increase clotting time via various mechanisms that disrupt production of clotting factors	• known thrombosis (e.g., PE or DVT) • prophylaxis of thrombosis (e.g., after A-fib, cardiac post-op procedures) • adjunct therapy in mechanical valve replacements, MI, and stroke	bleeding
Antidysrhythmics amiodarone, flecainide, procainamide, sotalol	suppress cardiac dysrhythmias and restore normal cardiac conduction	• dysrhythmias (hemodynamically stable)	bradycardia liver dysfunction
Beta-adrenergic antagonists (beta blockers) metoprolol, carvedilol, atenolol, propranolol, labetalol	lower BP and heart rate, decrease CO, and slow AV node conduction	• medical management post-MI (first line) • chronic angina • hypertension (second line) • cardiac dysrhythmias (A-fib, SVT)	bradycardia fatigue

Category	Action	Indications	Common Side Effects
Calcium channel blockers amlodipine, nicardipine, diltiazem, verapamil	cause coronary vasodilation, which slows cardiac conduction, decreases heart rate, and decreases myocardial contraction	• hypertension • variant (Prinzmetal) angina • artery vasospasm	pedal edema facial flushing
Cardiac glycosides digoxin	increase myocardial contraction, decrease heart rate, slow cardiac conduction, and increase CO	• atrial dysrhythmias (e.g., A-fib) • paroxysmal SVT conversion • HF (although not first line treatment)	vision changes (halos) renal impairment
Central alpha2 agonists clonidine, methyldopa	causes vasodilation, resulting in decreased SVR, HR, and contractility	• hypertension (as adjunct therapy) • hypertension in pregnancy	bradycardia drowsiness
Loop diuretics furosemide, torsemide, bumetanide	increase excretion of water and electrolytes	• hypertension • volume management in HF • edema	hypokalemia
Nitrates nitroprusside, nitroglycerin	cause vasodilation, which decreases preload, afterload, and CO; reduces work effort of LV	• ACS • hypertension	hypotension headache
inotropic/ vasodilator agents milrinone	vasodilator; increase SV and CO	• emergent HF	chest pain headache tremors

continued on next page

TABLE 1.5. Cardiovascular Medications (continued)

Category	Action	Indications	Common Side Effects
Sympathomimetics epinephrine, norepinephrine, dobutamine, dopamine	alpha- and beta-adrenergic agonists that cause vaso-constriction, increased force of cardiac contraction, or increased rate of cardiac conduction (depending on the affected receptors)	• hypotension • HF • cardiogenic shock • cardiac arrest, asystole, PEA • acute bronchospasm • anaphylaxis	tachycardia headache nausea/vomiting
Thiazide diuretics hydrochlorothiazide, chlorothiazide, chlorthalidone, metolazone	increase excretion of sodium and water	• hypertension (first-line) • fluid volume management	hypokalemia dizziness
Thrombolytics (fibrinolytics) tPA or alteplase, tenecteplase	promote destruction of fibrin clots	• MI when coronary angiography is unavailable • acute CVA • massive PE	bleeding

QUICK REVIEW QUESTIONS

7. Why are beta blockers contraindicated for patients with second-degree AV blocks?

_____

8. What hemodynamic response should the nurse expect to observe in a patient after administration of diltiazem IV push?

_____

Cardiac Interventions

- **Synchronized electrical cardioversion** uses electrical current supplied by external electrode pads placed on the chest to reset the heart to a normal sinus rhythm.
  - Current is supplied during the R wave of the QRS complex.
  - Indicated for narrow or wide QRS complex tachycardias (per ACLS guidelines), SVT, V-tach with a pulse, A-fib, and atrial flutter.
- During **defibrillation**, also known as **unsynchronized cardioversion**, electrical current is used to reset the heart to a normal sinus rhythm.
  - The electrical current is supplied randomly during the cardiac cycle, disrupting the heart's electrical rhythm and allowing the SA node's impulse to return to normal sinus rhythm.
  - indicated for pulseless V-tach and V-fib
- An **implantable cardioverter-defibrillator (ICD)** can be programmed to provide cardioversion or defibrillation to prevent sudden cardiac death in patients at high risk for V-tach or V-fib (e.g., structural heart disease, LVEF < 35%).
- A **pacemaker** is a device that uses electrical stimulation to regulate the heart's electrical conduction system and maintain a normal heart rhythm.
  - **Temporary pacemakers** can include transvenous leads or transcutaneous adhesive pads attached to the chest (**transcutaneous pacing [TCP]**). Temporary pacemakers are controlled by an external pulse generator.
  - **Permanent pacemakers** are implanted subcutaneously, and the leads are then run through the subclavian vein into the heart. The device is battery operated and allows the physician to continuously monitor the patient's cardiac rhythm.
  - The electrical activity of the pacemaker appears on the ECG as a **pacing spike**, a sharp vertical line that may appear below or above the isoelectric line.

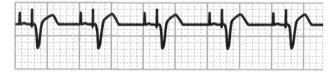

Figure 1.7. Pacing Spikes (AV Pacing)

- In a **coronary angiogram procedure** (also called **cardiac catheterization** or **left heart catheterization**), a catheter is inserted into a large blood vessel to diagnose and treat damage in the arteries, heart muscles, and valves.

☐ During an **angioplasty,** a balloon is placed in the stenotic artery via a catheter and is inflated to open the artery. A **stent** may be placed to hold the artery open.

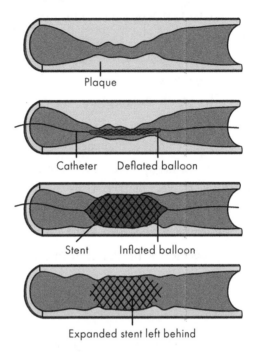

Plaque

Catheter   Deflated balloon

Stent   Inflated balloon

Expanded stent left behind

Figure 1.8. Angioplasty with Stent

☐ **Percutaneous coronary intervention (PCI)** (also called coronary angioplasty) is used to revascularize the coronary arteries in patients with ACS.

■ A **coronary artery bypass graft (CABG)** revascularizes ischemic heart tissue by bypassing blocked coronary arteries. Blood is diverted from the left internal mammary artery to a patent portion of a coronary

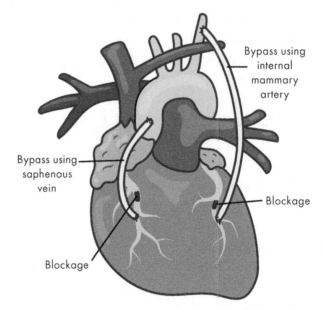

Bypass using internal mammary artery

Bypass using saphenous vein

Blockage

Blockage

Figure 1.9. Coronary Artery Bypass Graft (CABG)

artery or by grafting a section of the great saphenous vein from the aorta to below the blocked vessel.

- **Intra-aortic balloon pump (IABP) therapy** is used in patients with cardiogenic shock to increase coronary artery perfusion and cardiac output. The intra-aortic balloon is inserted into the ascending aortic arch via the femoral artery.

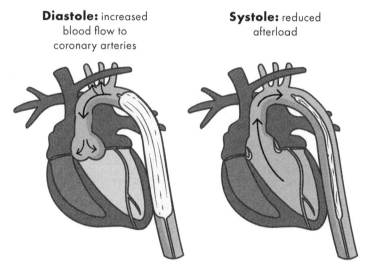

Diastole: increased blood flow to coronary arteries

Systole: reduced afterload

Figure 1.10. Intra-Aortic Balloon Pump (IABP) Therapy

- **Left ventricular assist devices (LVADs)** provide support for a severely weakened left ventricle in patients with end-stage HF. An implanted mechanical pump in the left ventricle moves blood from the left ventricle to the ascending aortic branch, so that blood can be pumped to the rest of the body.

QUICK REVIEW QUESTION

9. A patient presents to the ED with chest pain, dyspnea, and diaphoresis. The nurse finds a narrow complex tachycardia with a heart rate of 210 bpm, blood pressure of 70/42 mm Hg, and a respiratory rate of 18. The nurse should anticipate which priority intervention?

Acute Coronary Syndrome

Pathophysiology

Acute coronary syndrome (ACS) is an umbrella term for cardiac conditions in which thrombosis impairs blood flow in coronary arteries. **Angina pectoris** (commonly called just angina) is chest pain caused by narrowed coronary arteries and presents with negative troponin, an ST depression, and T wave changes.

- **Stable angina** usually resolves in about 5 minutes. It is resolved with medications or rest and can be triggered by exertion, large meals, and extremely hot or cold temperatures.

- **Unstable angina** can occur at any time and typically lasts longer (> 20 minutes). The pain is usually rated as more severe than stable angina and is not easily relieved with nitrates.

- **Variant angina** (also called Prinzmetal angina or vasospastic angina) is episodes of angina and temporary ST elevation caused by spasms in the coronary artery. Chest pain is easily relieved with nitrates.

A **myocardial infarction (MI),** or ischemia of the heart muscle, occurs when the coronary arteries are partly or completely occluded. An MI is diagnosed via positive troponin and ECG changes; it is classified by the behavior of the ST wave. A **non-ST-elevation myocardial infarction (NSTEMI)** includes an ST depression and a T wave inversion. _**An ST-elevation myocardial infarction (STEMI) includes an elevated ST (≥ 1 mm), indicating a complete occlusion of a coronary artery.**_

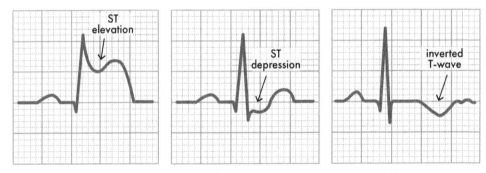

Figure 1.11. ECG Changes Associated with ACS

Signs, symptoms, and diagnostic findings for MI vary according to which coronary artery is occluded.

- **Septal/Anterior wall MI** is occlusion of the LAD artery, which supplies blood to the anterior of the left atrium and ventricle. **Septal MI** may occur alongside anterior wall MI (but is rarely diagnosed in isolation).
  - _ST changes in V1 – V4_
  - _increased risk of left ventricular failure (and subsequent cardiogenic shock)_
  - increased risk of second-degree, type II heart block and BBB
  - increased risk of ventricular septal rupture (usually 2 – 7 days post MI)

- **Inferior wall MI** is occlusion of the RCA, which supplies blood to the right atrium and ventricle, the SA node, and the AV node.
  - ST changes in II, III, aVF
  - presents with bradycardia and hypotension
  - increased risk of AV heart blocks (because of the proximity to the SA/AV nodes)
  - increased risk for papillary muscle rupture
  - beta blockers and nitrates used cautiously to avoid reducing preload
- **Right ventricular infarction** may occur with inferior wall MI.
  - ST changes in V4R – V6R
  - presents with tachycardia, hypotension, and JVD
  - treat with positive inotropes
  - ***avoid preload-reducing medications (beta blockers, diuretics, morphine, nitrates)***
- **Lateral wall MI** is occlusion of the left circumflex artery, which supplies blood to the left atrium and the posterior/lateral walls of the left ventricle. Changes in ST may be seen in I, aVL, V5, or V6.
- **Posterior wall MI** is occlusion of the RCA or left circumflex artery, with ST elevation in V7 – V9 and ST depression in V1 – V4. Posterior wall MI is rare but may be missed or read as an NSTEMI on a 12-lead ECG.

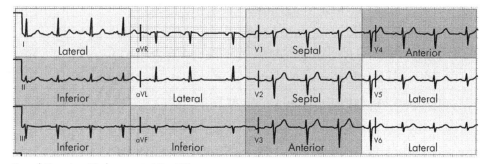

Septal/Anterior: ST changes in V1 – V4
Inferior: ST changes in II, III, aVF
Right Ventricular: ST changes in V4R – V6R
Lateral-wall: ST changes in I, aVL, V5, V6
Posterior-wall: ST elevation in V7 – V9 and ST depression in V1 – V4

Figure 1.12. ECG Leads Changes in STEMI by Location

Physical Examination

- continuous chest pain that may radiate to the back, arm, or jaw (possible Levine's sign)

- upper abdominal pain (more common in adults > 65, people with diabetes, and women)
- dyspnea
- nausea or vomiting
- dizziness or syncope
- diaphoresis and pallor
- palpitations

Diagnostic Tests

- elevated troponin (> 0.01 ng/mL)
- elevated CK-MB (> 2.5%)

Management

- An early invasive strategy with coronary angiogram is the gold standard treatment for STEMI.
  - *__Anticipate patient transfer to cath lab for diagnostic evaluation with possible PCI.__*
  - Treat with fibrinolytic agents (alteplase) if cath lab services are not available.
    - goal for door to balloon time: 90 minutes
    - goal for door to fibrinolytics: 30 minutes
  - Post-procedure antithrombotic therapy may include aspirin, clopidogrel, abciximab, eptifibatide, and/or heparin.
- NSTEMI is initially treated with medication (may require PCI).
- pharmacological management for ACS
  - nitroglycerin
  - antiplatelets: aspirin 325 mg (chewable) and platelet P2Y12 inhibitors (e.g., clopidogrel or ticagrelor)
  - supplemental oxygen
  - anticoagulant (heparin or low molecular weight heparin)
  - beta blocker (usually metoprolol as first choice)
  - morphine (only for severe pain not relieved by nitroglycerin)
- isolated right ventricular infarction
  - IV fluids
  - antiplatelets and anticoagulants
  - cautious use of nitrates, beta blockers, and morphine

HELPFUL HINT:

Contraindications for beta blocker use during STEMI include bradycardia, hypotension, cardiogenic shock, and heart block.

Aneurysm and Dissection

Pathophysiology

An **abdominal aortic aneurysm (AAA)**, often called a triple A, occurs when the lower aorta is enlarged. Other common aneurysms include thoracic aneurysms and thoracoabdominal aortic aneurysms.

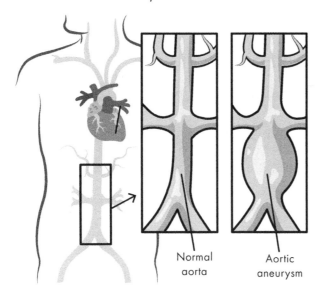

Normal aorta

Aortic aneurysm

Figure 1.13. Abdominal Aortic Aneurysm (AAA)

An **aortic rupture**, a complete tear in the wall of the aorta, rapidly leads to hemorrhagic shock and death. An **aortic dissection** is a tear in the aortic intima; the tear allows blood to enter the aortic media. Both aortic rupture and dissection will lead to hemorrhagic shock and death without immediate intervention.

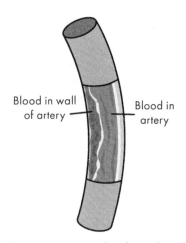

Blood in wall of artery

Blood in artery

Figure 1.14. Aortic Dissection

Risk Factors

- hypertension

- heart disease

- lifestyle factors (smoking, poor diet, lack of exercise)

- genetic syndromes in which connective tissues are weakened (e.g., Marfan syndrome)

- trauma

HELPFUL HINT:

Approximately 75% of aortic aneurysms occur in men.

Physical Examination

- _sharp, severe pain in the chest, back, abdomen, or flank; often described as "tearing"_

- rapid, weak, or absent pulse

- _a blood pressure difference of [3] ≥ 20 mm Hg between the left and right arms_

- new-onset murmur

- diaphoresis

- nausea and vomiting

- pallor

- hypotension

- orthopnea

Diagnostic Tests

- CT scan, TEE, angiogram, or chest MRI

Management

- pain management (usually morphine)
- beta blockers; nitroprusside may also be given
- hemodynamically unstable patients: immediate surgical repair usually required

HELPFUL HINT:

Positive inotropes are contraindicated in patients with aortic dissection because the medications increase stress on the aortic wall.

HELPFUL HINT:

Torsades de pointes, a type of V-tach with irregular QRS complexes, occurs with a prolonged QT interval. It can be congenital or caused by antidysrhythmics, antipsychotics, hypokalemia, or hypomagnesemia.

Cardiopulmonary Arrest

Pathophysiology

Ventricular tachycardia (V-tach) is tachycardia originating below the bundle of His, resulting in slowed ventricular activation. During V-tach, ≥ 3 consecutive ventricular beats occur at a rate > 100 bpm. V-tach is often referred to as a **wide-complex tachycardia** because of the width of the QRS complex.

Because the ventricles cannot refill before contracting, patients in this rhythm may have reduced cardiac output, resulting in hypotension. V-tach may be short and asymptomatic, or it may precede V-fib and cardiac arrest. Pulse-less V-tach is unstable and should be treated the same as V-fib.

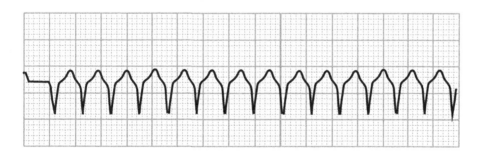

Figure 1.15. ECG: Monomorphic Ventricular Tachycardia

During **ventricular fibrillation (V-fib)** the ventricles contract rapidly (300 – 400 bpm) with no organized rhythm. There is no cardiac output. The ECG will initially show **coarse V-fib** with an amplitude > 3 mm. As V-fib continues, the amplitude of the waveform decreases, progressing through **fine V-fib** (< 3 mm) and eventually reaching asystole.

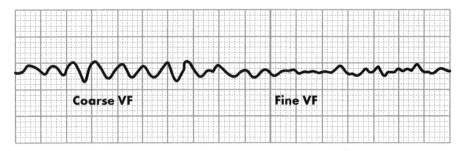

Figure 1.16. ECG: Ventricular Fibrillation

Pulseless electrical activity (PEA) is an organized rhythm in which the heart does not contract with enough force to create a pulse. **Asystole**, also called a "flat line," occurs when there is no electrical or mechanical activity within the heart. Both PEA and asystole are nonshockable rhythms with a poor survival rate.

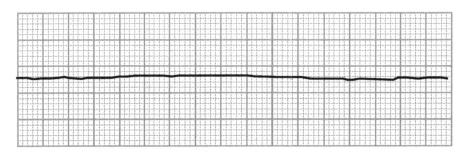

Figure 1.17. ECG: Asystole

Management

- priority intervention for V-tach: check for pulse
  - □ V-tach with a pulse, patient stable: administer amiodarone
  - □ V-tach with a pulse, patient unstable: synchronized cardioversion
- *follow the advanced cardiovascular life support (ACLS) protocols for patients in pulseless V-tach, V-fib, PEA, and asystole*

QUICK REVIEW QUESTIONS

15. What intervention should the nurse anticipate for a hemodynamically unstable patient in V-tach with a pulse?

_____

16. What is the first-line medication for patients whose V-fib is unresponsive to defibrillation?

_____

17. A patient is found in bed unresponsive to commands. The patient appears cyanotic, and the nurse determines there is no pulse and no breathing present. What should the nurse do first?

_____

18. What medication is administered to patients in asystole?

_____

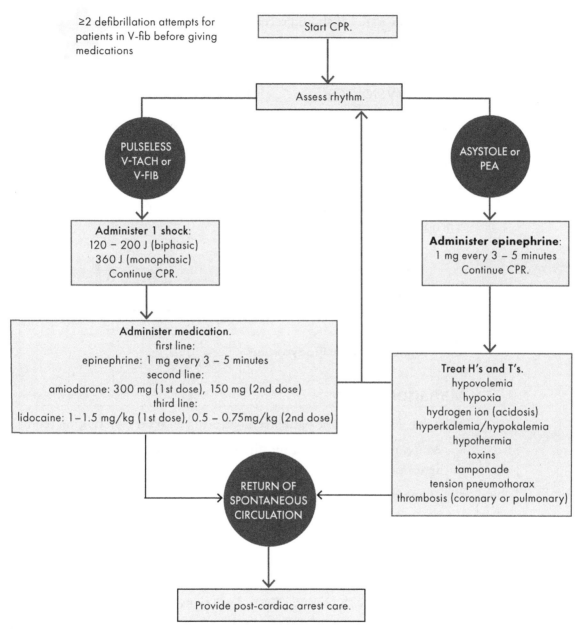

Figure 1.18. ACLS Cardiac Arrest Algorithm (Simplified)

Dysrhythmias

A cardiac **dysrhythmia** is an abnormal heartbeat or rhythm. Dysrhythmias are typically caused by a malfunction in the heart's cardiac conduction system. Most dysrhythmias of clinical importance are caused by **reentry**: the re-excitation of the heart by an electrical impulse that did not die out. Reentry dysrhythmias include A-fib, atrial flutter, V-tach, and V-fib.

HELPFUL HINT:

When treating dysrhythmias, medical staff should always consider a hypotensive patient unstable.

Treatment is based on whether the patient is deemed hemodynamically stable or unstable.

- Stable patients can receive noninvasive interventions or drugs as a priority intervention to correct an abnormal rhythm.

- Unstable patients should receive the appropriate electrical therapy.

BRADYCARDIA

Pathophysiology

Bradycardia is a heart rate of < 60 bpm. It results from a decrease in the sinus node impulse formation (automaticity). Bradycardia is normal in certain individuals and does not require an intervention if the patient is stable or asymptomatic. Symptomatic patients, however, need immediate treatment to address the cause of bradycardia. Symptoms of bradycardia may include hypotension, syncope, confusion, or dyspnea.

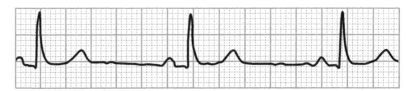

Figure 1.19. ECG: Bradycardia

Management

- stable, asymptomatic patients: monitoring with no intervention required
- symptomatic, hemodynamically stable patients: monitor while determining underlying cause
- symptomatic, hemodynamically unstable patients: medication
  - first line: atropine 0.5 mg for first dose, with a maximum of 3 mg total
  - second line: dopamine or epinephrine if atropine is ineffective or if maximum dose of atropine already given and patient is still stable
  - patients with bradycardia and who have had a heart transplant: administer isoproterenol (atropine is ineffective in these patients)
- unstable patients who do not respond to medication: TCP (first line), transvenous cardiac pacing (second line)

QUICK REVIEW QUESTIONS

19. A patient presents with complaints of confusion, dizziness, and dyspnea. The patient's blood pressure is 72/40 mm Hg, with a heart rate of 32 bpm and O$_2$ saturation of 92% on room air. What priority intervention should the nurse prepare for?

NARROW-COMPLEX TACHYCARDIAS

Pathophysiology

Narrow-complex tachycardias (also called **supraventricular tachycardias [SVT]**) are dysrhythmias with > 100 bpm and a narrow QRS complex (< 0.12 seconds). The dysrhythmia originates at or above the bundle of His (supraventricular), resulting in rapid ventricular activation. Specific SVT rhythms include AV nodal reentrant tachycardia (AVNRT), AV reentrant tachycardia (AVRT), and atrial tachycardia (AT).

Narrow-complex tachycardias are often asymptomatic. Symptomatic patients may have palpitations, chest pain, hypotension, and dyspnea.

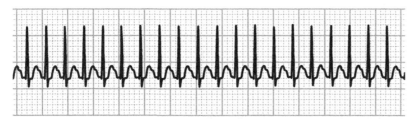

Figure 1.20. ECG: Supraventricular Tachycardia

Management

- first line: vagal maneuvers
- second line: medication
  - rapid bolus dose of adenosine 6 mg
  - second dose of adenosine 12 mg given if chemical cardioversion does not occur within 1 – 2 minutes
- refractory SVT
  - stable patients: calcium channel blockers (e.g., diltiazem), beta blockers, or digoxin
  - unstable patients and patients for whom medications are ineffective: synchronized cardioversion

ATRIAL FIBRILLATION AND FLUTTER

Pathophysiology

Atrial fibrillation (A-fib) is an irregular narrow-complex dysrhythmia. During A-fib, the atrium does not contract normally, which may cause blood clots to form in the left atrium (on the left atrial appendage), increasing stroke risk. The irregular atrial contractions also decrease cardiac output.

In **atrial fibrillation with rapid ventricular response (A-fib with RVR)**, the ventricular rate is > 100 bpm. The ECG in A-fib will show an irregular ventricular rhythm with no clear P waves and an undeterminable atrial rate.

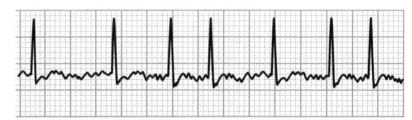

Figure 1.21. ECG: Atrial Fibrillation

During **atrial flutter**, the atria beat regularly but too fast (240 – 400 bpm), causing multiple atrial beats in between the ventricular beat. Atrial flutter can be regular or irregular. The ECG in atrial flutter will show a saw-toothed flutter and multiple P waves for each QRS complex.

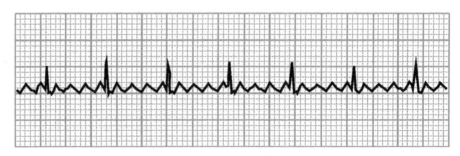

Figure 1.22. ECG: Atrial Flutter

Management

- _**adenosine: slows the rhythm so that it may be identified (i.e., discern between atrial dysrhythmia and SVT), but will not convert dysrhythmia to a sinus rhythm**_
- hemodynamically stable patients: medication

- calcium channel blockers (diltiazem), beta blockers, or cardiac glycoside to slow the rhythm
- antidysrhythmics (amiodarone) to convert to sinus rhythm
- hemodynamically unstable patients: cardioversion
- anticoagulation to lower risk of stroke
- cardiac ablation may be used to correct A-fib and atrial flutter

Myocardial Conduction System Defects

Atrioventricular Blocks

Pathophysiology

An **atrioventricular (AV) block** is the disruption of electrical signals between the atria and ventricles. The electrical impulse may be delayed (first-degree block), intermittent (second-degree block), or completely blocked (third-degree block).

A **first-degree AV block** occurs when the conduction between the SA and the AV nodes is slowed, creating a prolonged PR interval. A first-degree AV block is a benign finding that is usually asymptomatic, but it can progress to a second-degree or third-degree block.

The ECG in a first-degree AV block will show a prolonged PR interval of > 0.20 seconds.

HELPFUL HINT:

If the R is far from P, then you have a *first degree.*
Longer, longer, longer, *drop,* this is how you know it's a *Wenckebach.*
If some Ps just don't go *through,* then you know it's a *type 2.*
If Ps and Qs don't agree, then you have a *third degree.*

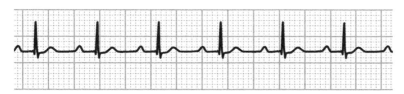

Figure 1.23. ECG: First-Degree Atrioventricular (AV) Block

A **second-degree AV block, type 1** (Wenckebach or Mobitz type 1), occurs when the PR interval progressively lengthens until the atrial impulse is completely blocked and does not produce a QRS impulse. This dysrhythmia occurs when the atrial conduction in the AV node or bundle of His is either slowed or blocked. This type of block is cyclic; after the dropped QRS complex, the pattern will repeat itself.

The ECG in second-degree AV block, type 1, will show progressively longer PR intervals until a QRS complex completely drops.

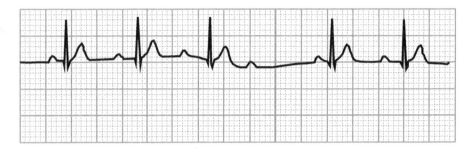

Figure 1.24. ECG: Second-Degree AV Block, Type 1

A **second-degree AV block, type 2** (Mobitz type 2), occurs when the PR interval is constant in length but not every P wave is followed by a QRS complex. This abnormal rhythm is the result of significant conduction dysfunction within the His-Purkinje system.

The ECG in second-degree AV block, type 2, will show constant PR intervals and extra P waves, with dropped QRS complexes.

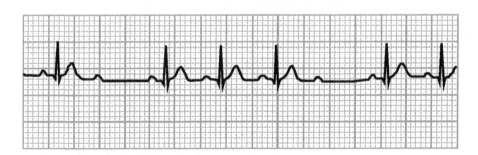

Figure 1.25. ECG: Second-Degree AV Block, Type 2

A **third-degree AV block**, sometimes referred to as a complete heart block, is characterized by a complete dissociation between the atria and the ventricles. There are effectively 2 pacemakers within the heart, so there is no correlation between the P waves and the QRS complexes. The most common origin of the block is below the bundle of His, but the block can also occur at the level of the bundle branches of the AV node.

The ECG for third-degree AV block will show regular P waves and QRS complexes that occur at different rates. There will be more P waves than QRS complexes, with P waves possibly buried within the QRS complex.

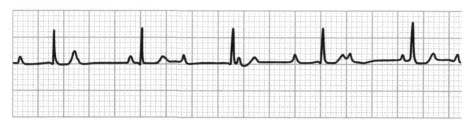

Figure 1.26. ECG: Third-Degree AV Block

Physical Examination

- first- and second-degree AV blocks usually asymptomatic
- may show symptoms of reduced cardiac output (e.g., hypotension, dyspnea, chest pain)
- bradycardia

Management

- symptomatic patients: TCP possibly needed to manage symptoms
- implantable pacemaker if underlying cause cannot be resolved
- hypotensive patients: dopamine or epinephrine may be needed
- discontinue medications that slow electrical conduction in the heart (e.g., antidysrhythmtics, beta blockers)

QUICK REVIEW QUESTION

25. A patient begins to complain of dizziness and weakness and appears diaphoretic. The nurse notes from the telemetry monitor that the patient has a third-degree AV block. BP is 71/55 mm Hg, and HR is 30 bpm. What interventions does the nurse expect?

HELPFUL HINT:

Atropine is ineffective for Mobitz type 2 and third-degree AV blocks. It only increases the firing of the SA node, and the block prevents the SA node from influencing ventricular contraction.

BUNDLE BRANCH BLOCK

- **Right bundle branch block (RBBB)** and **left bundle branch block (LBBB)** are interruptions in conduction through a bundle branch.

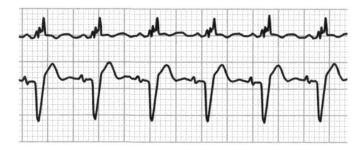

Figure 1.27. ECG: Bundle Branch Blocks

- Ischemic heart disease is the most common cause of both RBBB and LBBB.
  - LBBB can also arise from other heart diseases, hypertension, digoxin, or cardiomyopathy.
  - Other causes of RBBB include cor pulmonale, pulmonary embolism, and COPD.
  - Both RBBB and LBBB may occur in the absence of heart disease.
- LBBB in particular is associated with progressive underlying structural heart disease and is associated with poor outcomes post MI.
- If the patient with a BBB is asymptomatic, no treatment is necessary.
- Patients with syncopal episodes may need to have a pacemaker inserted.

QUICK REVIEW QUESTION

26. A patient with HF develops a new-onset LBBB. What medication would be important to consider as a possible cause of the LBBB?

CONGENITAL CONDUCTION DEFECTS

- **Long QT syndrome** is a cardiac electrical disturbance that causes a prolonged ventricular repolarization (seen as a QT interval > 0.44 seconds on ECG).
  - may be asymptomatic or present with dysrhythmias (especially torsades de pointes), syncope, seizure, or sudden cardiac death
  - management: beta blockers may be used; placement of an ICD; stop medications likely to prolong the QT interval

- **Wolff-Parkinson-White syndrome,** caused by an early excitation of an extranodal accessory pathway, results in tachycardia.
  - Patient may be asymptomatic or present with sudden A-fib or paroxysmal tachycardia with HR > 150.
  - ECG shows short PR interval (< 0.12 seconds) with a slurred QRS upstroke and a wide QRS (> 0.12 seconds).
  - Treatment is synchronized cardioversion. Unstable patients may require catheter ablation.
  - Contraindicated medications include adenosine, digoxin, amiodarone, beta blockers, and calcium channel blockers.
- **Brugada syndrome** is a genetically inherited cardiac electrical pathway syndrome that is linked to 4% – 12% of all sudden cardiac deaths.
  - It is diagnosed by characteristic ECG findings with sudden cardiac arrest, ventricular tachydysrhythmias, or syncopal episodes.

- The ECG shows pseudo-RBBB and persistent ST-segment elevation.
- The ECG abnormalities may be unmasked by sodium channel blockers.
- It is treated with medication (quinidine or flecainide) or ICD placement.
- Medications likely to prolong the QT interval are contraindicated.

QUICK REVIEW QUESTION

27. A combative patient with schizophrenia develops torsades de pointes in the ED. What medications may have caused this dysrhythmia?

Endocarditis

Pathophysiology

Infective endocarditis occurs when an infection causes inflammation of the endocardium. The inflammation impairs valve function and may also disrupt the electrical conduction system. Infective endocarditis can occur secondary to surgical valve replacement; these cases have a high mortality rate.

Risk Factors

- more common in women and immunocompromised individuals
- heart valve problems or surgery involving heart valves
- poor dental health or recent dental work
- central venous line access
- rheumatic heart disease
- history of illegal IV drug use

Physical Examination

- chest pain
- flu-like symptoms (chills, fatigue)
- fever
- murmur
- petechiae
- Janeway lesions

- Osler's nodes
- Roth spots
- joint pain
- dyspnea
- splinter hemorrhages under fingernails
- hematuria
- night sweats
- weight loss

Diagnostic Tests

- blood cultures showing bacteria present in the bloodstream
- WBC; may be elevated because of infection
- elevated C-reactive protein and sedimentation rate due to inflammation
- echocardiogram and TEE showing any possible heart valve damage and vegetations

Management

- aggressive treatment with IV antimicrobials
- pharmacologic management of symptoms: antipyretics, diuretics, or dysrhythmics
- surgical repair of valves if necessary

QUICK REVIEW QUESTIONS

28. A 39-year-old patient presents to the ED with general achiness, fever, and reddened spots on the palms. The patient recently underwent dental surgery. What diagnostic tests would likely be ordered?

_____

29. What is the primary risk factor for infective endocarditis?

_____

Heart Failure

Pathophysiology

Heart failure (HF) is a clinical syndrome caused by a variety of pathophysiologic processes; it is important to know the cause (i.e., ischemic, infiltrative, congenital) for better long-term management. **Acute decompensated heart failure** is the sudden onset or worsening of HF symptoms usually manifested by fluid volume overload.

HF is classified according to the left ventricular ejection fraction. Impairment of systolic function results in **heart failure with reduced ejection fraction** (**HFrEF**, or **systolic HF**), classified as an ejection fraction of < 50%. **Heart failure with preserved ejection fraction (HFpEF, or diastolic HF)** is characterized by an ejection fraction of > 50% and diastolic dysfunction.

TABLE 1.6. Systolic Versus Diastolic Heart Failure (HF)	
Systolic HF (HFrEF)	**Diastolic HF (HFpEF)**
<ul><li>reduced ejection fraction (< 40%)</li><li>dilated left ventricle</li><li>S3 heart sound</li><li>hypotension</li><li>impaired contractility; reduced SV and cardiac output</li></ul>	<ul><li>normal ejection fraction</li><li>no enlargement of heart</li><li>S4 heart sound</li><li>hypertension</li><li>elevated LV filling pressures</li></ul>

HF can also be categorized as left-sided or right-sided, depending on which ventricle is affected. **Left-sided HF** is usually caused by cardiac disorders (e.g., MI, cardiomyopathy) and produces symptoms related to pulmonary function. **Right-sided HF** is caused by right ventricle infarction or pulmonary conditions (e.g., PE, COPD) and produces symptoms related to systemic circulation. Unmanaged left-sided HF can lead to right-sided HF.

Risk Factors

- coronary artery disease, history of MI, and/or hypertension
- lifestyle factors (smoking, poor diet, lack of exercise)
- diabetes
- obesity
- congenital heart disease

HELPFUL HINT:

Cor pulmonale, or impaired functioning of the right ventricle, is caused by pulmonary disease or pulmonary hypertension.

→
CONTINUE

Physical Examination

TABLE 1.7. Physical Examination of Right- and Left-Sided Heart Failure (HF)

Left-Sided HF	Right-Sided HF
increased pulmonary capillary wedge pressure	increased right ventricular end-diastolic pressure (RVEDP) and right atrial pressures
increased PAP	increased CVP
dyspnea or orthopnea	increased PAP
pulmonary edema	dependent edema (usually in lower legs); ascites
tachycardia	JVD
bibasilar crackles	hepatomegaly
cough, frothy sputum, hemoptysis	right-sided S3 sound
left-sided S3 sound	weight gain
diaphoresis	nausea, vomiting, abdominal pain
pulsus alternans	nocturia

Diagnostic Tests

- BNP > 100 pg/mL
- echocardiogram to assess ejection fraction, ventricular hypertrophy, valve dysfunction
- CXR to show cardiomegaly or pulmonary congestion
- right heart catheterization to assess filling pressures and hemodynamics

Management

- Pharmacological, dietary, and surgical interventions vary depending on the patient's type and degree of HF.
- Managing decompensated HF:
  - Treatment goal is to improve cardiac output, CI, and respiratory status.
  - Administer supplemental oxygen (e.g., nasal cannula, BIPAP).
  - Keep patient upright (sitting or semi-Fowler's position).
  - First-line medication is a loop diuretic (e.g., furosemide or bumetanide).
  - If severe, reduce afterload and preload with nitroprusside or hydralazine.
  - If CI remains low, start inotropes (e.g., milrinone, dopamine).

- ☐ Consider IABP placement if severely decompensated.
- ☐ For hemodynamically stable patients, start or resume medication (e.g., ACE-Is, ARBs, beta blockers).
- ☐ Patient should be on fluid/salt restriction.
- ☐ ICD/pacemaker, VAD, or heart transplant are long-term possible interventions.

QUICK REVIEW QUESTIONS

30. A patient presents with sudden onset dyspnea, JVD, and peripheral edema. What laboratory test would confirm a diagnosis of acute decompensated heart failure?

_____

31. A patient with acute-on-chronic heart failure presents to the ED with JVD and pitting edema and reports a 5 kg weight gain within the last week. Heart failure on which side should be suspected?

_____

Hypertensive Crisis

Pathophysiology

Hypertensive crises include hypertensive urgency and hypertensive emergencies. **Hypertensive urgency** occurs when blood pressure is > 180/110 mm Hg without evidence of organ dysfunction. A **hypertensive emergency** occurs when systolic blood pressure is > 180 mm Hg or when diastolic blood pressure is >120 mm Hg and when either of these is accompanied by evidence of impending or progressive organ dysfunction (e.g., elevated kidney function, abnormal liver enzymes). Hypertensive crises increase the risk of cerebral infarction, and prolonged hypertension can lead to heart or renal failure.

Risk Factors

- history of hypertension (particularly with medication noncompliance or inadequate treatment)
- kidney disease
- endocrine conditions (e.g., Cushing disease)
- use of sympathomimetic drugs (e.g., amphetamines)

Physical Examination

- headache
- blurred vision

- dizziness
- dyspnea
- retinal hemorrhages
- epistaxis
- chest pain

Management

- blood pressure reduction
  - *limited to a decrease of ≤ 25% within the first 2 hours to maintain cerebral perfusion*
  - goal of SBP of 140 – 160 mm Hg or DBP less than 105 mm Hg
- first-line medications: IV antihypertensives (e.g., labetalol, hydralazine, nicardipine)
- quiet, non-stimulating environment
- O_2 administration

QUICK REVIEW QUESTIONS

32. A patient is found to be alert and oriented with a blood pressure of 200/100 mm Hg and is asymptomatic. What is the priority intervention for this patient?

_____

33. Why is it important to slowly lower BP in patients in hypertensive crisis?

_____

HELPFUL HINT:

Constrictive pericarditis is fibrosis of the pericardial sac. It is usually chronic and is often caused by radiation therapy. Definitive treatment is a pericardiectomy.

Cardiac Tamponade

Pericarditis is the inflammation of the **pericardium**, the lining that surrounds the heart. When inflammation occurs, fluid can accumulate, resulting in **pericardial effusion**.

Pericardial tamponade (also called cardiac tamponade) occurs when the effusion is large enough to impair the ability of the heart to pump blood sufficiently. The increased pressure reduces chamber compliance and filling. With enough pressure, venous return is reduced and cardiac output drops, causing hemodynamic compromise.

The onset of cardiac tamponade may be acute (usually due to trauma) or subacute. The most common etiologies of subacute cardiac tamponade are infection, MI, and malignancy.

Symptoms and Physical Findings

- Beck's triad
  - *low arterial BP*
  - *dilated neck veins*
  - *muffled heart sounds*
- sudden and severe chest pain
  - increases with movement, lying flat, and inspiration
  - decreases by sitting up or leaning forward
- tachycardia (usually the earliest sign)
- hypotension
- pulsus paradoxus
- pericardial rub
- dyspnea

Diagnostic Tests

- ECG
  - ST elevation possible, usually in all leads except aVR and V1
  - tall, peaked T waves
- CXR showing "water bottle" silhouette in pericardial effusion.
- Echocardiogram may show pericardial effusion, thickening, or calcifications.

HELPFUL HINT:

Positive pressure ventilation should be avoided in patients with cardiac tamponade because the pressure further limits venous return.

Management

- definitive treatment: pericardiocentesis or surgical drainage
- Hemodynamically stable patients may be monitored while underlying condition is treated:
  - maintain fluid volume
  - manage pain (positioning, analgesics)

QUICK REVIEW QUESTIONS

34. What is Beck's triad and what diagnosis is it associated with?

_____

35. A patient with acute pericarditis complains of sudden chest pain, and a pericardial friction rub can be heard on auscultation. What interventions should the nurse expect to perform?

_____

Peripheral Vascular Disease

- **Atherosclerosis**, also called atherosclerotic cardiovascular disease (ASCVD), is a progressive condition in which **plaque** builds up in the tunica intima of arteries.

- The presence of advanced atherosclerosis places patients at a high risk for several cardiovascular conditions, including stenosis, aneurysms, and arterial/venous occlusions.

- Atherosclerosis can occur in any artery and is categorized according to the location of the plaque buildup.

  - **peripheral vascular disease** (also called peripheral artery disease): narrowing of the peripheral arteries
  - **coronary artery disease (CAD)**: narrowing of the coronary arteries
  - **renal artery stenosis**: narrowing of the renal arteries
  - **carotid artery occlusive disease (CAOD)**, or **stenosis**: narrowing or hardening of the carotid arteries

- Risk factors for atherosclerosis include:
  - age (some degree of atherosclerosis is common in people > 65)
  - dyslipidemia
  - hypertension
  - lifestyle factors (smoking, poor diet, lack of exercise)
  - obesity
  - diabetes

HELPFUL HINT:

Carotid artery stenosis may be asymptomatic and is usually diagnosed after a CVA. It is the cause of most ischemic strokes.

HELPFUL HINT:

75% of all acute MIs are caused by plaque rupture.

QUICK REVIEW QUESTION

36. A patient diagnosed with peripheral vascular disease asks the nurse what to do to prevent further buildup of plaque in the arteries. What should the nurse tell the patient?

Thromboembolic Disease

ARTERIAL OCCLUSION

Pathophysiology

Acute peripheral vascular insufficiency (also **acute arterial occlusion**) occurs when a thrombus or an embolus occludes a peripheral artery, causing ischemia. This condition is a medical emergency requiring prompt treatment to prevent tissue necrosis.

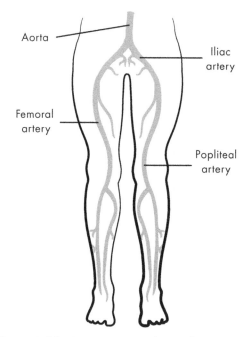

Figure 1.28. Common Locations of Acute Arterial Occlusion

Physical Examination

- the 6 Ps (hallmark signs) of an arterial occlusion
  - □ pain (intermittent claudication)
  - □ pallor
  - □ pulselessness
  - □ paresthesia
  - □ paralysis
  - □ poikilothermia
- petechiae (visible with microemboli)
- ankle-brachial index (ABI) < 0.30: indicates low likelihood of limb survivability

Diagnostic Tests

- duplex ultrasonography, CT angiography, or catheter-based arteriography
- elevated D-dimer

Management

- medications: IV anticoagulants (usually heparin), thrombolytics, and/ or antiplatelet agents

- surgical/catheter intervention: catheter-directed thrombolysis, bypass surgery, or embolectomy
- nursing considerations
  - frequent pulse and neurovascular checks
  - do not elevate extremity
  - monitor for signs and symptoms of bleeding following use of anticoagulants or thrombolytics

VENOUS OCCLUSION

Pathophysiology

A **deep vein thrombosis (DVT)** is the most common form of acute venous occlusion and occurs when a thrombus forms within a deep vein. DVT is most common in the lower extremities.

Risk Factors

- Virchow's triad
  - hypercoagulability (e.g., due to estrogen, contraceptive use, or malignancy)
  - venous stasis (bed rest or any other activity that results in decreased physical movement)
  - endothelial damage (damage to the vessel wall from trauma, drug use, inflammatory processes, or other causes)
- pregnancy, hormone replacement therapy, or oral contraceptives
- recent surgery

Physical Examination

- pain localized to a specific area (usually the foot, ankle, calf, or behind the knee)
- unilateral edema, erythema, and warmth
- positive Homan's sign

Diagnostic Tests

- elevated D-dimer

- venous duplex ultrasonography

Management

- pharmacological management: anticoagulants (first line), thrombolytics (second line)

- surgical or endovascular thrombectomy (if medication is ineffective or contraindicated)

- *inferior vena cava (IVC) filter: may be placed to avoid a PE in patients who cannot tolerate anticoagulants*

QUICK REVIEW QUESTIONS

39. A patient with unilateral edema in the lower extremities has elevated D-dimer results. What diagnostic imaging should be ordered?

40. A patient with a history of a cerebral hemorrhage is diagnosed with a DVT in the right lower extremity (RLE). What procedure should be expected?

Cardiac Trauma

- **Cardiac trauma** occurs when an outside force causes injury to the heart. Cardiac trauma can cause rupture of heart chambers, dysrhythmias, damage to the heart valves, or cardiac arrest.

- **Blunt cardiac injury (BCI)** occurs when an object forcefully strikes the chest. Damage due to BCI may be caused by compression of the heart between the sternum and spine, pressure fluctuations in the thoracic cavity, or shearing forces. Because the right side of the heart is anteriorly positioned, it is typically the most affected.

  - **Cardiac contusion** is a general term used to describe damage to the heart from blunt trauma.

  - Common consequences of BCI include dysrhythmias; damage to chamber walls, septa, or valves; and decreased contractility and SV.

  - Management of BCI may include antidysrhythmic drugs, temporary pacemakers, medications to manage heart failure, and surgery to repair damaged heart tissues.

  - Fluid and electrolytes should be monitored closely to preserve myocardial conduction and cardiac output.

HELPFUL HINT:

The most common cause of blunt cardiac trauma is MVC. Any patient who experiences rapid deceleration forces during an MVC should be assessed for BCI.

- **Blunt aortic injury (BAI)** is a tear in the aorta resulting from compression of the aorta between the vertebrae and anterior chest wall. Patients with BAI are administered antihypertensives (sodium nitroprusside IV infusion) to maintain SBP < 90 mm HG and usually require surgery.
- **Penetrating cardiac trauma** involves the puncture of the heart by a sharp object or a broken rib. The penetration causes blood to leak into the pericardial space or mediastinum.
  - □ The most frequently affected area is the right ventricle (due to its anterior position).
  - □ Blood leakage can result in cardiac tamponade, and blood loss from penetrating injuries can also result in shock.
  - □ Penetrating objects should be stabilized and the patient prepped for surgery.

Cardiogenic Shock

Pathophysiology

Cardiogenic shock is a cyclical decline in cardiac function. It results in decreased cardiac output, impaired oxygen delivery, and reduced tissue perfusion. A lack of coronary perfusion causes or escalates ischemia/infarction by decreasing the ability of the heart to pump effectively. HR increases to meet myocardial oxygen demands. However, the reduced pumping ability of the heart decreases cardiac output. Demands for coronary or tissue perfusion are not met. LVEDP increases, leading to stress in the left ventricle and an increase in afterload. This distress results in lactic acidosis.

Cardiogenic shock is most common after an MI but can be associated with trauma, pericardial tamponade, or dysrhythmia.

HELPFUL HINT:

When assessing patients with suspected BCI, BP in both arms should be measured; a tear in the aortic arch may create a pressure gradient between the upper extremities. An aortic disruption may also cause upper extremity hypertension and lower extremity relative hypotension.

HELPFUL HINT:

Left ventricular dysfunction caused by an anterior MI is the most common cause of cardiogenic shock.

Physical Examination

- tachycardia and sustained hypotension (SBP < 90 mm Hg)
- oliguria (< 30 mL/hr or < 0.5 mL/kg/hr output)
- crackles
- tachypnea and dyspnea
- pallor
- JVD
- altered LOC
- cool, clammy skin
- S3 heart sound possible

Diagnostic Tests

- CI < 2.2 L/min/m²
- PAOP > 15 mm Hg
- elevated SVR, CVP, PCWP
- MAP < 60 mm Hg
- elevated lactate
- ABG shows metabolic acidosis and hypoxia

Management

- immediate goal: reduce cardiac workload and improve myocardial contractility
- initial, careful administration of intravenous fluids
- medications given based on hemodynamic status
  - vasopressor (usually norepinephrine) for hypotensive patients
  - inotrope (usually dobutamine) and vasodilator for normotensive patients
- other interventions
  - IABP to reduce afterload and increase coronary perfusion
  - cardiac catheterization with PCI (if cause is thought to be ischemic) to improve myocardial perfusion
  - LVAD
- monitor patient for cardiac dysrhythmias

Obstructive Shock

Pathophysiology

Obstructive shock is reduced cardiac output caused by extracardiac mechanical obstruction or compression of the vasculature. Obstruction of the pulmonary vasculature (e.g., pulmonary embolism, pulmonary hypertension) increases pulmonary vascular resistance and decreases cardiac output. Compression of the heart (e.g., tension pneumothorax, pericardial tamponade) prevents atrial filling, reducing preload and cardiac output.

Physical Examination

- hypotension (may initially be moderate)
- visible JVD
- nonspecific signs and symptoms of shock
    - tachycardia
    - oliguria
    - tachypnea or dyspnea
    - altered mental status
    - cool, mottled extremities

Diagnostic Tests

- ECG and CXR
- CT or ultrasound based on suspected etiology

Treatment and Management

- immediate management of underlying condition
- IV fluids and vasopressors as needed

QUICK REVIEW QUESTIONS

45. After being admitted for dyspnea, a patient becomes tachycardic and hypotensive with signs of shock. The patient mentions having recently been on a long flight. What diagnostic test should the nurse prepare the patient for?

_____

46. An X-ray returns on a patient who was injured in a stabbing to the left upper quadrant. The patient has had increasing dyspnea and tachycardia, and a CXR shows mediastinal shift. What immediate action should the nurse take?

_____

ANSWER KEY

1. Blood from the lungs is returned to the left side of the heart. When the left side cannot pump this blood back out to the body, fluid builds up in the lungs. Blood from the body is returned to the right side of the heart, so right-sided failure causes fluid to build up in the abdomen and extremities.

2. The nurse should focus on CVP because CVP is an indirect measure of right ventricular pressure and is highly influenced by fluid status. In sepsis, CVP is <2 mm Hg, because of profound systemic vasodilation. Both treatments would be expected to increase preload, thereby increasing CVP.

3. Elevated troponin (> 0.01 ng/mL) and elevated CK-MB (> 2.5%) are indicators of myocardial injury.

4. An S3 gallop is a common sign of systolic heart failure.

5. The highlighted area is the QRS complex.

6. The P wave shows atrial depolarization. If a rhythm shows abnormalities in the P waves, then the SA node (which controls atrial contraction) is not functioning properly.

7. Beta blockers depress conduction through the AV node; the reduced conduction may exacerbate an underlying AV block, resulting in severe bradycardia or third-degree AV block.

8. The nurse should anticipate a slower HR and lower BP because of the negative dromotropic, chronotropic, and inotropic effects.

9. The patient is experiencing an unstable SVT (with BP of 70/42 mm Hg) and requires immediate synchronized cardioversion.

10. ST depression in the precordial leads suggests a STEMI of the posterior wall. Finding can be confirmed with a posterior ECG.

11. The priority intervention for patients diagnosed with STEMI is transfer to the cath lab for PCI or fibrinolytic therapy.

12. The symptoms indicate inferior wall MI, which puts the patient at risk for right ventricular infarctions. For patients with right ventricular infarction, medications that reduce preload (e.g., beta blockers, nitrates, diuretics, morphine) should be avoided.

13. The chest/back pain experienced by patients with an aortic dissection is often described as "tearing."

14. Because the patient describes the pain as tearing, the nurse should take the blood pressure in the other arm. A difference of ≥ 20 mm Hg can be a strong indicator that the patient is experiencing an aortic rupture or dissection.

15. A hemodynamically unstable patient in V-tach requires synchronized cardioversion.

16. Epinephrine is the first-line medication for patients whose V-fib is unresponsive to defibrillation.

17. The nurse should activate the code team and begin high-quality compressions immediately.

18. Epinephrine is administered to patients in asystole.

19. This patient is hemodynamically unstable because of bradycardia. The nurse should prepare to push IV atropine.

20. Unstable patients with bradycardia that cannot be managed with medication require TCP.

21. The first-line intervention for stable patients with SVT is vagal maneuvers.

22. If the patient in SVT does not respond to vagal maneuvers, the patient will likely be administered 6 mg of adenosine to terminate the dysrhythmia.

23. The nurse should expect a hemodynamically stable patient with A-fib to receive calcium channel blockers, beta blockers, or cardiac glycosides to decrease the heart rate.

24. When adenosine is administered to a patient with atrial flutter, the heart rate will slow, but the dysrhythmia will not convert to sinus rhythm.

25. The nurse should prepare the patient for TCP. Atropine may be an appropriate medication to administer for a third-degree block as it will increase the overall heart rate.

26. Digoxin, often administered for treatment of HF, has a narrow therapeutic index. Digoxin toxicity may manifest itself as an LBBB. Labs would need to be drawn to assess for digoxin toxicity.

27. There is a strong association between antipsychotic medication use and torsades de pointes in patients with prolonged QT. The patient may have been administered haloperidol, which is one of the most commonly used medications in the ED associated with torsades de pointes.

28. WBC, blood cultures, and an echocardiogram should be ordered to rule out infective endocarditis.

29. The primary risk factor for infective endocarditis is heart valve problems or surgery involving the heart valves.

30. A BNP lab value of > 100 pg/mL indicates HF.

31. The patient has symptoms of right-sided HF.

32. The priority for this patient is to administer an antihypertensive medication.

33. Decreasing BP too quickly (or too low) can decrease cerebral perfusion.

34. Beck's triad is hypotension, JVD, and muffled heart tones occurring simultaneously. It is associated with pericardial tamponade.

35. The nurse should expect to obtain a 12-lead ECG. To alleviate pain, the nurse should have the patient sit up and lean forward; NSAIDs may be administered.

36. The nurse should tell the patient that some lifestyle choices can slow the progression of atherosclerosis. Topics to discuss with the patient include a healthy diet and exercise regimen, smoking cessation, and the management of dyslipidemia.

37. The nurse should assess for pain (intermittent claudication), pallor, pulselessness, paresthesia, paralysis, and poikilothermia.

38. IV anticoagulants (usually heparin), thrombolytics, and/or antiplatelet agents are ordered for acute arterial occlusion.

39. Venous duplex ultrasonography should be ordered to confirm presence of a DVT.

40. Patients with a history of hemorrhage will likely not be given anticoagulants. They will instead require placement of an IVC filter to prevent a PE.

41. The object should be stabilized, and bleeding controlled. Two large-bore IVs should be placed for the administration of IV fluids and blood if needed. The patient should be prepped for surgery to have the object removed and to be assessed for underlying damage to organs and surrounding areas.

42. The nurse should prepare to administer an inotropic medication to increase contractility and cardiac output.

43. Cardiogenic shock is more likely to occur in an anterior MI because the LAD is usually the occluded vessel.

44. Cardiogenic shock is characterized by signs and symptoms of hypoperfusion combined with a systolic BP of < 90 mm Hg, a CI of < 2.2 L/min/m², and a normal or elevated PAOP (> 15 mm Hg).

45. The patient's symptoms and history suggest a pulmonary embolism. The nurse should prepare the patient for a spiral CT or pulmonary angiogram.

46. Mediastinal shift indicates a tension pneumothorax. The patient should be prepared for an emergent needle decompression and chest tube insertion site to relieve positive pressure.

2 RESPIRATORY EMERGENCIES

Respiratory Anatomy and Physiology

- The **respiratory system** is responsible for the exchange of gases between the human body and the environment.
  - Air is drawn in through the **nose** and **mouth**, then into the throat, where cilia and mucus filter out particles before the air enters the **trachea**.

□ Air then passes through either the left or right bronchi and smaller bronchioles into the left or right **lung**.

□ Eventually, air enters the **alveoli**—tiny air sacs where gases exchange with the blood.

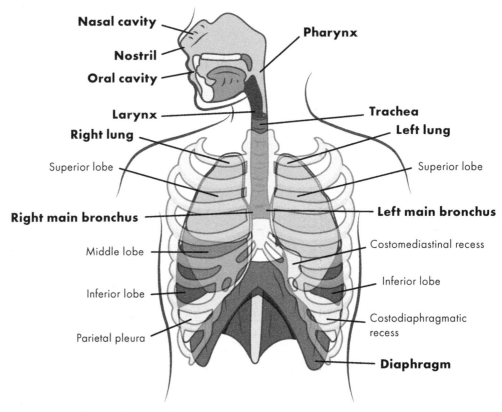

Figure 2.1. The Respiratory System

■ The primary functions of the respiratory system are ventilation and respiration.

□ **Ventilation** is the inhalation and exhalation of air by the lungs.

□ **Respiration** is the exchange of gas within the lungs.

■ **Ventilation/perfusion (V/Q)** ratio is the amount of air that reaches the alveoli (ventilation, V) divided by the amount of blood flow in lung capillaries (perfusion, Q).

□ Normal V/Q ratio is 0.8.

□ A **V/Q mismatch** occurs when either perfusion or ventilation is inadequate.

□ A low V/Q ratio (perfusion with low ventilation) causes **intrapulmonary shunting**. Common causes of low V/Q include asthma, ARDS, and pulmonary edema.

□ A high V/Q ratio (ventilation with low perfusion) causes increased **dead space** (the volume of air that does not participate in gas exchange). The most common cause of a high V/Q ratio is pulmonary embolism.

HELPFUL HINT:

Administering O_2 to patients with severe intrapulmonary shunting (very low V/Q) will have little effect on PaO_2 because air is not reaching the area where perfusion occurs.

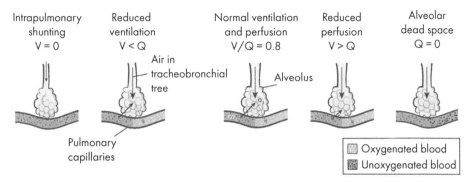

Figure 2.2. Ventilation/Perfusion (V/Q) Ratio

- **Hypoxemia** is a decreased level of oxygen (O_2) in the blood (as measured by SaO_2, PaO_2, or A-a gradient). It can be caused by several different underlying pathophysiological processes.
  - □ V/Q mismatch (e.g., PE)
  - □ shunting (e.g., pneumonia, ARDS)
  - □ hypoventilation (e.g., sedation, brain injury)
  - □ impaired diffusion (e.g., pulmonary fibrosis)

- **Hypoxia** is a deficiency in oxygenation at the tissue or cellular level. It may be caused by hypoxemia or other processes, including hypoperfusion (e.g., MI) or the inability of tissues to metabolize O_2 (e.g., cyanide poisoning).

- **Lung volumes and capacities** are measured by spirometry at bedside for clinical application in pulmonary management.
  - □ **Tidal volume (VT)** is the volume of air exhaled after a normal resting inhalation. Normal value is 7 mL/kg.
  - □ **Vital capacity (VC)** is the maximal volume of air that can be exhaled after a maximal inhalation. It increases with height and decreases with age; the normal value is 60 – 70 mL/kg.
  - □ **Inspiratory capacity (IC)** is the maximal volume of gas that can be inspired from the resting expiratory level.
  - □ **Functional residual capacity (FRC)** is the volume of gas retained in the lungs when the patient is at rest and at the end of expiration.
  - □ **Total lung capacity (TLC)** is the volume of gas contained in the lungs at the end of a maximal inspiration.
  - □ **Normal resting minute ventilation** is the volume of air inhaled or exhaled per minute. Normal is 5 – 8 L/min.

QUICK REVIEW QUESTION

1. A patient who has tested positive for COVID-19 is admitted with lethargy, dyspnea, and hypoxemia. The blood gas levels return at PaO_2 of 61 mm Hg and $PaCO_2$ of 45 mm Hg. The patient is on 3 L high-flow nasal cannula. Why would increasing the high-flow nasal cannula to 4 L likely not help this patient?

_____

Respiratory Assessment

- Start the respiratory assessment by evaluating **airway patency**. The airway must be patent before any other assessments or interventions are performed.

- **Respirations** should be evaluated for rate, rhythm, depth, and quality.

TABLE 2.1. Normal Respiratory Rate	
Age	**Breaths per Minute**
Adult	12 to 20
Child 11 – 14 years	12 to 20
Child 6 – 10 years	15 to 30
Child 6 months – 5 years	20 to 30
Infant 0 – 6 months	25 to 40
Newborn	30 to 50

- Disruptions to the respiratory system can result in abnormal breathing patterns.
  - **eupnea**: normal breathing
  - **tachypnea**: rapid breathing
  - **bradypnea**: slow breathing
  - **dyspnea**: difficulty breathing
  - **apnea**: not breathing
  - **hyperventilation**: increase in rate or volume of breaths, which causes excessive elimination of CO_2
  - **agonal breathing**: irregular gasping breaths accompanied by involuntary twitching or jerking. Agonal breathing is associated with severe hypoxia and is a sign the patient requires immediate medical treatment.
  - **Biot's breathing**: alternating rapid respirations and apnea. Causes include stroke, trauma, and opioid use.
  - **Cheyne-Stokes breathing**: deep breathing alternating with apnea or a faster rate of breathing; associated with left heart failure or sleep apnea
  - **Kussmaul breathing**: type of hyperventilation characterized by deep, labored breathing that is associated with metabolic acidosis

- Listen for abnormal breath sounds.

TABLE 2.2. Lung Sounds

Sound	Description	Etiology
Normal	air heard moving through the lungs with no obstructions	normal function of the lungs
Wheezes	continuous musical-like sound; can occur on inspiration or expiration	air being forced through narrowed passages in the airway (e.g., asthma, COPD)
Rhonchi	low-pitched, coarse rattling lung sounds	secretions in the airway (e.g., pneumonia, cystic fibrosis)
Stridor	high-pitched wheezing sound	air moving through narrowed or obstructed passages in the upper airway (e.g., aspiration, laryngospasm)
Rales (crackles)	crackling, rattling sound that can be coarse or fine	fluid in the small airways of the lung (e.g., pulmonary edema, pneumonia)
Pleural friction rub	grating, creaking sound	inflamed pleural tissue (e.g., pleuritis, pulmonary embolism)
Diminished or absent breath sounds	decreased intensity of breath sounds due to lack of air in lung tissues	air or fluid around the lungs (e.g., pleural effusion, pneumothorax) or blocked airway

- **Pulse oximetry** (SpO_2) measures the percentage of red blood cells that are carrying oxygen.
  - Pulse oximetry can provide false readings in patients who have suffered carbon monoxide poisoning: the actual oxygenation saturation will be lower.
  - Pulse oximetry may not work well on patients with cold hands, anemia, or nail polish.
- $PEtco_2$ is the measure of **end-tidal carbon dioxide** (partial pressure of CO_2 at the end of exhalation) and is often displayed graphically as a waveform.
  - Normal $PEtco_2$ in adult patients is between 35 and 45 mm Hg.
  - If a patient is in cardiac arrest and CPR is in progress, high-quality chest compressions will result in $PEtco_2$ between 10 and 20 mm Hg.
- An **arterial blood gas (ABG)** test measures the pH (acidity) and amount of dissolved CO_2 and O_2 in the blood. ABG tests provide information on acid-base balance and pulmonary gas exchange.

TABLE 2.3. Normal Values for ABG

Elements of an ABG	Normal Value
pH	7.35 – 7.45
Partial pressure of oxygen (PaO_2)	75 – 100 mm Hg
Partial pressure of carbon dioxide ($PaCO_2$)	35 – 45 mm Hg
Bicarbonate (HCO_3^-)	22 – 26 mEq/L
Oxygen saturation (SaO_2)	94% – 100%

- The following tic-tac-toe method is one of many tools available for understanding the pathophysiology behind the ABG result in critically ill patients.

1. Identify the normal, acidic, and basic values.

Lower	Normal	Higher
	pH	
Acidic ←	7.35–7.45	→ Basic
	$PaCO_2$	
Basic ←	35–45 mm Hg	→ Acidic
	HCO_3^-	
Acidic ←	22–26 mEq/L	→ Basic

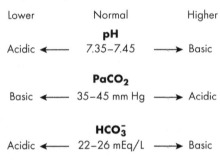

Figure 2.3. Normal ABG Values

2. Draw tic-tac-toe grid.

Acid	Normal	Base

Figure 2.4. ABG Tic-Tac-Toe Grid

3. Plug in the given values in the appropriate column.

Acid	Normal	Base
HCO_3^- 19		pH 7.5
		$PaCO_2$ 26

Figure 2.5. Example of a Completed ABG Tic-Tac-Toe Grid

4. Name the acid-base result by finding the "tic-tac-toe/3-in-a-row."
   □ If PaCO₂ is in the tic-tac-toe, the imbalance is respiratory.
   □ If HCO₃⁻ is in the tic-tac-toe, the imbalance is metabolic.

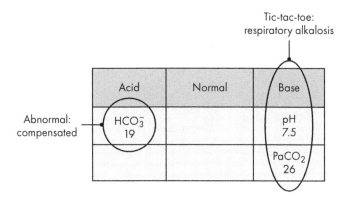

Figure 2.6. Analysis of an ABG Tic-Tac-Toe Grid

5. Determine if uncompensated, partially compensated, or fully compensated.
   □ If pH is normal, ABG is fully compensated; the body has done its job.
   □ If pH is abnormal and the remaining value (not the tic-tac-toe/3-in-a-row) is abnormal, then the ABG is partially compensated: the body is trying but is not able to maintain acid-base balance.
   □ If pH is abnormal and the remaining value is normal, then the ABG is uncompensated: the body isn't doing anything to fix the problem.

6. Consider possible causes of acid-base imbalance to implement plan of care.

TABLE 2.4. Common Causes of Changes in ABG Values			
Abnormality	**pH**	**ABG**	**Etiology**
Respiratory acidosis	decreased	PaCO₂ increased	• asthma (late stage) • cardiac arrest • COPD • Guillain-Barre syndrome, ALS, myasthenia gravis • respiratory depressant drugs
Respiratory alkalosis	increased	PaCO₂ decreased	• asthma (early stage) • cirrhosis • CNS disorders • hypoxemia • salicylate overdose • sepsis

continued on next page

TABLE 2.4. Common Causes of Changes in ABG Values (continued)			
Abnormality	pH	ABG	Etiology
Metabolic alkalosis	increased	HCO_3^- increased	• blood transfusions • GI: vomiting • hypokalemia
Metabolic acidosis	decreased	HCO_3^- decreased	• DKA • GI: diarrhea • lactic acidosis • renal failure • rhabdomyolysis

QUICK REVIEW QUESTION

2. A patient is in the critical care unit post-cardiac arrest with the following ABG values:

   pH: 7.30

   PaO_2: 95

   $PaCO_2$: 48

   HCO_3^-: 28

   How should the nurse interpret these results?

HELPFUL HINT:

Asynchrony occurs when ventilator gas-flow delivery is not efficiently matched to the patient's needs. Machine-delivered breaths may be early or late, or the flow rate may not meet the patient's needs.

Mechanical Ventilation

- **Invasive mechanical ventilation** uses an advanced invasive airway.
  - □ **Endotracheal tube (ETT)** placement (oral or nasal) should be checked after intubation.
  - □ **Tracheostomy tubes** are placed emergently for obstruction and used for long-term ventilator support.
- Volume-limited ventilation delivers a set volume.
  - □ **Assist-control (AC)** ventilation always delivers a set V_T and set respiratory rate (RR).
  - □ **Synchronized intermittent mandatory ventilation (SIMV)** always delivers a set V_T and a set RR.
- During **pressure-support ventilation (PSV)**, patient-initiated breaths receive positive pressure support on inspiration.
- Ventilator settings
  - □ RR: 8 – 20 breaths/min

□ V_T: customized to the patient's predicted body weight (as part of lung-protective ventilation [LPV] bundles) to prevent volutrauma (6 – 8 mL/kg of patient's body weight)

□ The lowest tolerated FiO_2 should be used to maintain SaO_2 without oxygen toxicity.

□ **Positive end-expiratory pressure (PEEP)** is positive pressure applied at the end of exhalation to prevent the passive emptying of the lung, which causes end-expiratory alveolar collapse. For most patients, extrinsic PEEP is set at 5 cm H_2O.

□ The normal inspiratory-expiratory (I:E) ratio is 1:2.

□ The inspiratory flow rate is usually set with a peak rate of 60 L/min.

■ **Noninvasive ventilation (NIV)** uses a noninvasive interface such as a face mask or mouthpiece.

■ **Continuous positive airway pressure (CPAP)** delivers a single level of pressure for both inspiration and expiration. It is primarily used for obstructive sleep apnea and cardiogenic pulmonary edema.

■ **Bilevel positive airway pressure (BiPAP or BPAP)** delivers two levels of positive airway pressure, IPAP and EPAP.

□ **Inspiratory positive airway pressure (IPAP)** enhances airflow and augments patient's V_T; corresponds to pressure support.

□ **Expiratory positive airway pressure (EPAP)** reduces amount of pressure to ease expiratory effort; corresponds to PEEP.

QUICK REVIEW QUESTION

3. What is PEEP, and what are the complications of this therapy?

Aspiration

Pathophysiology

Pulmonary aspiration is the entry of foreign bodies, or material from the mouth or gastrointestinal tract, into the upper and/or lower respiratory tract. Aspiration may lead to **aspiration pneumonia**, inflammation of lung tissue caused by infection or a reaction to the aspirated substances.

Risk Factors

■ age > 65 years

■ difficulty swallowing/neurological dysfunction

■ intoxication/sedation/altered LOC

HELPFUL HINT:

Volutrauma is injury due to mechanical settings that deliver excessive volume to the alveoli. Ventilated patients with ARDS are at high risk for volutrauma and should receive a lower V_T.

HELPFUL HINT:

Complications of PEEP include barotrauma, decreased blood pressure and cardiac output, and air-leak disorders.

Physical Examination

- coughing or choking
- dyspnea
- fever
- abnormal lung sounds
    - □ possible wheezing, rhonchi, or crackles
    - □ diminished lung sounds in the lobe where the aspiration has settled

Diagnostic Tests

- CXR showing infiltrates after the aspiration
- WBC and blood cultures may show infection

Management

- manage airway
- oxygen and antibiotics as needed

QUICK REVIEW QUESTIONS

4. What risk factors should lead a nurse to consider aspiration as a cause of dyspnea and crackles?

_____

5. A patient presents to the ED with pleuritic chest pain, difficulty breathing, fevers, chills, and an altered LOC. Three days ago, the patient was found in a pool of vomit after an overdose. What test should the nurse anticipate will be ordered to diagnose aspiration?

_____

HELPFUL HINT:

Aspirin-exacerbated respiratory disease (aspirin-sensitive asthma) is asthma that develops after taking aspirin or other NSAIDs. It is a pseudoallergic reaction, meaning it is not antibody-mediated, seen in around 14% of people with severe asthma.

Asthma

Pathophysiology

Asthma is a chronic obstructive pulmonary disease characterized by airway inflammation and bronchoconstriction. Asthma exacerbations may be triggered by allergens, infections, exercise, aspirin, and GERD. When the triggered response occurs, the airway becomes obstructed by a combination of bronchospasm, thick mucus, mucosal edema, and airway inflammation.

Status asthmaticus is a severe, progressively worsening asthma event that does not respond to bronchodilator therapy; the condition may develop into acute respiratory failure.

Physical Examination

- tachypnea and severe dyspnea
- bronchoconstriction
  - □ expiratory wheeze (early stage); inspiratory and expiratory wheeze (late stage)
  - □ wheezes may disappear with fatigue or if obstruction prevents wheezing
- increased use of accessory respiratory muscles
- decreased breath sounds in all lung fields (ominous sign, as patient is not moving enough air)
- hypoxia (early); hypercapnia (late)
- tachycardia and hypertension
- pulsus paradoxus >20 mm Hg
- with progression of disease
  - □ decreased cardiac output
  - □ hypotension and bradycardia
  - □ seizure
  - □ coma

HELPFUL HINT:

During severe asthma exacerbations, lactate overproduction occurs in respiratory muscles, resulting in respiratory and metabolic acidosis.

Diagnostic Tests

- peak expiratory flow rate (PEFR) showing 20% drop from expected response to treatment or baseline best effort
- ABG
  - □ *initial: respiratory alkalosis with hypoxemia*
  - □ *worsening: respiratory acidosis with hypercapnia*
- ECG may show peaked P wave and right-axis deviation
- CXR to rule out other underlying diseases (e.g., pneumonia, pneumothorax)

Management

- high-flow O_2 to keep SpO_2 >92%, or heliox to decrease airway resistance
- medications
  - □ *inhaled bronchodilators (beta 2 agonists)*
  - □ anticholinergics (synergistic effect with beta 2 agonists)
  - □ corticosteroids
- mechanical ventilation required if patient is unresponsive to medication

Chronic Obstructive Pulmonary Disease (COPD)

Chronic obstructive pulmonary disease (COPD) is characterized by a breakdown in alveolar tissue (emphysema), chronic productive cough (chronic bronchitis), and long-term obstruction of the airways. The condition worsens over time.

COPD is characterized by low expiratory flow rates. Acute exacerbations of COPD are characterized by increased sputum production and hypoxia or hypercapnia, which may require emergent treatment.

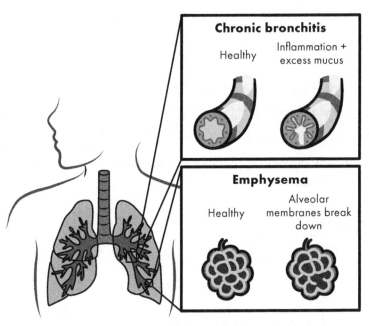

Figure 2.7. Chronic Obstructive Pulmonary Disease (COPD)

Risk Factors

- smoking (> 30 pack years [pack-years = packs per day × years])
- passive exposure to cigarette smoke
- exposure to inhaled chemicals or pollution
- severe childhood respiratory illness

Diagnosis

- chronic, productive cough
- dyspnea and wheezing
- prolonged expiration
- barrel chest (late sign)
- spirometry
  - forced expiratory volume in one second (FEV_1) and forced vital capacity (FVC) used to measure airflow limitations
  - FEV_1/FVC less than 0.7 after bronchodilator administration generally diagnostic of COPD

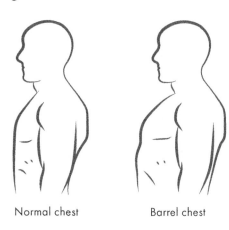

Normal chest   Barrel chest

Figure 2.8. Barrel Chest

Management

- first-line management
  - bronchodilators (*not* inhaled corticosteroids) such as short-acting beta-agonists (e.g., albuterol)
  - anticholinergics: inhaled ipratropium
- administer oxygen
  - cautious use of oxygen (***titrated to SpO₂ 88 – 92%*** or PaO_2 of 60 mm Hg)
  - monitor for hypercapnia when administering oxygen
- BiPaP if SpO_2 does not improve

HELPFUL HINT:

In COPD, inflammation is mainly caused by neutrophils. In asthma, inflammation is caused by eosinophils and activated T cells. Corticosteroids are highly effective against eosinophilic inflammation but mostly ineffective against neutrophilic inflammation.

- chest physiotherapy and comfortable positioning
- teach smoking cessation at discharge

> **QUICK REVIEW QUESTIONS**
>
> **9.** What medication should the nurse expect to administer to a patient admitted with an acute exacerbation of COPD?
>
> _____
>
> **10.** Why is O_2 administered to patients with acute exacerbations of COPD titrated to SpO_2 88% – 92%?
>
> _____

Respiratory Infections

- **Pneumonia** is a lower respiratory tract infection that can be caused by bacteria, fungi, protozoa, or parasites. The infection causes inflammation in the alveoli and can cause them to fill with fluid.
    - Diagnosis and treatment of community-acquired pneumonia (CAP), hospital-acquired pneumonia (HAP), and aspiration pneumonia are similar.
    - Signs and symptoms include cough, dyspnea, hemoptysis, pleuritic chest pain, and fever. Abnormalities in affected lung/lobe include decreased lung sounds, inspiratory crackles, and dull percussion.
    - CXR will show infiltrates; WBC and blood cultures will show infection.
    - Management is antibiotics and oxygen as needed.

- **Croup** is an upper airway obstruction caused by subglottic inflammation that results from viral illness (although rarely it can be caused by bacterial infection). The inflammation results in edema in the trachea and adjacent structures. Additionally, thick, tenacious mucus further obstructs the airway.
    - Croup is associated with a **_barking cough_** and characteristic high-pitched stridor.
    - Management may include oxygen, cool mist therapy, corticosteroids (dexamethasone) and **_nebulized racemic epinephrine_**.

- **Bronchitis** is inflammation of the bronchi. Most cases (> 90%) are caused by a viral infection, but bronchitis can also result from bacterial infection or environmental irritants.
    - Signs and symptoms may include nonproductive cough that evolves into a productive cough, sore throat, and congestion.
    - Acute bronchitis will usually spontaneously resolve without intervention.

HELPFUL HINT:

In patients with unilateral lung disease (e.g., right lung pneumonia), the patient should be positioned with the "good" lung down to promote blood flow and perfusion in the healthy lung.

- Discharge instructions should include home symptom management (e.g., adequate hydration, use of humidifiers, and OTC antitussives)
- Fluids, antitussives, analgesics, or antibiotics may be administered.

- **Bronchiolitis** is inflammation of the bronchioles, usually because of infection by RSV or human rhinovirus. The inflammation and congestion lead to a narrowing of the airway, resulting in dyspnea. Bronchiolitis is seen in children younger than 2 years and will usually spontaneously resolve.

QUICK REVIEW QUESTIONS

11. A patient with bronchitis is being discharged. What should the nurse recommend to the patient to assist with symptom management?

12. A 1-year-old patient arrives at triage. The parent says that the child has had a barking cough and difficulty breathing. The nurse notes a hoarse cry and that the child seems to be fatigued. What interventions should the nurse anticipate for this patient?

13. An 18-month-old patient is diagnosed with bronchiolitis following a negative CXR and a positive RSV antigen test. The physician determines that the patient does not require pharmacological intervention, but the parent believes that the child has pneumonia and refuses to allow the patient to be discharged. How should the nurse respond?

Inhalation Injuries
Pathophysiology

Inhalation injuries fall into three categories differentiated by the mechanism of the injury.

- Exposure to asphyxiants such as carbon monoxide (CO) can cause injuries. In the case of CO poisoning, the CO displaces the oxygen on the hemoglobin molecule, leading to hypoxia and eventual death of tissue.

- Thermal or heat inhalation injuries can be caused by steam, heat from explosions, or the consumption of very hot liquids. The resulting edema and blistering of the airway mucosa lead to airway obstruction.

- Smoke exposure from fire or toxic gases causes damage to pulmonary tissue and causes mucosal edema and the destruction of epithelia cilia. Pulmonary edema is a late development, one to two days after the injury.

Risk Factors

- occupational exposure to asphyxiants or toxic gases
- proximity to fire
- intentional inhalation of toxic gases

Diagnosis

- depends on what irritant the patient is exposed to
- mucosal and pulmonary edema possible up to 48 hours after exposure
- general s/s of respiratory distress (e.g., dyspnea, wheezing, etc.)
- may be signs of injury at mouth, nose, or oral mucosa

Management

- manage airway
    - intubate for burns in or around mouth
- oxygen as needed
- administer antidote if available
- vigorous pulmonary hygiene with patient (including suctioning of airways, blow bottles, and nasotracheal suction)

QUICK REVIEW QUESTIONS

14. A nurse is discharging a patient who was rescued from a house fire. The patient's respiratory status is WNL and the patient is stable. What should the nurse educate the patient to be aware of for the next 2 days?

15. EMS arrives with a patient who was rescued from a house fire. The patient is unconscious, but the airway is clear and intact. Assessment of the airway reveals black soot at the opening of the mouth and at the nares. What is the next nursing consideration for this patient?

Obstruction

Pathophysiology

Airway obstruction, or blockage of the upper airway, can be caused by a foreign body (e.g., teeth, food, marbles), the tongue, vomit, blood, or other secretions. Possible causes of airway obstruction include traumatic injuries to the face, edema in the airway, peritonsillar abscess, and burns to the airway. Small children may also place foreign bodies in their mouths or obstruct their airway with food.

Risk Factors

- age < 2 years and > 65 years
- upper airway burn or inhalation injury
- severe facial trauma
- seizures
- infections or inflammation of the upper airway
- difficulty swallowing

Diagnosis

- visually observed obstruction in airway
- dyspnea or gasping for air
- stridor
- excessive drooling in infants
- agitation or panic
- loss of consciousness, altered LOC, or respiratory arrest

Management

1. inspect the airway
2. suction out any visible foreign bodies
3. reassess the patency of the airway
4. if the airway is still obstructed, view with a laryngoscope
5. if all else fails, cricothyrotomy to open the airway; suction mouth and upper airway

QUICK REVIEW QUESTIONS

16. A 3-year-old is brought into the ED choking on a piece of food. What should be done before suctioning or attempting to digitally clear the airway?

_____

17. After unsuccessfully attempting to intubate a patient with a pharyngeal swelling, what should the nurse prepare for?

_____

CONTINUE

Pleural Effusion

Pathophysiology

Pleural effusion is the buildup of fluid around the lungs in the pleural space. The fluid can displace lung tissue and inhibit adequate ventilation and lung expansion. There are two types of pleural effusions.

- **Transudative pleural effusions** are fluid leakages caused by increased systemic pressure in the vessels or low serum protein levels. The most common causes of transudative pleural effusions are heart failure (due to increased pulmonary capillary pressure) or cirrhosis (currently believed to be the result of fluid movement from the peritoneal cavity to the thorax).

- **Exudative pleural effusions** are the result of changes in capillary permeability resulting in exudate. They have widely varying etiologies, including malignancy (especially lung cancer), pulmonary embolism, and infections.

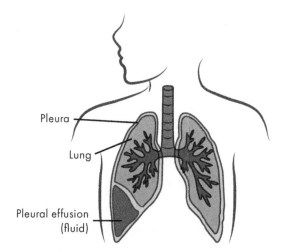

Figure 2.9. Pleural Effusion

Physical Examination

- dyspnea
- dullness upon percussion of the lung area
- asymmetrical chest expansion
- decreased breath sounds on affected side
- cough (dry or productive)
- pleuritic chest pain

Diagnostic Tests

- CXR showing white areas at the base of the lungs (unilaterally or bilaterally)
- CT scan to further diagnose the severity of the condition
- thoracentesis to determine the mechanism of effusion

Management

- stable, asymptomatic patients: monitoring and treatment of underlying condition
- symptomatic patients: drainage of excess pleural fluid (usually via thoracentesis)
  - multiple thoracenteses necessary for reaccumulated fluid
  - pleurodesis or indwelling pleural catheter for recurrent effusions
- medications based on underlying condition (e.g., diuretics, antibiotics)

> **QUICK REVIEW QUESTIONS**
>
> **18.** A patient with heart failure comes to the ED with complaint of dyspnea and chest pain and is diagnosed with a pleural effusion. What intervention should the nurse expect?
>
> _____
>
> **19.** What interventions should the nurse anticipate for a patient with an asymptomatic pleural effusion secondary to pneumonia?
>
> _____

Pneumothorax

Pathophysiology

Pneumothorax is the collection of air between the chest wall and the lung (pleural space). It can occur from blunt chest-wall injury, medical injury, underlying lung tissue disease, or hereditary factors. Pneumothorax is classified according to its underlying cause.

- **Primary spontaneous pneumothorax (PSP)** occurs spontaneously in the absence of lung disease and often presents with only minor symptoms.
- **Secondary spontaneous pneumothorax (SSP)** occurs in patients with an underlying lung disease and presents with more severe symptoms.
- **Traumatic pneumothorax** occurs when the chest wall is penetrated.
- **Tension pneumothorax**, the late progression of a pneumothorax, causes significant respiratory distress in the patient and requires immediate intervention for treatment.

HELPFUL HINT:

Removal of greater than 1000 mL effusion fluid will increase negative intrapleural pressure and lead to **re-expansion pulmonary edema** if lung does not re-expand to fill the now-available pleural space. Signs of re-expansion pulmonary edema include severe cough and dyspnea.

Risk Factors

- for PSP: more common in men 20 – 40 years old who are tall and underweight
- underlying lung tissue disease
- medical procedures
- blunt chest-wall injuries
- changes in atmospheric pressure
- smoking

HELPFUL HINT:

Pneumothorax presents with tracheal deviation *toward* affected side. Tension pneumothorax presents with tracheal deviation *away from* unaffected side.

Physical Examination

- sudden unilateral chest pain
- dyspnea
- tachycardia
- hypoxia and cyanosis
- hypotension
- tension pneumothorax:
  - ☐ **_decreased breath sounds on the affected side_**
  - ☐ increased percussion note
  - ☐ tracheal deviation away from the side of the tension
  - ☐ distended neck veins

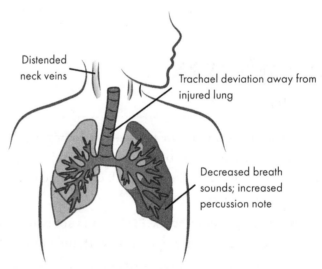

Distended neck veins

Trachael deviation away from injured lung

Decreased breath sounds; increased percussion note

Figure 2.10. Physical Examination of Tension Pneumothorax

Diagnostic Tests

- CXR will show lung tissue separated from the chest wall

Management

- pneumothorax < 15%: supplemental oxygen and monitoring

- pneumothorax > 15%: percutaneous needle aspiration of air from pleural space and insertion of chest tube

- emergent treatment of tension pneumothorax: immediate percutaneous placement of large-bore needle (insertion at second intercostal space mid-axillary line on affected side) and chest-tube insertion

QUICK REVIEW QUESTIONS

20. What are the signs and symptoms of a tension pneumothorax?

21. A patient with blunt thoracic trauma has been diagnosed with pneumothorax and was alert and oriented upon arrival via EMS. On reassessment, the nurse finds the patient restless and anxious. The patient also has tachypnea and tachycardia, with visually distended neck veins. What intervention should the nurse anticipate?

Noncardiac Pulmonary Edema

Pathophysiology

Noncardiac pulmonary edema (NPE) is when fluid collects in the alveoli of the lungs, but the condition is not due to heart failure. This fluid inhibits gas exchange.

Acute respiratory distress syndrome (ARDS) is a sudden and progressive form of noncardiogenic NPE in which the alveoli fill with fluid following damage to the pulmonary endothelium. ARDS is the systemic response to lung injury and is initiated by the inflammatory-immune system, which releases inflammatory mediators from the site of injury within 24 – 48 hours. Inflammation causes alveoli to stiffen and collapse, resulting in NPE with refractory hypoxemia. Left- and right-sided heart failure may follow.

Risk Factors

- ARDS
  - □ gastric aspiration, pneumonia
  - □ toxic inhalation
  - □ pulmonary contusion
  - □ sepsis
  - □ DIC
  - □ pancreatitis

- fluid overload
- CNS injury (**neurogenic pulmonary edema**)
- removal of airway obstruction (**postobstructive pulmonary edema**)
- rapid increase in altitude (**high-altitude pulmonary edema**)
- reexpansion of the lung (**reexpansion pulmonary edema**)

Physical Examination

- tachycardia and hypotension
- tachypnea with increased accessory-muscle usage for work of breathing
- productive cough with frothy sputum (may be pink)
- wheezes, crackles, and rhonchi
- progressive hypoxemia
- other signs and symptoms of heart failure

HELPFUL HINT:

Historically, respiratory distress with a P/F ratio between 200 and 300 was referred to as acute lung injury (ALI). That term is generally no longer used; instead, ARDS has been divided into mild, moderate, and severe, based on the P/F ratio.

Diagnostic Tests

- CXR showing pulmonary infiltrates, ground-glass opacity, and an elevated diaphragm
- *Decreasing P/F ratio*
  - □ <300 = mild ARDS
  - □ <200 = moderate ARDS
  - □ <100 = severe ARDS
- ABG findings
  - □ refractory hypoxemia
  - □ increasing hypercapnia

Management

- high-flow oxygen
- inhaled bronchodilator
- positive inotropic therapy and other vasoactive medications to maintain cardiac output
- mechanical ventilation required for severe ARDS
  - □ *set PEEP at lowest possible amount (10 – 15 cm H2O)*
  - □ low V_T (4 – 6 mL/kg) to reduce barotrauma and volutrauma
  - □ permissive hypercapnia with arterial pH ≥7.20
- treat underlying condition

Pulmonary Embolus

Pathophysiology

A **pulmonary embolus (PE)** is a thromboembolus that occludes a pulmonary artery. The most common embolus is a blood clot caused by deep vein thrombosis (DVT), but fat emboli, tumor emboli, and amniotic fluid emboli can also reach the lungs.

Damage to the lungs during PE follows several pathways. The occlusion increases pulmonary dead space and causes V/Q mismatch, resulting in pulmonary shunting and hypoxemia. PE may also trigger bronchoconstriction and disrupt surfactant functioning, resulting in atelectasis and worsening hypoxemia.

Pulmonary hypertension develops from both the mechanical obstruction (clot) and the release of an injury-site mediator that causes pulmonary vasoconstriction. These processes elevate pulmonary vascular resistance (PVR), which in turn increases right ventricular workload and eventually results in right ventricular failure. Left ventricular preload decreases, cardiac output drops, hypotension follows, and shock occurs.

Risk Factors

- trauma (high risk with fracture)
- surgery
- A-fib
- immobility
- hypercoagulability states

Physical Examination

- pleuritic chest pain
- tachycardia
- tachypnea and dyspnea
- hemoptysis

- increased pulmonary S2
- sudden onset
  - increased PA pressures
  - right-sided HF

Diagnostic Findings

- *__ABG showing low PaO$_2$__*
- *__pulmonary angiogram: definitive diagnosis but with long study time__*
- V/Q scan (25% – 30% accuracy)
- spiral CT scan: a 30-second study with >90% sensitivity/specificity
- ultrasound for DVT in lower extremities
- 12-lead ECG
  - tall, peaked T waves in II, III, aVF
  - transient RBBB
  - right-axis deviation
- D-dimer positive
- ETCO$_2$ value ≥36 rules out PE with high reliability

Management

- supportive treatment for symptoms
  - *__O$_2$ therapy__*
  - analgesics
  - vasopressors to manage blood pressure
- IV fluid resuscitation
- IV anticoagulants once diagnosis is confirmed
- thrombolytics for unstable patients with no contraindications

---

QUICK REVIEW QUESTIONS

24. Why would a patient with a suspected PE receive a CXR?

_____

25. What medication should the nurse expect to administer to a patient with a confirmed PE?

_____

26. A 52-year-old patient arrives at the ED with tachycardia, tachypnea, hemoptysis, and chest pain. The patient is currently hemodynamically stable, and a diagnosis of a PE is suspected. What diagnostic study should the nurse expect to be ordered?

_____

Respiratory Trauma

Pathophysiology

Chest trauma, whether from blunt injury, sharp, invasive penetration, or thoracic surgical procedures, creates a wide range of respiratory complications.

TABLE 2.5. Thoracic Injuries		
Injury	**Pathophysiology**	**Clinical Presentation**
Pulmonary contusion	Bruising of the parenchyma of the lung. Capillary rupture causes blood and other fluid to leak into lung tissue, causes localized edema, and may result in hypoxia from diminished gas exchange. Fluid accumulation in alveoli and decreased pulmonary secretion clearance put patients at risk for ARDS and pneumonia.	• signs and symptoms may be delayed 24 – 72 hours until edema develops • hemoptysis (pink, frothy sputum) • crackles • tachypnea and tachycardia • hypoxia • chest wall bruising • pain • decreased $PaCO_2$ • decreased P/F ratio
Rib fractures	Commonly caused by traumatic crushing injury to chest or cancer; leads to altered ventilation and perfusion status. Most common fractures are ribs 4 – 8. Ribs 9 – 12 may cause splenic rupture and tears to the diaphragm and liver.	• pain with breathing • shallow breaths • splinting
Hemothorax	Blood in the pleural space, usually resulting from blunt or penetrating trauma to the chest wall. Damage to the lung parenchyma and great vessels causes alveoli collapse. May also present with pneumothorax (pneumo-hemothorax).	• symptomatic with blood volume >400 mL • absence of breath sounds on affected side • tracheal deviation toward unaffected side • dullness to percussion • tachypnea • hypovolemia • shock

continued on next page

TABLE 2.5. Thoracic Injuries (continued)

Injury	Pathophysiology	Clinical Presentation
Tracheal rupture (or perforation)	Occurs when there is injury to the structure of the trachea. The perforation can be caused by forceful or poor intubation efforts or by traumatic injury to the trachea such as in crush injuries or hanging injuries.	• hemoptysis • dyspnea • ***diffuse subcutaneous emphysema***
Ruptured diaphragm	Injury to the diaphragm creates a negative pressure gradient, allowing abdominal viscera to enter the thoracic cavity. The shift compresses the lungs and mediastinum, causing decreased venous return and cardiac output.	• respiratory distress • ***bowel sounds in chest on auscultation*** • tracheal deviation
Flail chest	Multiple anterior and posterior fractures to 3 or more ribs.	• ***paradoxical movement of the chest wall*** (flail segment moves inward during inspiration and outward during exhalation)

HELPFUL HINT:

A sudden crush injury to the chest wall produces **traumatic asphyxia**. This specific crush injury results in an "ecchymotic mask" characterized by subconjunctival hemorrhage, facial edema, and petechiae and cyanosis of the head, neck, and upper extremities.

Management

- pain management as needed (intercostal nerve blocks, thoracic epidural analgesia, opioids, or NSAIDs)
- small contusions: heal in 3 – 5 days, often without treatment
- severe contusions: aggressive pulmonary care (e.g., ambulation, turning, incentive spirometry) and fluid management with possible mechanical ventilation
- hemothorax: chest-tube insertion or thoracotomy (if bleeding cannot be managed)
- tracheal perforation: maintain airway and prepare for surgical repair
- ruptured diaphragm: prep patient for immediate surgical intervention
- flail chest: aggressive management with analgesics, pulmonary hygiene, and noninvasive positive pressure ventilation

QUICK REVIEW QUESTIONS

27. What signs and symptoms should lead the nurse to suspect a diagnosis of hemothorax?

28. A patient is admitted to the ED with a tracheal rupture following a suicide attempt by hanging. What intervention should the nurse anticipate?

_____

29. A 46-year-old patient with A-fib who is on anticoagulant medication suffered a fall at home with no head injury or loss of consciousness. The following day, the patient presents to the ED with pink frothy sputum, crackles in the lung fields, tachypnea, tachycardia, and pain. Ecchymosis is evident over ribs 4 – 8. ABG shows hypoxia. CXR has ruled out rib fractures but is not remarkable. The patient is sent for a chest CT scan. What diagnosis should the nurse expect, and why was a chest CT scan ordered?

_____

Pulmonary Hypertension

Pathophysiology

Pulmonary hypertension, elevated blood pressure in the arteries to the lungs (> 20 mm Hg), is caused by occlusions or narrowing of the arteries. Because blood cannot pass through the arteries, extra strain is placed on the heart, reducing its ability to pump effectively.

There is currently no cure for pulmonary hypertension; treatment is focused on reducing symptoms through medications.

Risk Factors

- can be idiopathic
- hereditary
- chronic conditions (e.g., lupus, liver disease, HIV)
- stimulant drug use (e.g., cocaine, methamphetamines)

Physical Examination

- dyspnea
- signs of right-ventricular failure

Diagnostic Tests

- CXR may show enlarged arteries or ventricles
- CT scan of the chest may show pulmonary hypertension
- echocardiogram necessary to ascertain pressures within the pulmonary arteries

Management

- emergent management: oxygen and medications (vasodilators, diuretics, and/or anticoagulants)

QUICK REVIEW QUESTION

30. A patient with a history of pulmonary hypertension presents to the ED and has not taken her medications for a month. Which types of intervention and medications will this patient probably need?

ANSWER KEY

1. COVID-19 can cause fluid to build up in the alveoli, resulting in shunting. Because the hypoxemia is a result of low ventilation (less air reaching the alveoli), increasing O_2 delivery will not sufficiently improve PaO_2.

2. The patient has respiratory acidosis that is partially compensated, meaning the body is attempting unsuccessfully to restore acid-base balance.

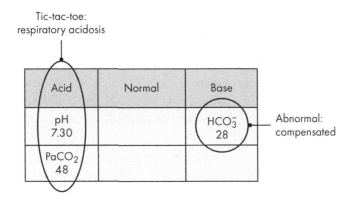

3. PEEP, or positive end-expiratory pressure, allows for more effective gas exchange by keeping the alveoli open especially at end expiration. Complications include barotrauma to the lungs, decreased blood pressure and cardiac output, and air-leak syndromes.

4. Risk factors for aspiration include age >65, difficulty swallowing or neurologic dysfunction, intoxication, sedation, and altered LOC.

5. A CXR will be ordered to diagnose aspiration.

6. The nurse should administer O_2 via nonrebreathing mask.

7. The nurse should expect to administer an inhaled beta 2 agonist, inhaled ipratropium, and a corticosteroid to a patient experiencing an acute asthma exacerbation.

8. Signs of worsening asthma exacerbation include inspiratory and expiratory wheezes, decreased breath sounds in all lung fields, and respiratory acidosis with hypercapnia.

9. The nurse should expect to administer an inhaled beta 2 agonist and inhaled ipratropium to patient with an acute exacerbation of COPD.

10. O_2 is titrated to SpO_2 88% – 92% in patients with COPD to avoid hypercapnia.

11. Patients can manage bronchitis with adequate hydration, humidification of air in the home, and OTC antitussives.

12. The nurse should expect to administer O_2 therapy and corticosteroids (for management of croup).

13. The nurse should explain that the medical team performed a CXR and labs to rule out pneumonia.

14. The nurse should educate the patient to monitor for mucosal and pulmonary edema. The patient should seek emergent care for any shortness of breath, excessive coughing, or respiratory distress in the next 48 hours.

15. The nurse should administer O_2 and place the patient on monitors.

16. The nurse should visualize the back of the throat to prevent lodging a foreign body further into the airway.

17. The nurse should prepare for an emergent cricothyrotomy.

18. The nurse should expect to assist with a thoracentesis.

19. The nurse should anticipate administering antibiotics and monitoring the patient.

20. The signs and symptoms of a tension pneumothorax include tracheal deviation away from the side of the tension, decreased breath sounds on the affected side, increased percussion note, and distended neck veins.

21. The nurse should anticipate that the patient will need a needle thoracostomy.

22. ABG for patients with ARDS will show decreasing P/F ratio, refractory hypoxemia, and increasing hypercapnia.

23. The patient will require intubation and mechanical ventilation.

24. A patient with a suspected PE will receive a CXR to rule out other conditions.

25. A patient with a confirmed PE will be administered an anticoagulant.

26. The nurse should expect a pulmonary angiogram to be ordered.

27. Signs and symptoms of hemothorax include absence of breath sounds on affected side, tracheal deviation toward unaffected side, dullness to percussion, and signs and symptoms of hypovolemia.

28. The nurse should maintain the patient's airway and prepare the patient for surgical repair.

29. The nurse should expect a diagnosis of a pulmonary contusion; a CT scan is more sensitive than CXR.

30. The patient will require oxygenation and vasodilators.

3 NEUROLOGICAL EMERGENCIES

Neurological Anatomy and Physiology

- The **nervous system** coordinates the processes and action of the human body.
- The functions of the nervous system are broken down into the somatic nervous system, which controls skeletal and voluntary muscles, and the **autonomic nervous system**, which controls involuntary muscle actions.
- The autonomic nervous system is further broken down into the sympathetic nervous system and parasympathetic nervous system.

□ The **sympathetic nervous system** is responsible for the body's reaction to stress and induces a "fight or flight" response to stimuli.

□ The **parasympathetic nervous system** is stimulated by the body's need for rest or recovery.

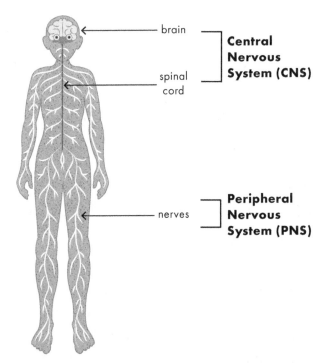

Figure 3.1. Divisions of the Nervous System

■ The **peripheral nervous system (PNS)** is the collection of nerves that connect the central nervous system to the rest of the body.

■ The **central nervous system (CNS)** is made up of the **brain** and **spinal cord**.

■ Each area of the brain has specific functions that are affected by localized tissue damage.

□ frontal lobe: thinking, speaking, movement, memory

□ parietal lobe: touch, language

□ temporal lobe: emotions, hearing, learning

□ occipital lobe: vision, color perception

□ cerebellum: balance, coordination

□ brainstem: breathing, heart rate, temperature regulation

□ thalamus: sleep, alertness, sensory processing

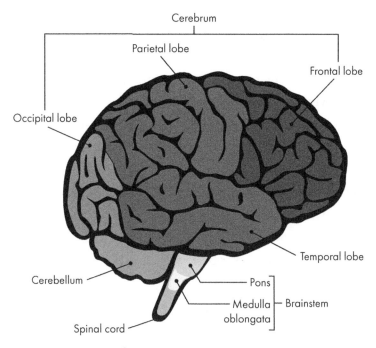

Figure 3.2. Areas of the Brain

- Blood supply to the brain comes by two arterial sources: the **internal carotid artery** and the **vertebral arteries**. Blockage in any of these arteries causes intense temporary or permanent damage to each area of the brain they supply.

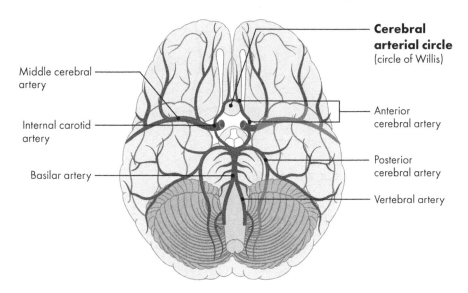

Figure 3.3. Vasculature in the Brain

- The **meninges** form a protective coating over the brain and spinal cord. They consist of three layers:

□ The outermost layer is the **dura mater**. The epidural space (above the dura) and the subdural space (below the dura) contain vasculature that can bleed following injury to the brain.

□ The **arachnoid mater** is below the dura mater.

□ The **pia mater** is the innermost layer that is attached to the CNS.

■ **Cerebral spinal fluid (CSF)** is a clear, colorless fluid that circulates around the brain and spinal cord. It cushions the brain and transports nutrients and waste.

■ The **vertebral column** is made up of twenty-four vertebrae.

□ the cervical, or the neck vertebrae (C1 – C7)

□ the thoracic, or the chest vertebrae (T1 – T12)

□ the lumbar, or the lower back vertebrae (L1 – L5)

□ sacrum and coccyx

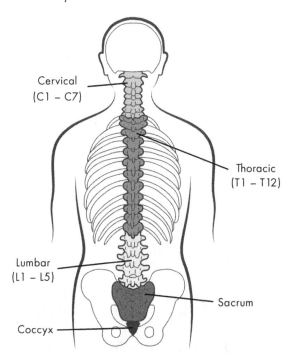

Figure 3.4. The Vertebral Column

QUICK REVIEW QUESTION

1. What type of focal neurological deficits would indicate likely damage to the occipital lobe?

Neurological Assessment

- Neurological assessment should be done continuously to obtain baseline data and to assess for neurological deterioration or improvements related to treatment.
  - □ level of consciousness (LOC): earliest indication of neurological deterioration
  - □ pupillary response: late indication of neurological deterioration
  - □ mental status
  - □ motor function
  - □ sensation/touch perception
  - □ vision changes
  - □ speech changes
  - □ Glasgow Coma Scale (GCS) (Table 3.1)
  - □ cranial nerve assessment (Table 3.2)

TABLE 3.1. Scoring on the Glasgow Coma Scale

Eye Opening (E)	Verbal Response (V)	Motor Response (M)
4 = spontaneous 3 = to sound 2 = to pressure 1 = none	5 = oriented 4 = confused 3 = inappropriate words 2 = incomprehensible sounds 1 = no response	6 = obeys command 5 = localizes 4 = normal flexion 3 = abnormal flexion 2 = extension 1 = none
15: fully awake <8: severe brain injury 3: coma or death		

TABLE 3.2. Cranial Nerve Function and Assessment

Cranial Nerve	Function
I. Olfactory	sense of smell
II. Optic	central and peripheral vision
III. Oculomotor	constriction of pupils
IV. Trochlear	downward eye movement
V. Trigeminal	facial sensation and motor control of mouth
VI. Abducens	sideways eye movement

continued on next page

TABLE 3.2. Cranial Nerve Function and Assessment (continued)

Cranial Nerve	Function
VII. Facial	movement and expression
VIII. Vestibulocochlear	hearing and balance
IX. Glossopharyngeal	tongue and throat
X. Vagus	sensory and motor
XI. Accessory	head and shoulder movement
XII. Hypoglossal	tongue position
Other Cranial Nerve Assessments	
Doll's eyes reflex	assessment of oculocephalic function (cranial nerves III, IV, VI) in an unconscious patient: **normal** (both eyes roll/move to opposite side of head position) **abnormal** (eyes roll/move in opposite directions of each other): indicates a brainstem injury **absent** (eyes remain midline/move with head position): indicates significant brainstem injury
Consensual response	assessment of CN II and III: constriction of pupil when light shined into opposite eye

- postural indicators of brain damage
  - **decorticate** (patient brings arms to the CORE of the body): damage to cerebral hemispheres (CORtex)
  - **decerebrate** (extended position): ominous sign of brainstem damage and possible brain herniation

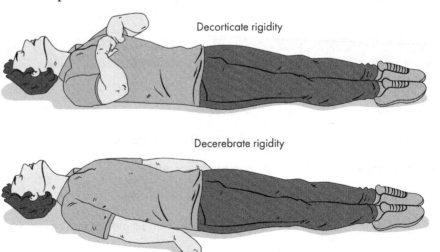

Decorticate rigidity

Decerebrate rigidity

Figure 3.5. Decorticate and Decerebrate Postures

- medical signs of possible brain damage
  - □ **Kernig's sign** (indicator of meningitis): patient in supine position with the hips and knees flexed, unable to straighten leg due to hamstring pain
  - □ **Brudzinski's sign** (indicator of meningitis): passive flexion of the neck elicits automatic flexion at the hips and knees
  - □ **nuchal rigidity** (indicator of meningitis): inability to place the chin on the chest (neck flexion) due to muscle stiffness
  - □ **Babinski sign** (indicator of damage to corticospinal tract): a single, firm stroking of the sole of the foot from the heel to toes causes big toe to point up and toes to fan out
- **Cushing's triad** is a late, ominous sign of increased ICP and possible brain herniation.
  - □ widening pulse pressure (elevated SBP and decreased DBP)
  - □ bradycardia
  - □ decreased/abnormal RR (Cheyne-Stokes respiration)

QUICK REVIEW QUESTION

2. A patient is being assessed with the GCS. There is a slight reaction to pressure, incoherent verbal responses, and decorticate positioning. What would the GCS result be, and what does it indicate?

Neurological Disorders

TABLE 3.3. Diagnosis and Management of Neurological Disorders		
Disorder	**Diagnosis**	**Management**
Alzheimer's disease a cognitive deterioration caused by beta-amyloid deposits and neurofibrillary tangles in the cerebral cortex and subcortical gray matter of the brain; most common cause of dementia in U.S.	loss of short-term memory impaired reasoning and judgment language dysfunction inability to recognize faces and common objects behavioral disturbances: wandering, agitation, yelling	supportive treatment for symptoms most common cause for ED visit is agitation or aggression assess for the most common causes of agitation and aggression: UTI, pain, underlying medical condition, medications olanzapine (Zyprexa): preferred medication for geriatric patients in acute crises lorazepam (Ativan) or diphenhydramine (Benadryl) may be given

continued on next page

TABLE 3.3. Diagnosis and Management of Neurological Disorders (continued)

Disorder	Diagnosis	Management
Amyotrophic lateral sclerosis (ALS) (Lou Gehrig's disease) a neurodegenerative disorder that affects the neurons in the brain stem and spinal cord; symptoms progressively worsen until respiratory failure occurs	**_progressive asymmetrical weakness_**; can affect both upper and lower extremities difficulty swallowing, walking, or speaking muscle cramps	supportive treatment for symptoms respiratory support high risk of aspiration
Multiple sclerosis (MS) a neurodegenerative disorder caused by patches of demyelination in the brain and the spinal cord; has periods of both remission and exacerbation of symptoms, gradually growing disability	paresthesia weakness of at least one extremity visual, motor, or urinary disturbance vertigo fatigue mild cognitive impairment increased deep tendon reflexes positive Babinski sign clonus	corticosteroids for inflammation baclofen (Lioresal) or tizanidine (Zanaflex) for spasticity gabapentin (Neurontin) or tricyclic antidepressants for pain
Muscular dystrophy (MD) a genetic disorder in which a mutation in the recessive dystrophin gene on the X chromosome causes muscle fiber degeneration; results in progressive proximal muscle weakness	first noted at 2 – 3 years of age steady progression of weakness limb flexion and contraction scoliosis dilated cardiomyopathy, conduction abnormalities, or dysrhythmias respiratory insufficiency	prednisone or deflazacort monitor CO_2 levels; noninvasive ventilator support may be needed supportive treatment of symptoms related to falls, cardiovascular disorders

Disorder	Diagnosis	Management
Myasthenia gravis (MG) autoimmune disorder that causes cell-mediated destruction of acetylcholine receptors, resulting in episodic muscle weakness and fatigue **Myasthenic crisis** an emergent condition in which MG symptoms rapidly worsen; weakening of the bulbar and respiratory muscles can cause respiratory dysfunction	weakened eye muscles and visual disturbances dysphagia fatigue myasthenic crisis: dyspnea, respiratory failure, tachycardia, hypertension, no cough or gag reflex, urinary and bowel incontinence ***diagnosed with Tensilon (edrophonium) test***	IV fluids IV immunoglobulin anticholinesterase (e.g., edrophonium) respiratory support long-term medications: pyridostigmine (Mestinon), steroids, muscle relaxants
Guillain-Barré syndrome an autoimmune disorder in which the immune system attacks healthy cells within the nervous system, rapidly affecting motor function; muscle weakness may lead to respiratory dysfunction	***neuropathy and weakness ascending from lower extremities and advancing symmetrically upward*** paresthesia in extremities unsteady gait absent or diminished deep tendon reflexes dyspnea autonomic dysfunction: hypertension, bradycardia, asystole	analgesics IV immunoglobulins treatment of dysrhythmias respiratory support

HELPFUL HINT:

Patients with MG are at risk for a cholinergic crisis if they are given high doses of anticholinesterase medications.

HELPFUL HINT:

Antipsychotic medications, especially Haloperidol lactate (Haldol), are used cautiously in geriatric patients with dementia because they increase the risk of stroke, MI, and death.

QUICK REVIEW QUESTIONS

3. A patient presents to the ED with a recent diagnosis of ALS. What type of weakness would the ED nurse expect the patient to exhibit?

_____

4. A patient is being treated for proximal weakness related to MD. The most recent ABG values show a CO_2 level of 32 mmol/L. What intervention should the nurse anticipate?

Headaches

TABLE 3.4. Diagnosis and Management of Headaches	
Condition	**Management**
Cluster headaches characterized by intense unilateral pain in the peri-orbital or temporal area, with ipsilateral autonomic symptoms happens at the same time each day, often waking the patient at night episodic, lasting from 1 to 3 months, with more than 1 episode of headaches a day can go into remission for months to years	usually resolves within 30 minutes to 1 hour 100% oxygen via non-rebreather triptans (e.g., sumatriptan)
Migraine a neurovascular condition caused by neurological changes that result in vasoconstriction or vasodila-tion of the intracranial vessels intense or debilitating headache (typically unilat-eral) lasting from 4 hours to several days accompanied by nausea, vomiting, and sensitivity to light and sound may be preceded by aura	analgesics (NSAIDs) triptans (e.g., sumatriptan) dihydroergotamine antiemetics limit sensory triggers and apply ice packs to painful area
Temporal arteritis headache caused by inflamed or damaged arteries in the temporal area severe, throbbing headache in the temporal or forehead region, combined with scalp pain that is exacerbated with touch muscle pain in the jaw or tongue small period of full or partial blindness in one eye; may progress to both eyes fever definitive diagnostic test: biopsy of the temporal artery rare in patients < 50 years old	glucocorticoids (e.g., prednisone, methylpred-nisolone): early interven-tion to prevent permanent blindness methotrexate if glucocorti-coid contraindicated

Condition	Management
Tension headaches	
headaches characterized by generalized mild pain without any of the symptoms associated with migraines, such as nausea or photophobia	NSAIDs
can be either episodic or chronic	barbiturates or opioids (Fioricet [butalbital, acet-aminophen, and caffeine] or morphine) for severe pain
pain is mild to moderate, often described as a vise pressing on the head	
originates in the occipital or frontal area bilaterally	

QUICK REVIEW QUESTIONS

5. A patient in the ED is diagnosed with temporal arteritis and is experiencing temporary episodes of blindness in the left eye. What intervention would the nurse anticipate?

   _____

6. A patient presents to the ED with a headache. What signs and symptoms would be indicative of a migraine and would most likely not be present in a patient with a more serious neurological injury?

   _____

HELPFUL HINT:

Post-traumatic headaches start within 7 days of a traumatic injury and typically resolve within 3 months. They may resemble migraines or tension headaches and can be treated similarly.

Increased Intracranial Pressure

Pathophysiology

Intracranial pressure (ICP) is the pressure within the intracranial compartment (the area enclosed by the cranium). A normal adult cranium encloses a fixed volume of around 1500 mL divided between brain tissue (80% of volume), CSF (10%), and blood (10%). Since the cranium does not expand or otherwise move, insults to brain tissue that increase intracranial volume will increase ICP.

Normal ICP is 5 – 15 mm Hg. An ICP >20 mm Hg is a neurological emergency that requires immediate treatment.

When ICP increases, immediate interventions must be implemented to maintain **cerebral perfusion pressure (CPP)**, the net pressure gradient that drives oxygen delivery to brain tissue. CPP is defined as the difference between MAP and ICP (i.e., MAP – ICP), and should be maintained at 50 – 70 mm Hg.

Risk Factors

- trauma (TBI, brain contusion)
- mass displacement of brain tissue by tumor, hematoma, or abscess
- hypoxic-ischemic brain injury

HELPFUL HINT:

Increased ICP may also cause brain tissue to herniate downward through the tentorial notch and foramen magnum into the brainstem; herniation is rapidly fatal.

- intracranial hemorrhage
- increased CSF production (meningitis)
- blockages to CSF flow/reabsorption (hydrocephalus, meningeal disease)
- seizures
- hyperthermia (core temperature > 37.5°C)

Physical Examination

- change in LOC
- headache
- vomiting
- Cushing's triad
- irritability
- photophobia
- lethargy and impaired/slowed decision-making

Diagnostic Tests

- _**ICP > 20 mm Hg**_
- abnormal ICP waveform
  - An elevated tidal wave (P2) indicates reduced intracranial compliance and increased ICP.
  - A single wave with a lack of distinct peaks indicates a critical increase in ICP that requires immediate intervention.

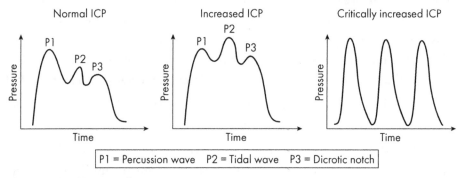

P1 = Percussion wave   P2 = Tidal wave   P3 = Dicrotic notch

Figure 3.6. ICP Waveform

Management

- hyperosmolar/hypertonic fluid therapy
  - _**mannitol 20%**_
  - loop diuretics (assess for hypokalemia)
  - hypertonic saline

- patient positioning: elevate HOB 30 – 35° with midline head alignment, and avoid hip flexion
- maintain normal body temperature
- limit activities that may raise ICP, including coughing, sneezing, vomiting, suctioning, PEEP, restraint use, and the Valsalva maneuver
- stabilize blood glucose: maintain blood glucose ≤140 mg/dL
- decrease environmental stimuli, and minimize nursing care
- higher-level interventions for refractory ICP: mechanical ventilation, IV opioids, sedation, and decompressive craniotomy

QUICK REVIEW QUESTIONS

7. When is treatment for ICP usually initiated for adults?

_____

8. What medication is administered to decrease ICP?

_____

HELPFUL HINT:

Hypotonic solutions (D5W, 0.45% NaCl) should be avoided in patients with ICP. They decrease plasma osmolality and move water from extracellular to intracellular spaces in the brain, increasing ICP.

Meningitis

Pathophysiology

Meningitis, an acute inflammation of the meninges, is caused by bacterial, viral, or fungal pathogens that invade the subarachnoid space. The infection triggers WBC accumulation and tissue damage, leading to swelling and purulent exudate within the cranium.

Viral infection is the most common cause of meningitis. Bacterial meningitis is a medical emergency because of the rapidity of deterioration and the high mortality rate.

Physical Examination

- headache
- nuchal rigidity
- _positive Brudzinski's and Kernig's signs_
- fever
- altered mental status
- rash
- photophobia

HELPFUL HINT:

Each 1°C increases cerebral O_2 demand by 7 – 10%, which in turn increases CBF and ICP.

Diagnostic Tests

- lumbar puncture to confirm
  - CSF finding for viral meningitis: elevated protein and lymphocytes; _clear fluid_
  - CSF finding for bacterial meningitis: very elevated protein, elevated WBCs and neutrophils, _low glucose, cloudy fluid_

Management

- standard and droplet isolation precautions until specific cause is determined
- _empirical IV antibiotic therapy_
- corticosteroids
- antivirals (as appropriate)
- monitor for sepsis, increased ICP, and SIADH/DI

QUICK REVIEW QUESTIONS

9. An 18-year-old college student comes into the ED complaining of a severe headache and fever; due to stiffness, he cannot turn his head. The patient complains of extreme pain when attempting to move the head forward. What test should the nurse anticipate preparing the patient for?

10. A patient with suspected meningitis is awaiting transfer to the floor. A lumbar puncture was completed and CSF results are pending. What precautions should the nurse initiate before the patient leaves the ED?

Seizure Disorders

Seizure disorders are caused by abnormal electrical discharges in the brain. During a seizure, brain neurons abnormally or excessively fire because the membrane potential is altered in a way that makes those neurons hypersensitive to stimuli. Seizures may be **focal** (limited to one part of the brain) or **generalized.**

Status epilepticus is a medical emergency in which seizure activity continues or recurs for more than 5 minutes. It has a high mortality rate (20 – 30%) and requires immediate intervention.

Risk Factors

- trauma
- drug toxicity or withdrawal
- fluid or electrolyte imbalances
- hypoglycemia
- hypoxic-ischemic events
- cerebral edema
- sepsis
- tumors

Physical Examination

- convulsive: tonic-clonic (grand mal) seizure
    - tonic phase: loss of consciousness, rigidity of extremities, dilated pupils
    - clonic phase: rhythmic shaking, violent alternating contraction/relaxation, tachycardia, mouth frothing
    - postictal: impaired mental status and focal neurological deficits (Todd paralysis common)
- status epilepticus: seizure activity lasting longer than 5 minutes or repeat seizures with no regaining of consciousness between

Management

- manage ABCs
- prevent injury
    - roll patient on the left side to avoid aspiration
    - loosen clothes around the neck
    - lace a pillow under patient's head and remove objects near head
- finger-stick blood glucose: administer 50 mL D50W IV push if blood glucose <60 mg/dL
- prompt pharmacological treatment
    - *first-line drugs: IV lorazepam, IV diazepam, or IM midazolam*
    - *second-line drugs (after 20 minutes of nonresponse to treatment): IV fosphenytoin, IV valproate, or IV levetiracetam*

QUICK REVIEW QUESTIONS

11. What are the diagnostic criteria for status epilepticus?

12. A patient with a history of seizures is brought into the ED in status epilepticus. What medication should the nurse prepare to administer?

Stroke (Hemorrhagic)

Pathophysiology

A **hemorrhagic stroke**, the disruption of CBF, is caused by bleeding. The resulting hypoxia rapidly leads to brain cell death, and the excess blood in the cranium also increases ICP, increasing the risk of brain herniation. Bleeding may be caused by the spontaneous rupture of a blood vessel, head trauma, a brain mass, or uncontrolled anticoagulation conditions. The hemorrhage is classified by location as intracerebral or subarachnoid.

An **intracerebral hemorrhage (ICH)** is arterial bleeding directly into cerebral tissue. An ICH is most commonly caused by hypertensive rupture of a cerebral artery that has become damaged over time by atherosclerosis. The burst of blood from such a break in the artery causes a hematoma in the brain tissue around the rupture site. Patients with an ICH often present to EMS as unconscious and require immediate intubation for ventilatory support.

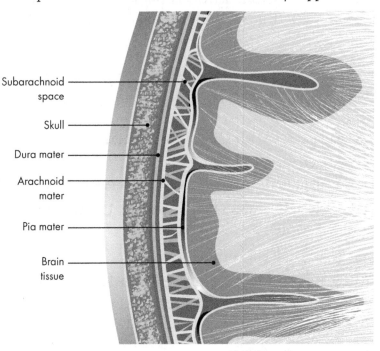

Figure 3.7. Anatomy of the Subarachnoid Space

A **subarachnoid hemorrhage (SAH)** is bleeding into the subarachnoid space. About 85% of spontaneous SAHs are due to the rupture of a saccular **cerebral aneurysm**, most commonly located at the circle of Willis. When age-related or long-term hypertension places stress on the weakened arterial blood vessel, the dome of the outpouching aneurysm thins and ruptures.

Risk Factors

- hypertension
- arteriovenous malformation (AVM)
- smoking
- diabetes
- A-fib

Diagnosis

TABLE 3.5. Diagnosis of Hemorrhagic Stroke		
	Intracerebral hemorrhage	**Subarachnoid hemorrhage**
Physical Examination	acute onset of symptoms that gradually worsen over minutes or hours sudden loss of consciousness (hallmark differentiation from ischemic stroke) sudden focal deficit (determined by site of bleed) severe headache nausea and vomiting severe hypertension (200/100 – 250/150 mm Hg) seizures	abrupt onset of pain, often described as "the worst headache of my life" brief loss of consciousness that may progress to coma nausea and vomiting focal neurological deficits, especially CN III palsy nuchal rigidity meningeal irritation: positive Kernig's and Brudzinski's signs

continued on next page

TABLE 3.5. Diagnosis of Hemorrhagic Stroke (continued)

	Intracerebral hemorrhage	Subarachnoid hemorrhage
Diagnostic Tests	priority (interpreted in < 45 minutes): noncontrast CT scan of head to differentiate ischemic from hemorrhagic stroke	noncontrast CT scan: blood visualized in subarachnoid space if scan obtained within 48 hours of hemorrhage lumbar puncture (if initial CT scan is negative): CSF bloody with RBC >1000 cells/µL CT angiogram to locate cause of hemorrhage (for surgical intervention) Hunt and Hess Grading Scale • 1: asymptomatic, mild headache, slight nuchal rigidity • 2: moderate to severe headache, nuchal rigidity, no neurological deficit other than cranial nerve palsy • 3: drowsiness, confusion, mild focal neurological deficit • 4: stupor, moderate to severe hemiparesis • 5: coma, decerebrate posturing

HELPFUL HINT:

Patients with SAH may describe sudden onset of headaches with vomiting in preceding weeks. These symptoms are the result of small amounts of blood leaking from aneurysms ("warning leaks" from preruptured aneurysms).

Management

- *__priority goal: management of ABCs and reduction of BP__*
- intubation and mechanical ventilation usually necessary for ICH
- moderate BP reduction to reduce bleeding
  - □ MAP = 110 – 130 mm Hg
  - □ CPP > 70 mm Hg
  - □ vasopressor therapy after fluid replacement if SBP <90 mm Hg
- treat increased ICP (per above)
- reverse or stabilize anticoagulation state
- management of seizures (possibly with prophylactic medication)
- DVT prophylaxis
- surgical intervention based on location of bleed and neurological condition

HELPFUL HINT:

Nimodipine is administered to lower risk of cerebral vasospasm, a common cause of death after cerebral aneurysm rupture. (It is less common in SAH due to AVM rupture).

QUICK REVIEW QUESTIONS

13. What symptom, when reported by the patient, should always lead to assessment to rule out hemorrhagic stroke?

_____

14. What is the nursing priority for a patient admitted with a hemorrhagic stroke?

_____

15. A CT scan has determined a patient with stroke symptoms has had an intracerebral hemorrhage. The patient has a history of hypertension and A-fib and is currently taking hydrochlorothiazide, lisinopril, and warfarin. The patient's SBP was initially 200 mm Hg but has been stabilized to 170/86 mm Hg on a nicardipine IV infusion at 10 mg/hr. Results of coagulation labs find that the INR is 4.5. What medication should the nurse expect to administer?

_____

Stroke (Ischemic)

Pathophysiology

During an **ischemic stroke**, blood flow to the brain is interrupted because of either a thrombotic or an embolic clot. Regardless of etiology, loss of CBF leads to hypoperfusion of brain cells, ischemic injury to a focal area, and brain death if anoxia is sustained.

A **transient ischemic attack (TIA)**, a sudden, brief neurological deficit resulting from brain ischemia, does not cause permanent damage or infarction. Symptoms depend on the area of the brain affected. Most TIAs last less than 5 minutes and are resolved within 1 hour. A majority are caused by emboli in the carotid or vertebral arteries.

HELPFUL HINT:

Hemiplegic migraine headaches and severe hypoglycemia can mimic stroke.

Risk Factors

- atherosclerosis or carotid artery disease
- history of A-Fib
- hypertension
- abdominal obesity
- diabetes
- sickle cell disease
- vasculitis
- tobacco use
- cocaine and amphetamine usage

Physical Examination

- sudden onset of severe headache
- focal neurological signs determined by location and size of the area of ischemia (lesion)
  - facial drooping, usually on one side
  - numbness, paralysis, or weakness on one side of the body
  - arm drift
  - slurred speech or inability to speak
  - confusion
  - vision changes
  - dizziness or loss of balance control

Diagnostic Tests

- *priority (interpreted in < 45 minutes): noncontrast CT scan of head to differentiate ischemic from hemorrhagic stroke*
- bedside glucose check to rule out hypoglycemia as cause of symptoms
- National Institute of Health Stroke Scale (NIHSS)
  - LOC
  - eye deviation (CN III, IV, VI)
  - visual field loss (tests hemianopia and extinction)
  - facial palsy
  - motor arm (drift)
  - motor leg (drift)
  - limb ataxia (tests for unilateral cerebellar lesion)
  - sensory
  - best language (tests for comprehension/aphasia)
  - dysarthria (tests for speech ability)
  - extinction and inattention (tests for visual/spatial "neglect")

Management

- *IV or intra-arterial fibrinolytic therapy (alteplase)*
  - dosage: 0.9 mg/kg to a maximum of 90 mg; first 10% as IV bolus dose over 1 minute, with remaining 90% given as IV infusion over 1 hour
  - *must be initiated within 3 hours from "last seen normal"; time window expanded to 4.5 hours for eligible patients* (<80 years old, no history of diabetes/stroke, NIHSS score <25)

- hypertensive patients: BP should be lowered to <185/110 with anti-hypertensive medication before administration
- aspirin administered >24 hours after alteplase administration
- monitor for side effects, including bleeding, angioedema, ICH, pulmonary edema, DVT, seizure, and sepsis
- mechanical thrombectomy for fibrinolytic-ineligible patients or fibrinolytic-eligible patients with high likelihood of stroke due to LVO; may be done in conjunction with tenecteplase administration
- cardiac monitoring for post-reperfusion dysrhythmias
- regular neurological checks and monitor ICP
- maintain normal body temperature
- maintain blood glucose of 140 – 180 mL/dL (do not administer D5W)
- supplemental O_2 for saturation below 94%
- DVT prophylaxis

QUICK REVIEW QUESTIONS

16. A patient presents to the ED with slurred speech and a left-sided facial droop. What is the priority diagnostic test for this patient?

_____

17. How long after onset of ischemic stroke can a patient be given tPA?

_____

18. What is the main side effect of tPA that requires monitoring?

_____

Head and Spinal Cord Trauma

ACUTE SPINAL CORD INJURIES

- **Spinal cord injuries (SCIs)** are injuries to the vertebral column.
  - The **primary injury** is caused by trauma, including compression, hyperextension, contusion, or shearing.
  - **Secondary injuries** are caused by resulting physiological processes such as hypoxia and ischemia; they may lead to neurological dysfunction that presents hours or days after the initial trauma.
- SCIs may be **complete** (meaning all sensory and motor function is lost below the level of injury) or **incomplete** (meaning some sensory and motor function is retained).

HELPFUL HINT:

Spinal shock refers to depressed or absent reflexes that result from SCIs. It is not related to the circulatory system.

- The location and severity of sensory/motor loss depends on the type of injury.
  - **Anterior spinal cord syndrome** occurs when the blood flow to the anterior spinal artery is disrupted, resulting in ischemia in the spinal cord and complete loss of motor and sensory function below the lesion.
  - **Brown-Séquard syndrome** is an SCI caused by complete cord hemitransection, typically at the cervical level. Symptoms include ipsilateral motor loss below the lesion and contralateral loss of sensation of pain and temperature.
  - **Cauda equina syndrome** is an SCI typically caused by compression of, or damage to, the cauda equina, the nerve bundle that innervates the lower limbs and pelvic organs, most notably the bladder. Symptoms include sensory loss in the lower extremities, bowel and bladder dysfunction, numbness in saddle area, and loss of reflexes in upper extremities.
  - **Central cord syndrome** is caused by spinal cord compression and edema, both of which cause the lateral corticospinal tract white matter to deteriorate. Symptoms include greater motor function loss in the upper extremities than in the lower extremities and paresthesia in the upper extremities.
- Respiratory compromise due to SCI is determined by lesion level.

TABLE 3.6. Respiratory Compromise in SCIs

Level of Lesion	Description
C1 or C2 (high cervical lesions)	• vital capacity 5% – 10% of normal • cough absent • ventilator dependent
C3 – C6	• vital capacity 20% of normal • ineffective cough • variable ventilator support/weaning ability
T2 – T4 (high thoracic lesions)	• vital capacity 30% – 50% of normal • cough weak • compromised respiratory function
Below T4 – T10	• vital capacity >50% of normal • respiratory function improved
T11	• vital capacity normal • cough strong • minimal respiratory dysfunction

- Management of SCIs
  - goals of management: prevent life-threatening complications, maximize organ system functions, prevent secondary spinal cord damage, and address neurological deficits
  - immediate spinal cord stabilization (tongs, halo traction braces, kinetic therapy beds, body casts)
  - methylprednisolone IV (bolus followed by 24 – 48 hour infusion)
  - monitor for, and treat, cardiac and respiratory complications (both common in SCIs)
  - temperature stabilization
  - urinary catheterization (to avoid bladder distension)
- **Autonomic dysreflexia** is the overstimulation of the autonomic nervous system after SCIs above the T6 level. A sympathetic stimulation to the lower portion of the body leads to vasoconstriction below the area of injury and vasodilation above the injury, resulting in bradycardia and hypertension. If left untreated, cardiac status quickly deteriorates, and MI or stroke may occur.
  - Symptoms: flushing and sweating above the level of injury; cold, clammy skin below the level of injury; bradycardia; sudden, severe headache; hypertension
  - Management: anti-hypertensives; elevate HOB to 90°; have patient empty bladder and bowel; remove tight, restrictive clothing

HELPFUL HINT:

The use of methylprednisolone following SCI remains controversial because of the high risk of infection in already compromised, sepsis-prone trauma patients.

QUICK REVIEW QUESTIONS

19. A patient with a T4 spinal cord injury suddenly becomes diaphoretic and bradycardic. What interventions should be initiated?

_____

20. What characteristics are evident in central cord syndrome?

_____

21. A patient with a gunshot wound to the right lower back would exhibit what characteristic sign of Brown-Séquard syndrome?

_____

TRAUMATIC BRAIN INJURIES

- **Traumatic brain injury (TBI)** results from a blunt or penetrating blow to the head or from a blast injury.
  - **Primary injuries** are caused by mechanical forces and can cause skull fractures, brain contusions and concussions, lacerations, hemorrhages, hematomas, or damage to white brain matter.

- □ **Secondary injuries** occur days or weeks after the TBI event as a result of neurochemical cascades leading to chronic inflammation and vascular changes in the brain.
- □ The goal of management of TBI is to maintain CPP and decrease secondary injury to the brain.
- ■ The level of care for **skull fractures** depends on the type and severity of fracture.
  - □ Nondisplaced fractures generally do well with conservative treatment.
  - □ No treatment is usually required for a linear fracture, especially as the dura mater usually remains intact in adults.
  - □ Surgical decompression for a depressed fracture is necessary only when the depression is greater than the thickness of the skull (if the depression is ≥6 mm).
  - □ Basilar skull fractures require critical care monitoring and intervention.
- ■ **Basilar skull fractures** affect the floor of the skull.

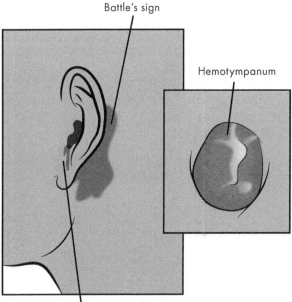

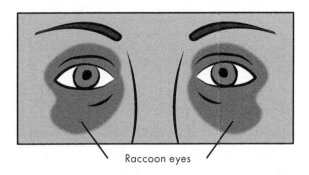

Figure 3.8. Physical Examination of Basilar Skull Fracture

- □ may cause rupture of meninges, resulting in pneumocephalus
- □ likely injury to CN I, III, VII, and VIII
- □ associated spinal cord injury common
- □ signs and symptoms: Battle sign, raccoon eyes, otorrhea, and rhinorrhea
- □ management: manage ABCs; manage ICP, hemorrhage, and meningeal injury (as described above); avoid NT and oral tube, oral suctioning, and positive-pressure support

- ■ **Diffuse axonal injury (DAI)** is a shearing injury that occurs during rapid acceleration–deceleration or rotational acceleration. These forces can shear axons in the brain and cause the death of the brain cells to which they were connected. Sufficient force will disconnect the cerebral hemisphere from the reticular activating system.
  - □ signs and symptoms: coma (GCS <8), decorticate or decerebrate posturing, cerebral edema, increased ICP, temperature elevation
  - □ management: manage ABCs; supportive treatment for symptoms; reduce secondary injury

- ■ An **epidural hematoma (EDH)** is a traumatic collection of blood between the dura mater and the skull, usually because of a temporal- or parietal-region skull fracture that causes a laceration of the middle meningeal artery.

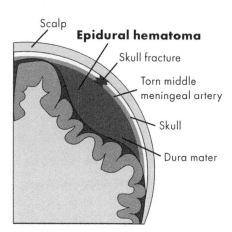

Figure 3.9. Epidural Hematoma

- □ EDH is a neurosurgical emergency: a rapidly expanding hematoma will increase ICP and quickly progress to uncal herniation of brain tissue.
- □ Diagnosis: unconsciousness followed by _lucid interval with continued deterioration_; agitation and confusion; nausea and vomiting; headache; ipsilateral pupil dilation; _Cushing's triad_; CT scan or MRI

□ Management: manage ABCs; craniotomy or trephination for hematoma evacuation

- A **subdural hematoma (SDH)** is low-pressure venous bleeding between the dura mater and the arachnoid space. SDH is generally caused either by trauma or by anticoagulation therapy.
  □ SDH is categorized as acute, subacute, or chronic, based on the rate of bleed, symptom appearance, and rebleeding subsequent to the initial trauma/event.
  □ Diagnosis: *progressive decrease in LOC*; headache; confusion; contralateral hemiparesis; increased ICP; ipsilateral pupil dilation; CT scan or MRI
  □ Management: manage ABCs; craniotomy or trephination for hematoma evacuation

QUICK REVIEW QUESTIONS

22. After management of ABCs, what is the priority for patients with TBI?

_____

23. What characteristic signs would the nurse expect to see in a patient with a basilar skull fracture?

_____

24. What type of head trauma can result in a diffuse axonal injury?

_____

Neurogenic Shock

Pathophysiology

Neurogenic shock is a form of distributive shock caused by an injury or trauma to the spinal cord, typically above T6. The injury causes a decrease in sympathetic tone, leading to vasodilation and rapid onset of hypotension. The resulting decrease in SVR causes blood to pool in the lower extremities, and cardiac output is greatly reduced. Bradycardia occurs because of unopposed vagal tone exacerbated by hypoxia and suctioning (common in spinal injury patients).

Unless rapidly recognized and treated, multisystem organ failure occurs with a very high mortality. This shock state may persist for more than a month from injury event.

Physical Examination

- hemodynamic triad: rapid onset of hypotension, bradycardia, hypothermia

- wide pulse pressure
- skin warm, flushed, and dry
- priapism

Diagnostic Tests

- spinal X-ray, CT scan, or MRI to diagnose spinal cord injury

Management

- *first-line treatment: IV fluids*
- vasopressors and/or inotropes if hypotension persists
- atropine (for bradycardia)
- spine immobilization

QUICK REVIEW QUESTIONS

25. What is the first-line treatment for neurogenic shock?

_____

26. What pathophysiological process leads to neurogenic shock?

_____

ANSWER KEY

1. Focal neurological deficits resulting from damage to the occipital lobe, which controls vision, include loss of vision, hallucinations, and cortical blindness.

2. The GCS score would be 7, indicating that the patient has severe brain injury (likely in the cerebral hemispheres, as suggested by decorticate positioning).

3. A patient with ALS presents with a progressive asymmetrical pattern of weakness that affects both upper and lower extremities.

4. The nurse should anticipate that the doctor will order noninvasive ventilator support.

5. The nurse should anticipate placing an IV and starting IV methylprednisolone.

6. A patient with a migraine typically will report a history of migraines, have unilateral pain, have photophobia, and experience auras prior to the pain.

7. Treatment for ICP is usually initiated for adults with ICP ≥20 mm Hg.

8. IV mannitol is administered to decrease ICP.

9. The patient will require a lumbar puncture to confirm a diagnosis of meningitis.

10. Meningitis requires standard and droplet precautions.

11. Status epilepticus is seizure activity lasting >5 minutes or repeat seizures with no regaining of consciousness between.

12. The first-line medication for status epilepticus is benzodiazepines.

13. A sudden severe headache should always lead to assessment to rule out hemorrhagic stroke.

14. The nursing priority for a patient admitted with a hemorrhagic stroke is to reduce BP and ICP.

15. Phytonadione (vitamin K) 1 mg IV would be administered to reverse the anticoagulation effects of warfarin and prevent further bleeding in the brain. The provider may also order 4-factor PCC or FFP to encourage clotting.

16. The priority intervention for a patient with a suspected ischemic stroke is to get a noncontrast CT scan of the head immediately.

17. tPA should be given within 3 – 4.5 hours of onset of ischemic stroke.

18. The main side effect of tPA is bleeding.

19. The nurse should expect to administer atropine for symptomatic bradycardia and to identify and correct underlying causes such as a full bladder, need for bowel movement, or restrictive clothing.

20. Central cord syndrome causes greater motor function loss in the upper extremities than in the lower extremities, weakness, and paresthesia in upper extremities.

21. Signs of Brown-Séquard syndrome include right-sided hemiparesis and decreased pain and temperature sensation on the left side.

22. The priority for patients with TBI is to maintain normotensive ICP.

23. The nurse would expect to see raccoon's eyes, Battle's sign, hemotympanum, otorrhea, and rhinorrhea in a patient with a basilar skull fracture.

24. A DAI occurs when the head is moved quickly in a back-and-forth motion. Patients with this type of injury have typically experienced trauma or been involved in a motor vehicle accident.

25. The first-line treatment for neurogenic shock is IV fluids.

26. Neurogenic shock occurs when an injury to the spinal cord causes massive vasodilation.

4 GASTROINTESTINAL EMERGENCIES

Gastrointestinal Anatomy and Assessment

- The **gastrointestinal system** is responsible for the breakdown and absorption of food necessary to power the body.

- Digestion occurs in the **gastrointestinal tract.**
  - □ Food enters the **mouth** and travel through the **esophagus** via **peristalsis,** the contraction of smooth muscles.
  - □ The esophagus leads to the **stomach,** which creates an acidic bolus of digested food known as **chyme.**
  - □ Chyme travels to the **small intestine,** where a significant amount of nutrient absorption takes place.
  - □ The small intestine then transports food to the **large intestine** which assists in water absorption, waste collection, and the production of **feces** for excretion.
  - □ At the end of the large intestine is the **rectum,** which stores feces; feces are expelled through the **anus.**

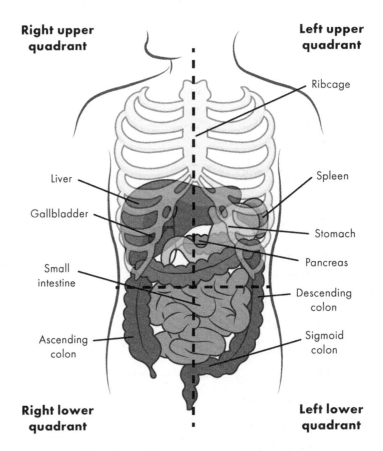

Figure 4.1. Abdominopelvic Anatomy and Quadrants

- The digestive system also includes accessory organs that aid in digestion:
  - □ **salivary glands:** produce saliva, which begins the process of breaking down starches and fats
  - □ **liver:** produces bile, which helps break down fat in the small intestine

- □ **gallbladder**: stores bile
- □ **pancreas**: produces pancreatic juice, which neutralizes the acidity of chyme, and digestive enzymes

■ Gastrointestinal assessment includes inspection, auscultation, percussion, and palpation.

1. Inspection: Look for distention, bulges, color, hernias, ascites, and/or pulsations.

2. Auscultation: High-pitched gurgling sounds are normal. Normal bowel sounds can be documented as normal, hypoactive, or hyperactive. Other types of bowel sounds include:

   - □ **Borborygmi** are loud, rumbling sounds caused by the shifting of fluids or gas within the intestines; these sounds are a normal finding.

   - □ **High-pitched bowel sounds** are often described as tinkling or rushing sounds and may indicate an early bowel obstruction.

   - □ **Absent bowel sounds** are an indication of an **ileus**, where no peristalsis is occurring. Bowel sounds may be temporarily absent in certain cases (e.g., after surgery), but their absence, combined with abdominal pain, indicates a serious condition.

3. Percussion: **Tympany** (air) sounds are normal, and **dull sounds** are heard over solid organs (liver and spleen).

4. Palpation: Check for guarding, rigidity, masses, and/or hernias.

TABLE 4.1. GI Signs		
Name	**Description**	**Indication**
Kehr sign	referred left shoulder pain caused when the diaphragm irritates the phrenic nerve	splenic rupture diaphragm irritation
Rovsing sign	pain in the RLQ with palpation of LLQ (indicates peritoneal irritation)	appendicitis
Cullen sign	a bluish discoloration to the umbilical area	retroperitoneal hemorrhage
Grey Turner sign	ecchymosis in the flank area	retroperitoneal hemorrhage
Psoas sign	abdominal pain when right hip is hyperextended	appendicitis, Crohn's disease
McBurney's point	RLQ pain at point halfway between umbilicus and iliac spine	appendicitis

continued on next page

TABLE 4.1. GI Signs (continued)

Name	Description	Indication
Murphy sign	pain and cessation of inspiration when RUQ is palpated	acute cholecystitis
Markle test (heel drop)	pain caused when patient stands on tiptoes and drops heels down quickly or when patient hops on one leg	appendicitis, peritonitis

- Diagnostic studies for GI assessment
  - A **focused assessment sonography for trauma (FAST)** exam is a quick bedside exam that uses ultrasound to assess for bleeding after trauma.
  - **Esophagogastroduodenoscopy (EGD or upper endoscopy)** is an endoscopic procedure that uses a scope to visualize the linings of the upper GI tract.
  - **Colonoscopy** is an endoscopic procedure that uses a scope to visualize the linings of the lower GI tract.
  - **Flexible sigmoidoscopy** is endoscopy of the rectum and sigmoid colon.
  - **Balloon-assisted enteroscopy** is used to assess areas of the GI tract that are hard to access, particularly the small intestine.
  - **Ultrasound** is frequently used to visualize the gallbladder, liver, pancreas, spleen, and abdominal aorta.
  - A **CT scan** is frequently used to diagnose or rule out a cause of abdominal pain.
  - **X-rays** are taken to visualize free air, gas, obstructions, foreign bodies, and dilatation.
- Common laboratory tests for GI conditions include liver function panels and tests for pancreatic enzyme levels.

TABLE 4.2. GI Laboratory Tests

Test	Description	Normal Range
Liver Function Tests		
Albumin	protein made in the liver; low levels may indicate liver damage	3.5 – 5.0 g/dL
Alkaline phosphatase (ALP)	enzyme found in the liver and bones; increased levels indicate liver damage	45 – 147 U/L

Test	Description	Normal Range
Liver Function Tests		
Alanine transaminase (ALT)	enzyme in the liver; helps metabolize protein; increased levels indicate liver damage	7 – 55 U/L
Aspartate transaminase (AST)	enzyme in the liver; helps metabolize alanine; increased levels indicate liver or muscle damage	8 – 48 U/L
Total protein	low levels may indicate liver damage	6.3 – 7.9 g/dL
Total bilirubin	produced during the breakdown of heme; increased levels indicate liver damage or anemia	0.1 – 1.2 mg/dL
Gamma-glutamyltransferase (GGT)	enzyme that plays a role in antioxidant metabolism; increased levels indicate liver damage	9 – 48 U/L
L-lactate dehydrogenase (LD or LDH)	enzyme found in most cells in the body; increased levels may indicate liver damage, cancer, or tissue breakdown	adults: 122 – 222 U/L
Pancreatic Enzymes		
Amylase	enzyme that breaks down carbohydrates	23 – 140 U/L
Lipase	enzyme that breaks down fats	<160 U/L

QUICK REVIEW QUESTION

1. A patient presents with severe upper GI bleeding. What diagnostic study will likely be ordered to locate the source of the bleeding?

_____

Acute Abdomen

Acute abdomen is sudden, severe abdominal pain. The physical examination of patients with acute abdomen should focus on pain location, history of GI

HELPFUL HINT:

Patients with acute abdomen may also have **referred pain** in other locations, such as the shoulders or hands. Referred pain is caused by the proximity of nerves carrying pain signals to and from the spinal cord.

symptoms, and palpation to assess for rigidity or guarding. Cardiovascular, genitourinary, and obstetrical conditions should also be considered when assessing acute abdomen.

TABLE 4.3 Causes of Acute Abdomen

Condition	Pathophysiology	Symptoms
Abdominal aortic aneurysm (AAA) *Discussed in detail in Ch. 1*	widening of the aorta in the abdomen	sharp, severe pain in the chest, back, abdomen, or flank; rapid, weak, or absent pulse; hypotension
Appendicitis *Discussed in detail below*	inflammation of the appendix	**_RLQ pain_**; rebound tenderness; positive psoas sign; fever
Cholecystitis *Discussed in detail below*	inflammation of the gallbladder	**_colicky RUQ pain_**, which can radiate to back or right shoulder; positive Murphy's sign
Kidney stones *Discussed in detail in Ch. 5*	blockage in the urethra leading to inflammation of the kidney	**_unilateral flank pain_** (can be severe); hematuria
Pancreatitis *Discussed in detail below*	inflammation of the pancreas	**_LUQ pain that may radiate to the back or shoulder_**; distension of abdomen
Peptic ulcer	erosion of the stomach by stomach acid	upper abdomen and back pain; heartburn
Ruptured ectopic pregnancy *Discussed in detail in Ch. 7*	rupture of the fallopian tube due to ectopic pregnancy	vaginal bleeding, abdominal pain, cessation of pregnancy s/s
Ruptured ovarian cyst *Discussed in detail in Ch. 7*	rupture of cyst in the ovary	sudden, severe, unilateral pelvic pain

QUICK REVIEW QUESTIONS

2. What type of pain would a patient with a ruptured ovarian cyst most likely report?

3. During assessment of a patient with acute abdomen, the nurse notes RLQ pain, rebound tenderness, and positive psoas sign. What condition should the nurse suspect?

_____

Appendicitis

Pathophysiology

Appendicitis is inflammation of the appendix. Obstruction of the appendiceal lumen results in a decrease in blood supply which can lead to necrosis and perforation.

Risk Factors

- more common in males under 30
- inflammatory bowel disease (e.g., Crohn's disease or ulcerative colitis)

Physical Examination

- abdominal pain
  - ☐ _**dull, steady periumbilical pain**_
  - ☐ _**RLQ pain that worsens with movement**_
  - ☐ _**pain in RLQ at McBurney's point**_
- positive Rovsing's sign and Psoas sign
- fever
- anorexia
- nausea and vomiting
- rebound tenderness
- abdominal rigidity

Diagnostic Tests

- CT scan, the most precise exam to diagnosis appendicitis
- WBCs may be elevated

Management

- surgical intervention required: keep the patient NPO and prep for surgery

- analgesics and antiemetics as needed
- antibiotics

Peritonitis

Pathophysiology

Peritonitis is inflammation of the peritoneum (the lining of the abdominal cavity). There are several common causes of peritonitis.

- **Perforation peritonitis** occurs when the perforation of an organ allows the contents to spill into the peritoneal cavity, causing infection.

- **Spontaneous bacterial peritonitis (SBP)** is infection of ascitic fluid in patients with cirrhosis. Mortality is high, and prompt intervention is required to prevent sepsis.

- Peritonitis is a common complication of peritoneal dialysis and is usually caused by contaminated equipment.

Physical Examination

- diffuse pain
  - □ usually worsens with movement
  - □ relieved by flexing the knees or bending right hip
- rigid abdomen
- guarding of abdomen and rebound tenderness
- fever
- ileus

Diagnostic Tests

- CT scan or acute abdominal series
- positive Markle test
- CBC and liver function tests
- possible paracentesis for fluid analysis

Management

- antibiotics (IV or intraperitoneal)
- analgesics and antiemetics as needed
- monitor for sepsis and follow facility sepsis protocols

QUICK REVIEW QUESTION

6. A patient presents to the ED with severe abdominal pain, guarding, and a fever (temperature, 38.6°C [101.5°F]). The CT scan shows peritonitis from a ruptured appendix. What should be the priority intervention for this patient?

Bowel Obstruction and Perforation

Pathophysiology

A **bowel obstruction** occurs when normal flow through the bowel is disrupted. **Mechanical obstructions** are physical barriers in the bowel. The most common mechanical obstructions in the small bowel are **adhesions**, **hernias**, and **volvuli** (twisting of the bowels). The most common obstruction in the large bowel are tumors.

Paralytic ileus is the impairment of peristalsis in the absence of mechanical obstruction. It is most common in postoperative patients and can also be caused by endocrine disorders or medications (e.g., opioids).

Increased pressure proximal to the obstruction can lead to **perforation** of the bowel wall. Other common causes of bowel perforation include surgery, abdominal trauma, and neoplasm (in large bowel).

Physical Examination

- nausea and vomiting
- diarrhea
- distended and firm abdomen
- abdominal pain (cramping and colicky)
- unable to pass flatus
- *high-pitched bowel sounds (early); absent bowel sounds (late)*
- tympanic percussion
- pain, often sudden onset (perforation)

Diagnostic Tests

- increased WBCs
- elevated BUN and decreased electrolytes from dehydration/vomiting
- abdominal X-ray may show dilated bowel loops
- CT scan to diagnose

Management

- bowel rest (NPO) or nutritional support distal to obstruction
- fluid resuscitation
- bowel decompression via tube (NG or Miller-Abbott) with low, intermittent suction for patients with severe vomiting or abdominal distention
- antibiotics as needed
- surgical intervention for obstructions that do not resolve within 48 hours
- surgical closure of perforation

QUICK REVIEW QUESTIONS

7. A patient presents with abdominal pain, nausea, and vomiting. A bowel obstruction is suspected and then confirmed by CT scan. What priority interventions should the nurse anticipate for this patient?

   _____

8. What intervention can be performed for patients with vomiting caused by bowel obstruction?

   _____

Cyclic Vomiting Syndrome

Pathophysiology

Cyclic vomiting syndrome (CVS) is characterized by a recurrent period of severe nausea and vomiting followed by periods of normal health. The etiology of CVS is unknown, but it has been linked to migraines, autonomic dysfunction, food sensitivities, and chronic cannabis use. It can occur in children and adults but is more common in children.

Physical Examination

- recurring vomiting that continues for hours or days (longer episodes more common in adults)

- episodes usually have patient-specific pattern (e.g., triggers, time of onset)
- prodrome: nausea, epigastric pain, headache

Management

- IV fluids
- antiemetic (usually IV ondansetron)
- sumatriptan or aprepitant may be given during prodrome or within first hour of symptom onset

---

QUICK REVIEW QUESTION

9. An 8-year-old patient previously diagnosed with cyclic vomiting syndrome is brought to the ED after vomiting six times during the preceding four hours. What medication should the nurse expect to administer?

Bleeding
UPPER GI BLEEDING
Pathophysiology

An **upper GI bleed** is bleeding that occurs between the esophagus and duodenum. Bleeding may be severe and require immediate hemodynamic management.

The etiology of upper GI bleed varies.

- **Peptic ulcers** and **esophagitis** (secondary to GERD) are the most common causes of upper GI bleeding.
- **Esophageal varices** _occur when veins in the esophagus rupture because of portal hypertension (usually caused by hepatic cirrhosis). Bleeding may be severe and is likely to recur_.
- **Esophageal perforation** or **rupture** may be iatrogenic, secondary to trauma, or caused by the severe effort of vomiting (**Boerhaave syndrome**).
- **Mallory-Weiss tears** occur at the gastroesophageal junction and result from forceful vomiting.
- NSAIDs and chronic gastritis can cause or worsen upper GI bleeding.

Physical Examination

- hematemesis (may be in nasogastric aspirate) or coffee-ground emesis
- hematochezia (if hemorrhaging)

- upper abdominal pain
- melena
- signs and symptoms of hypovolemia (after significant blood loss)

Diagnostic Tests

- decreased HgB, Hct, and platelets
- longer PT and aPTT
- electrolyte imbalances (due to hypovolemia)
- elevated BUN and BUN-creatinine ratio
- positive hemoccult
- diagnosed via appropriate endoscopy or angiogram (EGD to locate source of bleeding)

Management

- O$_2$ therapy
- *manage hemodynamic status: IV fluids, blood products, and management of coagulopathies*
- *medications to constrict vasculature: vasopressin, octreotides, and beta blockers*
- endoscopic or surgical repair if bleeding persists
  - □ esophageal varices: endoscopic variceal band ligation (EVL) or **esophageal balloon tamponade** (e.g., Sengstaken-Blakemore tube)
  - □ PPI to prevent post-procedure ulcers

HELPFUL HINT:

Elevated BUN-creatinine ratio is associated with decreased kidney function and increased breakdown of protein. It is often seen with upper GI bleeds (due to digestion of blood) but not with lower GI bleeds.

QUICK REVIEW QUESTIONS

10. What risk factors should a nurse assess for when taking a history on a patient with a suspected upper GI bleed?

11. Octreotide is an appropriate treatment for esophageal varices because it has what type of action?

LOWER GI BLEEDING
Pathophysiology

A **lower GI bleed** is any bleeding that occurs below the duodenum. Lower GI bleeds occur less frequently than do upper GI bleeds, are typically less emergent, and may stop on their own.

Risk Factors

- disease of the colon (e.g., diverticulitis, IBD, colitis)
- colon polyps, cancer, or tumors
- abscess or inflammation of rectum
- hemorrhoids
- anal fissures

Physical Examination

- hematochezia
- melena
- bleeding from rectum
- abdominal or chest pain
- signs and symptoms of hypovolemia (after significant blood loss)

Diagnostic Tests

- positive hemoccult
- decreased HgB and Hct
- PT and aPTT may be longer
- diagnosed via appropriate endoscopy, CT scan, or angiogram

Management

- manage hemodynamic status: IV fluids, blood products, and management of coagulopathies
- gastric lavage via NG tube
- endoscopic or surgical repair if bleeding persists

QUICK REVIEW QUESTIONS

12. A patient is being worked up for a possible lower GI bleed. What diagnostic imaging would be expected?

_____

13. Upon initial diagnosis of a GI bleed, what interventions are required to maintain hemostasis?

_____

★ Cholecystitis

Pathophysiology

Cholecystitis, acute or chronic inflammation of the gallbladder, usually results from impacted stone in the neck of the gallbladder or in the cystic duct. Cholelithiasis is the presence of gallstones in the gallbladder.

Risk Factors

- the 5 Fs for cholecystitis:
  - fair (more prevalent in the Caucasian population)
  - fat (BMI > 30)
  - female (occurs more often in females than in males)
  - fertile (one or more children) or pregnant
  - forty (age over 40)

Physical Examination

- RUQ pain, which can radiate to back or right shoulder; common after eating high-fat meal
- colicky pain
- positive Murphy's sign
- nausea and vomiting
- flatulence
- jaundice if obstruction is significant
- atypical symptoms in older patients and patients with type 2 diabetes: confusion, lack of pain

HELPFUL HINT:

Elevated amylase and/or lipase may indicate a stone blocking a duct and causing pancreatitis.

Diagnostic Tests

- ultrasound or CT scan

Management

- IV crystalloid
- antiemetic and analgesics as needed
- definitive treatment is cholecystectomy

QUICK REVIEW QUESTION

14. Where would a patient with cholecystitis most likely report pain?

Cirrhosis

Hepatic (liver) failure can be acute (onset <26 weeks) or chronic. Common causes of acute liver failure (also called **fulminate hepatitis**) include acetaminophen overdose and viral hepatitis; the most common cause of chronic liver failure is alcohol abuse.

Liver failure leads to dysfunction in multiple organ systems.

- **Hepatic encephalopathy** is impaired cognitive function caused by increased serum ammonia (NH_3) levels. Increased NH_3 levels may also cause neuromuscular symptoms, including asterixis and bradykinesia.

- Coagulopathies are caused by impaired synthesis of clotting factors in liver tissue.

- **Jaundice** is caused by hyperbilirubinemia.

- Acute kidney injury occurs in approximately 50% of patients with liver failure. (The mechanism is unknown.)

- Infections and sepsis develop secondary to decreased and defective WBCs.

- Metabolic imbalances may include hypokalemia, hyponatremia, and hypoglycemia.

- Lowered peripheral vascular resistance decreases BP and increases HR.

Chronic liver failure leads to **cirrhosis**—the development of fibrotic tissue in the liver. Cirrhosis in the liver increases resistance in the portal vein, causing **portal hypertension**. Common conditions that occur secondary to portal hypertension include esophageal varices, **ascites**, and **splenomegaly**.

Physical Examination

- cognitive changes or motor dysfunction
- jaundice
- petechiae or purpura
- spider angiomas
- ascites
- RUQ pain
- palmar erythema
- nausea and vomiting

Diagnostic Tests

- *elevated AST, ALT, and/or bilirubin*
- elevated NH_3 levels

HELPFUL HINT:

Sedatives should be used cautiously in patients with liver failure because of the liver's inability to clear them. Low doses of short-acting benzodiazepines should be used when sedation is necessary.

- decreased protein, albumin, and fibrinogen
- decreased WBCs, HgB, Hct, and platelets
- longer PT and PTT, and increased INR
- CT scan or MRI may show fibrosis of liver

HELPFUL HINT:

Alcoholic cirrhosis requires special considerations and the implementation of an alcohol withdrawal protocol. (See chapter 12, Medical Emergencies, for more information on alcohol withdrawal.)

Management

- IV fluid resuscitation
- *__lactulose and neomycin to reduce ammonia levels__*
- diuretics for ascites
- prophylactic treatment for stress ulcers
- monitor ICP
- tight glucose control for nonalcoholic fatty liver disease
- shunt to reduce portal hypertension

QUICK REVIEW QUESTIONS

15. A nurse is providing care to a patient with acute liver failure. What should the nurse expect to see in the patient's CBC and coagulation tests?

16. What medication will likely be administered to a patient with chronic liver failure to correct high ammonia levels?

Diverticulitis

Pathophysiology

Diverticulitis is inflammation of the diverticula (small outpouchings in the GI tract, usually in the sigmoid colon). The inflammation is usually caused by obstruction of diverticula by fecal material or undigested food. It may lead to infection, necrosis, or perforation.

Risk Factors

- age (more common in elderly patients)

Physical Examination

- LLQ abdominal pain
- rebound tenderness

- abdominal distention
- anorexia
- nausea and vomiting
- fever
- change in bowel habits (diarrhea or constipation)
- hematochezia

Diagnostic Tests

- CBC may show increased WBCs
- CT scan of abdomen to diagnose or rule out perforation
- electrolytes monitoring for imbalances

Management

- IV fluids
- keep patient NPO
- anticholinergics (to reduce spasms in colon)
- analgesics as needed
- patient education
  - □ stool softeners
  - □ *a liquid diet followed by a low-fiber diet until the inflammation is reduced, then a high-fiber diet to prevent straining*

QUICK REVIEW QUESTION

17. A patient diagnosed with diverticulitis has had multiple emergency visits over the past year. What information can the ED nurse implement at discharge to help prevent a reoccurrence?

Foreign Bodies in the GI System

Pathophysiology

A **foreign body** is any object that enters the GI system either intentionally or accidently. Foreign bodies within the GI system typically present as partial or full obstructions of the esophagus, although objects may also pass to other GI organs. These objects can cause damage, including tears, infection, and obstruction, to the GI system.

Physical Examination

- drooling or difficulty swallowing
- feeling of something "stuck" in throat
- subcutaneous emphysema present if esophageal perforation

Diagnostic Tests

- chest or neck X-rays to diagnose

Management

- maintain airway
- *glucagon to promote smooth muscle relaxation*
- endoscopy or surgery to remove objects that don't pass on their own
- emergent removal required
    - magnets anywhere in the GI tract
    - sharp objects or batteries in the esophagus

QUICK REVIEW QUESTIONS

18. A 2-year-old child is brought to the ED after swallowing a watch battery. Imaging shows the battery has lodged in the child's esophagus. What intervention should the nurse expect?

19. An 18-month-old child has swallowed several quarters which have passed into the stomach. The parents are upset that the medical team is not trying to remove the coins. How should the nurse respond?

Hepatitis

Pathophysiology

Hepatitis is inflammation of the liver. It can be caused by a systemic viral infection, autoimmune conditions, or by certain medications.

Physical Examination

- clay-colored stools
- *dark urine (foamy)*
- jaundice
- steatorrhea (excess fat in stool)

- flulike symptoms
- abdominal pain

Diagnostic Tests

- elevated liver enzymes (AST and ALT)
- elevated alkaline phosphatase
- elevated ammonia
- low albumin

Management

- manage symptoms of liver failure (detailed in the section Cirrhosis)
- treatment of underlying cause (e.g., antivirals, glucocorticoids)

HELPFUL HINT:

Hepatitis A and E are the 2 types transmitted through the fecal/oral route. Remember this mnemonic: the vowels hit your bowels.

TABLE 4.4. Types of Viral Hepatitis		
Type	**Route of Transmission**	**Prevention and Treatment**
A	Fecal/oral	Vaccine available Generally mild and requires only supportive care
B	Blood/body fluids	Vaccine available Generally mild and requires only supportive care Antivirals as needed
C	Blood/body fluids	No vaccine available Chronic infection may lead to liver failure Treat with antivirals
D	Blood/body fluids	Occurs simultaneously with hepatitis B Preventable with hepatitis B vaccine
E	Fecal/oral	More common in resource-limited countries in Asia and Africa No vaccine available Generally mild in patients who are not immunocompromised

QUICK REVIEW QUESTION

20. A patient presents to the ED with complaints of clay-colored stools; dark, foamy urine; abdominal pain; and flulike symptoms. What risk factors would suggest possible infection with hepatitis E?

Intussusception

Pathophysiology

Intussusception is a mechanical bowel obstruction caused when a loop of the large intestine telescopes within itself. This condition can cut off the blood supply, causing perforation, infection, and bowel ischemia. It usually occurs within the first 3 years of life and is more prevalent in males.

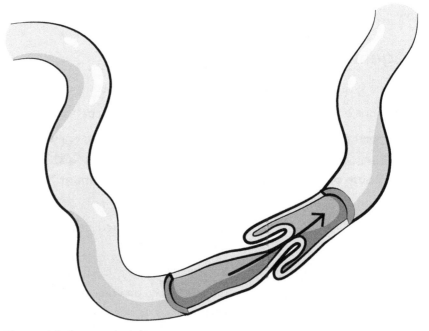

Figure 4.2. Intussusception

Physical Examination

- **_red currant-jelly–like stool_**
- sausage-shaped abdominal mass
- colicky pain
- inconsolable crying
- absence of stools

Diagnostic Tests

- abdominal X-rays to confirm diagnosis

Management

- keep patient NPO
- stable patients: hydrostatic or pneumatic enema
- unstable patients: surgery

Pancreatitis

Pathophysiology

Pancreatitis is caused by the release of digestive enzymes into the tissues of the pancreas. The condition causes autodigestion, inflammation, tissue destruction, and injury to adjacent structures and organs. Pancreatitis can be acute or chronic, but its onset is usually sudden.

The tissue damage caused by pancreatitis increases capillary permeability, resulting in fluid shifts into interstitial spaces that cause edema and systemic inflammatory responses (e.g., ARDS). Inflammation may also limit diaphragm movement and cause atelectasis. Severe damage to the pancreas may cause retroperitoneal bleeding.

Risk Factors

BAD HITS

- **b**iliary (e.g., gallstones blocking pancreatic duct)
- **a**lcohol
- **d**rugs (thiazide diuretics, sulfa drugs, pentamidine, antiretrovirals)
- **h**ypertriglyceridemia/hypercalcemia
- **i**diopathic causes
- **t**rauma
- **s**corpion sting or surgery (recent ERCP or abdominal surgery)

Physical Examination

- steady, severe pain abdominal pain; usually in the LUQ and may radiate to the back or shoulder
- guarding
- nausea and vomiting
- decreased bowel sounds

- steatorrhea
- fever
- tachycardia and hypotension
- dyspnea
- Cullen sign
- Grey Turner sign

Diagnostic Tests

- _**elevated amylase and lipase**_
- hypocalcemia
- decreased total protein
- hypoglycemia
- elevated Hct, BUN, and CRP
- increased WBCs
- imaging (MRI or CT scan with contrast) to diagnose

Management

- fluid resuscitation, including electrolyte replacement
- pain management (usually opioids) and antiemetics
- endoscopic retrograde cholangiopancreatography (ERCP) for gallstones and bile duct inflammation
- monitor for respiratory complications, including ARDS and atelectasis

---

QUICK REVIEW QUESTIONS

23. Labs for patients with acute pancreatitis will likely show large increases in which enzymes?

24. A patient with pancreatitis is complaining of sudden, severe abdominal pain in the mid-epigastric area that spreads to the left shoulder. What complications should the nurse assess for?

Gastrointestinal Trauma

Pathophysiology

GI trauma can be caused by a penetrating injury such as a gunshot or knife wound or can be caused by blunt trauma from a motor vehicle injury or a fall.

Diagnosis

Organ	Physical Examination	Diagnostic Tests and Findings
Spleen Most frequently injured abdominal organ	LUQ pain (referred to left shoulder) LUQ bruising Distended abdomen	CT scan or FAST exam may show splenic rupture
Liver Largest abdominal organ; injury most frequently caused by blunt trauma	RUQ pain (referred to right shoulder) RUQ bruising Rigid abdomen Labs consistent with liver damage	CT scan may show laceration or hemorrhage
Pancreas Most frequently missed abdominal injury with a high mortality rate	Epigastric pain Rebound tenderness Elevated pancreatic enzymes	CT for diagnosis Testing for elevated pancreatic enzymes can be delayed in bloodwork up to 6 hours
Stomach Most commonly caused by a penetrating injury	Hematemesis Rigid abdomen Rebound tenderness	Free air on chest X-ray

TABLE 4.5. Diagnosis of GI Trauma

HELPFUL HINT:

A hemodynamically unstable trauma patient with a positive FAST will likely require emergency surgery.

Management

- manage hypovolemia and monitor for hypovolemic shock
- surgery required for penetration injuries and unstable patients

QUICK REVIEW QUESTIONS

25. After blunt-force trauma to the stomach, a patient arrives at the ER. The patient states their pain is a 7/10 in the LUQ. What organ is this pain associated with?

26. Following an MVC, a patient reports acute pain in the RUQ and right shoulder, and the nurse notes a rigid abdomen during the physical examination. The patient's HR is 105 and BP is 85/60. What intervention should the nurse anticipate?

ANSWER KEY

1. EGD is the diagnostic study most commonly used to visualize sources of upper GI bleeding.

2. A ruptured ovarian cyst presents with sudden severe unilateral pelvic pain.

3. The nurse should suspect appendicitis.

4. Appendicitis presents with dull, steady periumbilical pain; RLQ pain that worsens with movement; and/or pain in RLQ at McBurney's point.

5. Priority interventions for a patient with appendicitis should be keeping the patient NPO, administering antiemetics, analgesics, and antibiotics, and preparing the patient for surgery.

6. Broad-spectrum antibiotics should be given.

7. Patients with bowel obstructions need IV fluids. During a bowel obstruction, severe vomiting and fluid sequestration in the bowel lumen lead to hypovolemia and electrolyte imbalances.

8. Bowel decompression via tube can be used to manage vomiting caused by bowel obstruction.

9. The nurse should expect to administer an antiemetic such as IV ondansetron.

10. Risk factors for upper GI bleeding include peptic ulcers or gastritis, alcohol abuse, cirrhosis, NSAID use, and recent forceful vomiting.

11. Octreotide constricts the dilated vessels in the esophagus and reduces bleeding.

12. Workup for a lower GI bleed may include endoscopy, CT scan, or angiogram.

13. Management of GI bleeds includes IV fluids, blood products, and management of coagulopathies.

14. Cholecystitis presents with RUQ pain possibly radiating to back or right shoulder.

15. Patients with liver failure will be pancytopenic with low levels of RBCs, platelets, and WBCs. They will also have prolonged PT and aPTT/PTT, an increased INR, and low fibrinogen.

16. Lactulose is administered to correct high ammonia levels.

17. Patients with acute diverticulitis should start with a liquid diet, with food items such as broth, popsicles, and gelatin, before slowly introducing low-fiber foods. After the acute stage has passed, patients should also be taught to routinely follow a high-fiber diet to help food pass through the colon and to prevent straining. High-fiber foods include fruits, vegetables, and whole grains.

18. The nurse should prepare for an emergent endoscopic removal.

19. The nurse should tell the parents that most coins pass through the GI tract on their own and reassure them that the child will be monitored and can be treated if symptoms develop.

20. Recent travel to resource-limited countries in Asia and Africa is a risk factor for hepatitis E infection.

21. Intussusception is most common in children 3 and under and is more prevalent in males.

22. The nurse should anticipate a hydrostatic or pneumatic enema to treat intussusception.

23. Amylase and lipase will be elevated in patients with acute pancreatitis.

24. The nurse should assess for atelectasis and other respiratory problems.

25. LUQ pain is usually associated with the spleen.

26. The nurse should anticipate an immediate surgery for suspected liver damage.

5 GENITOURINARY EMERGENCIES

Genitourinary Anatomy and Assessment

- The **urinary system** excretes water and waste from the body and is crucial for maintaining blood pressure, electrolyte balance, and acid-base balance.
  - **Nephrons** are the functioning portion of the kidney.
  - The **glomerulus**, the network of small capillaries within the nephron, is where filtration occurs.
  - **Urine** passes out of the kidneys through the **renal pelvis** and then through **ureters** to the **urinary bladder**. Urine exits the bladder through the **urethra**.
- Diagnostic studies for genitourinary assessment
  - pelvic or renal CT scan
  - **bladder scan:** noninvasive bedside ultrasound that provides quick assessment of the amount of urine in the bladder

- □ **cystoscopy**: visual exam of the bladder performed using a flexible cystoscope
- □ **kidney, ureter, bladder (KUB) X-ray**: used to assess size, shape, and position of the anatomical structures
- □ **IV pyelography (IVP)**: uses contrast to assess images of the kidneys, ureters, and bladder

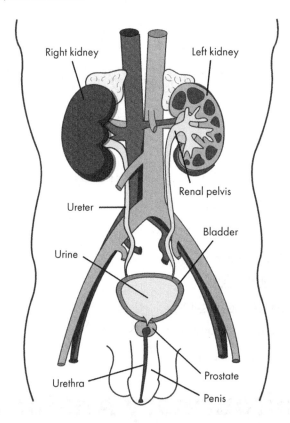

Figure 5.1. The Urinary System (Male)

QUICK REVIEW QUESTION

1. A patient with a history of bladder stones reports dysuria and pain. What diagnostic test should the nurse expect?

Genitourinary Infections

- **Epididymitis** is inflammation of the epididymis. It is usually the result of a bacterial infection secondary to a UTI or sexually transmitted disease.
  - □ Diagnosis: gradual onset pain posterior to testes; s/s lower UTI; positive Prehn sign; swelling and tenderness in testis; ultrasound showing enlarged epididymis; labs show infection

- Management: antibiotics; pain management (analgesics, ice packs, scrotal support or elevation); epididymectomy for severe infection
- **Orchitis** is inflammation of the testes usually caused by a bacterial or viral infection. It can occur secondary to epididymitis (epididymo-orchitis).
  - Diagnosis: _**unilateral, sudden onset of pain in testis**_; swelling and tenderness in testis; when associated with mumps, will appear 4 – 7 days after s/s of infection; ultrasound showing increased blood flow to the affected testis
  - Management: antibiotics; anti-inflammatories; pain management (analgesics, ice packs, scrotal support or elevation)
- **Prostatitis** is inflammation of the prostate, usually caused by bacterial infection (_E. coli_). Asymptomatic cases are often discovered during unrelated assessments and are not usually treated.
  - Diagnosis: urinary symptoms (e.g., frequent, urgent urination; dysuria); suprapubic, perineal, or low back pain; s/s of infection; labs show infection
  - Management: antibiotics; analgesics
- **Pyelonephritis** is infection of the kidneys. Symptoms can develop over hours or days, with some patients waiting weeks before seeking care.
  - Diagnosis: _**clinical triad (fever, nausea and vomiting, costovertebral pain)**_; cloudy, dark, foul-smelling urine; hematuria; dysuria; suprapubic, cervical, or uterine tenderness; urinalysis shows infection
  - Management: IV fluids (D5W); antibiotics; analgesics; antipyretics; antiemetics
- A **urinary tract infection (UTI)** is infection in the lower urinary tract (bladder and urethra) or in the upper urinary tract (kidneys and ureters).
  - Diagnosis: frequent small amounts of urine; cloudy, dark, foul-smelling urine; hematuria; dysuria; pelvic, suprapubic, abdominal, or lower back pain or pressure; s/s of infection; _**altered mental status in patients > 65 years old**_; urinalysis shows infection
  - Management: antibiotics; supportive treatment for symptoms

HELPFUL HINT:

Mumps is the most common cause of viral orchitis.

QUICK REVIEW QUESTIONS

2. What is the clinical triad associated with pyelonephritis?

_____

3. What symptoms are likely to be seen in a patient with a UTI?

_____

★ # Priapism

Priapism is an unintentional, prolonged erection that is unrelated to sexual stimulation and is unrelieved by ejaculation. **Nonischemic (high-flow) priapism** is the unregulated circulation of blood through the penis resulting from a ruptured artery in the penis or perineum. **Ischemic (low-flow) priapism** occurs when blood becomes trapped in the erect penis. Ischemic priapism is considered a medical emergency requiring immediate intervention to preserve function of the penis.

Risk Factors

- trauma (straddle injury or acute spinal cord injury)
- medications:
    □ antidepressants
    □ anticoagulants
    □ prostaglandin E1
    □ testosterone
- underlying disease (e.g., sickle cell disease, leukemia, malaria)
- recent urologic surgery
- cocaine use

Physical Examination

- ischemic priapism: rigid, painful erection unrelated to sexual activity lasting > 4 hours
- nonischemic priapism:
    □ recurrent episodes of persistent erections (may be partial)
    □ difficulty maintaining full erection
    □ no pain
    □ trauma (usually straddle injury)
    □ delay between injury and priapism

Diagnostic Tests

- ultrasound showing obstructed or decreased blood flow
- venous blood gas dark or black

Management

- *ischemic priapism: blood should be drained from the penis within 4 – 6 hours to prevent permanent damage*
  - □ first-line treatment: aspiration with intracavernosal phenylephrine injection
  - □ second-line treatment: a shunt (T-shunt, Al-Ghorab's shunt, or Ebbehoj's shunt)
  - □ penile prostheses for priapism lasting > 36 hours
- nonischemic priapism: the condition will often spontaneously resolve
  - □ monitor
  - □ first-line treatment, if needed: elective arterial embolization

---

QUICK REVIEW QUESTIONS

5. What is the first-line intervention for patients with ischemic priapism?

_____

6. A 22-year-old patient in the ED is diagnosed with nonischemic priapism resulting from a straddle injury and is currently under observation. The patient is becoming increasingly anxious and tells the nurse he wants to be treated so he won't lose function in his penis. How should the nurse explain to the patient why he is not receiving medical intervention?

_____

Renal Calculi ★

Pathophysiology

Renal calculi (kidney stones) are hardened mineral deposits (most often calcareous) that form in the kidneys. Renal calculi are usually asymptomatic but will cause debilitating pain and urinary symptoms once they pass into the urinary tract, where they are referred to as urinary calculi.

Physical Examination

- *severe, sharp, intermittent flank pain*
- urinary symptoms (e.g., dysuria, hematuria)
- signs and symptoms of infection

Diagnostic Tests

- CT scan to diagnose calculi

HELPFUL HINT:

Medications that may cause renal calculi include topiramate (Topamax), ciprofloxacin, sulfa antibiotics, diuretics, and decongestants.

Management

- small stones (< 5 mm) with minimal symptoms: will pass spontaneously
  - analgesics (may require opioids for severe pain)
  - alpha blockers (can help the stone pass)
  - encourage fluids
- large stones (> 5 mm) with symptoms: surgical intervention

QUICK REVIEW QUESTIONS

7.   A patient presents to the ED with complaints of bloody urine and severe side and back pain. What imaging study should the nurse anticipate will be ordered?

_____

8.   What medication should the nurse anticipate will be administered to a patient with small kidney stones?

_____

★ Testicular Torsion

Pathophysiology

Testicular torsion occurs when the spermatic cord, which supplies blood to the testicles, becomes twisted, leading to an ischemic testicle. The condition is considered a medical emergency that requires immediate treatment to preserve the function of the testicle. Most testicular torsion cases are caused by **bell-clapper deformity**, in which the testicle is not correctly attached to the tunica vaginalis.

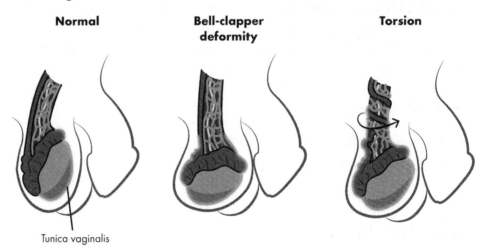

Figure 5.2. Testicular Torsion

Risk Factors

- male ages 10 – 25
- bell-clapper deformity
- cold weather (especially sudden shift from warm to cold)
- trauma

Physical Examination

- ***sudden, severe unilateral scrotal pain***
- high-riding testicle
- absent cremasteric reflex
- signs of inflammation in scrotal skin

Diagnostic Tests

- ultrasound showing reduced or absent blood flow to affected testicle

Management

- analgesics
- prep for immediate exploratory surgery

QUICK REVIEW QUESTIONS

9. What is the primary risk factor for testicular torsion?

_____

10. A patient with testicular torsion is likely to present with what symptoms?

_____

Genitourinary Trauma

Pathophysiology

Genitourinary (GU) trauma can cause injury to the kidneys, bladder, urethra, or external genitalia. GU trauma symptoms can be nonspecific and can be masked by or related to other injuries. Trauma may occur from blunt or penetrating injury.

- Renal: The majority of renal trauma occurs from blunt trauma such as direct impact into the seatbelt or steering wheel in frontal MVCs or from body panel intrusion in side-impact crashes. Renal injuries are ranked graded from 1 to 5 based on severity. Grade 5 renal injuries are referred to as **shattered kidney** and include severe renal vascular laceration.

- Bladder: The majority of bladder trauma occurs from blunt trauma, usually occurring with a pelvic fracture. Bladder rupture can also result from lap belt restraint. Leakage from ruptures may lead to peritonitis or sepsis.

- Urethral: Urethral injuries are more common in males and may result from trauma and pelvic fracture or from iatrogenic injuries resulting from catheterization.

- External genitalia: These injuries are more common in males due to anatomical presentation and greater participation in physical sports, acts of violence, and war. Up to two-thirds of all genitourinary traumas involve the external genitalia. Injuries to the penis and scrotum may occur from use of penile rings or other sexual pleasure devices.

Physical Examination

- pain (suprapubic, abdominal, groin/genital, or flank)
- urinary symptoms (e.g., hematuria, dysuria)
- bleeding at meatus
- ecchymosis
- distended bladder
- abdominal distention
- foul-smelling vaginal discharge

Diagnostic Tests

- urinalysis (for hematuria)
- decreased hemoglobin and hematocrit
- monitor for
  - elevated BUN and creatinine
  - fluid and electrolyte status
- diagnostic imaging (CT scan, KUB X-ray)

Management

- oxygen and IV fluids as needed
- analgesics as needed
- renal trauma may be admitted for monitoring (Hct, hemodynamic)
- keep bladder decompressed via Foley catheter (if no urethral injury present)

- manage sequalae (e.g., acute kidney injury, hemorrhage)
- penetrating injuries: surgical intervention

QUICK REVIEW QUESTIONS

11. A 16-year-old patient presents to the ED with complaints of nausea and genital pain after sustaining a straddle injury on a skateboard. What further signs and symptoms should the nurse assess to diagnose genitourinary trauma?

_____

12. After an MVC, a patient complains of hematuria and back pain. What diagnostic tests would be ordered?

_____

13. A confused 79-year-old patient who resides in a nursing home has been brought to the ED after traumatically pulling out a Foley catheter. What interventions should the nurse implement?

_____

Urinary Retention

Pathophysiology

Urinary retention is the inability to void the bladder. The condition can be acute or chronic and is most often caused by either an obstruction (e.g., prostatic hyperplasia, organ prolapse) or an infection (e.g., prostatitis, vulvovaginitis). Acute urinary retention is a medical emergency that can result in bladder injuries, kidney infections, and sepsis if left untreated.

Physical Examination

- inability to urinate
- urinary frequency or urgency
- pelvic pressure or pain

Diagnostic Tests

- renal/bladder ultrasound or CT scan to identify cause of retention

Management

- _**priority intervention: immediate voiding of bladder via catheter**_
- treatment for underlying cause of retention after bladder is voided

QUICK REVIEW QUESTIONS

14. A patient presents with severe pain and pressure in the lower abdomen and does not recall the last time they urinated. What should the nursing assessment include?

_____

15. A patient in the ED states that he has not voided for 16 hours, and a bladder scan shows 600 ml of urine in the bladder. What is the nurse's priority?

_____

ANSWER KEY

1. The nurse should expect the patient will require a bladder scan to assess for urinary retention.

2. The clinical triad associated with pyelonephritis consists of fever, nausea and/or vomiting, and costovertebral pain.

3. Symptoms of a UTI include frequent small amounts of urine; cloudy, dark, foul-smelling urine; hematuria; dysuria; and pelvic, suprapubic, abdominal, or lower back pain or pressure.

4. Orchitis is characterized by sudden onset of unilateral pain in a testis.

5. The first-line intervention for patients with ischemic priapism is aspiration with intracavernosal phenylephrine injection.

6. The nurse should explain that during episodes of nonischemic priapism, blood continues to move through the penis and the chance of permanent damage is very low. The nurse should further explain that this type of priapism usually resolves on its own but that treatment options are available if it does not.

7. The patient has symptoms of urinary calculi. A CT scan is the preferred imaging study to visualize the location, size, and composition of the calculi.

8. The patient will require analgesics for pain.

9. Bell-clapper deformity, a genetic condition in which the testicles are not attached to the scrotum, is found in 90 percent of testicular torsion cases.

10. Testicular torsion presents with sudden severe unilateral scrotal pain, high-riding testicle, and absent cremasteric reflex.

11. Common symptoms of straddle injuries, in addition to nausea and genital pain, include suprapubic or abdominal pain and dysuria.

12. Urinalysis, CT scan, and/or an ultrasound will be ordered to diagnose and differentiate between bladder or renal injury.

13. The nurse should use a sitter or soft restraints to maintain patient safety, administer ordered analgesics for pain control, and keep the patient NPO in case of need for surgical repair.

14. A bladder scan should be used to assess for urinary retention.

15. The nurse should assist the patient with voiding by placing a straight catheter or a Foley catheter.

6 GYNECOLOGICAL EMERGENCIES

Dysfunctional Uterine Bleeding

Abnormal uterine bleeding (AUB) is any bleeding from the uterus that is abnormal in volume or timing. This includes menses that occur irregularly, last for an abnormal number of days, or produce excessive blood loss. It occurs most often in adolescents and people approaching menopause. Common underlying causes of bleeding can be remembered with the mnemonic PALM-COEIN:

- Polyp
- Adenomyosis
- Leiomyoma (fibroids)
- Malignancy
- Coagulopathy
- Ovulatory disorder

- Endometrial
- Iatrogenic (e.g., IUD insertion)
- Not otherwise classified

Dysfunctional uterine bleeding (DUB) is irregular uterine bleeding with no underlying illness. It is usually the result of anovulation. Because no egg is released, the ovaries do not produce progesterone, leading to heavy, irregular periods. DUB is most common in adolescents and during perimenopause.

Physical Examination

- metrorrhagia and/or menorrhagia
- full gynecological and OB history to estimate volume of blood loss
- indicators of high volume of blood loss
  - □ soaking more than 1 pad or tampon per hour
  - □ changing pad or tampon frequently at night
  - □ greater than 30 cc volume measured via menstrual cup
  - □ passing clots > 1 in.

Diagnostic Tests

- pregnancy test
- CBC and coagulation profile

Management

- fluids or blood products as needed
- _**estrogen-progestin contraceptives (usually taken for 7 days)**_
- IV estrogen or tranexamic acid for severe bleeding
- nonemergent presentations: referred to a gynecologist/obstetrics specialist

QUICK REVIEW QUESTIONS

1. A young female patient accompanied by the mother presents to the ED with a complaint of menorrhagia after experiencing amenorrhea for the past three months. What problem should the nurse anticipate when trying to obtain a truthful and complete history from the patient?

2. A 50-year-old patient presents to the ED with menstrual bleeding that is saturating more than one pad per hour and has lasted for 5 hours. What medications should be reviewed?

Gynecological Infections

- **Chlamydia** is an STI caused by the bacteria *Chlamydia trachomatis*; left untreated, it can lead to PID, infertility, and ectopic pregnancy in women.
  - Diagnosis: often asymptomatic, especially for men; discharge from site of infection; vaginal bleeding; dysuria; pruritis; NAAT performed on urine or swab
  - Management: antibiotics (azithromycin [Zithromax], doxycycline); supportive treatment for symptoms

- **Genital herpes** is an STI caused by the two strains of the herpes simplex virus (HSV-1 and HSV-2). The first outbreak after the initial infection is the most severe; recurrent outbreaks, which vary in frequency and duration, will generally be less severe.
  - Diagnosis: prodrome of itching, burning, or tingling at infection site; vesicles on genitalia, perineum, or buttocks; fever, adenopathy during initial infection; PCR on swab of open lesion
  - Management: antivirals; supportive treatment for symptoms

- **Gonorrhea** is an STI caused by the gram-negative diplococcus *Neisseria gonorrhoeae*; left untreated, it can lead to PID, infertility, and ectopic pregnancy.
  - Diagnosis: usually asymptomatic; discharge from site of infection; dysuria; metrorrhagia; oropharyngeal erythema; culture or NAAT of swab
  - Management: antibiotics (not fluoroquinolones); supportive treatment for symptoms

- **Pelvic inflammatory disease (PID)** is an infection of the upper organs of the female reproductive system, usually caused by a STI.
  - Diagnosis: cervical, uterine, or adnexal tenderness; vaginal discharge; abdominal or low back pain; right scapular pain (Fitz-Hugh–Curtis syndrome); postcoital bleeding; metrorrhagia; dyspareunia; pleuritic URQ pain; nausea and vomiting; fever; labs show infection
  - Management: antibiotics; supportive treatment for symptoms

- **Syphilis** is an STI caused by the bacteria *Treponema pallidum*. The infection progresses through four stages: primary (3 – 90 days after infection), secondary (4 – 10 weeks after infection), latent (3 months – 3 years after infection), and tertiary (> 3 years after infection).
  - Signs and Symptoms (primary stage): firm, round, and painless chancres lasting 3 – 6 weeks

HELPFUL HINT:

Chlamydia is the most commonly reported STI in the United States; gonorrhea is the second most common STI.

- □ Signs and Symptoms (secondary stage): rough, red rash on torso, hands, soles of feet; fever; lesions on mucous membranes; arthritis
- □ Signs and Symptoms (latent stage): asymptomatic
- □ Signs and Symptoms (tertiary stage): varies by affected system
- □ Diagnosis: positive VDRL, RPR, or specific treponemal antibody test
- □ Management: antibiotics; supportive treatment for symptoms
- **Vulvovaginitis** is inflammation of the vulva and vagina. It is usually the result of an infection by bacteria, yeast, or trichomoniasis (a protozoan parasite).
  - □ Signs and Symptoms (general): dyspareunia, dysuria, vulvovaginal pruritis
  - □ Signs and Symptoms (bacterial vaginosis): malodorous white-grey vaginal discharge
  - □ Signs and Symptoms (vulvovaginal candidiasis): thick, white vaginal discharge with no odor (often described as "cottage cheese" like)
  - □ Signs and Symptoms (trichomoniasis): frothy, green-yellow vaginal discharge; vaginal inflammation ("strawberry cervix")
  - □ Diagnosis: culture or wet mount
  - □ Management: antibiotic, antifungal, or antiprotozoal as indicated

QUICK REVIEW QUESTIONS

3. A patient with PID may present with what symptoms?

_____

4. What medication is used to treat chlamydia?

_____

5. A 22-year-old female patient presents to the ED with white, foul-smelling vaginal discharge but no itching or urinary symptoms. What medication will the patient most likely require?

_____

Ovarian Disorders

Pathophysiology

Ovarian cysts form in the ovaries, usually a result of an unreleased egg (follicular cyst) or failure of the corpus luteum to break down (corpus luteum cyst). Ovarian cysts are usually asymptomatic and are often found during assessments related to other conditions. However, the cysts can **rupture**, causing intense pain. Symptoms of rupture are usually self-limiting, but rupture of corpus luteum cysts may lead to severe bleeding.

Ovarian torsion is twisting of the ovary or fallopian tube twists, usually secondary to ovarian cysts. It is a medical emergency that requires surgery to prevent further ischemia.

Risk Factors

- endometriosis
- infertility treatment
- hormonal imbalances
- hypothyroidism
- tubal ligation
- pelvic infection or inflammation
- smoking

Physical Examination

- cyst
  - often asymptomatic
  - pelvic pain, feeling of fullness, or discomfort
  - dyspareunia
  - irregular menstrual cycle
- _**rupture: sudden, severe, unilateral pelvic pain**_
- torsion
  - acute, unilateral pelvic pain
  - nausea and vomiting
  - low fever

Diagnostic Tests

- transvaginal ultrasound to diagnose

Management

- analgesics
- fluids or blood products (for severe hemorrhage)
- surgical intervention in rare cases of continued bleeding or large cyst
- torsion: surgical intervention required

6. A patient arrives at the ED with vaginal bleeding and pain on the right side of the abdomen. The pregnancy test is negative, and the nurse suspects an ovarian cyst. What produced should the nurse expect to be ordered to diagnose an ovarian cyst?

   _____

7. A patient with a history of ovarian cysts presents with severe unilateral, pelvic pain. What conditions should the nurse suspect?

   _____

Sexual Assault and Battery

Sexual assault is any unwanted sexual or physical contact or behavior that occurs without the explicit consent of the recipient. Victims of sexual assault can be male or female, adult or pediatric. It is a significantly underreported crime, and many victims know the assailant. Any patient presenting with a report of sexual assault should be treated with respect and dignity.

Management

- Assess for serious or emergent conditions that may require immediate treatment.

- For female patients, take a complete OB/GYN history.

- The physician or a certified **sexual assault nurse examiner (SANE)** may perform a sexual assault medical forensic exam (also called a sexual assault forensic exam or "rape kit") to document injuries and collect evidence.

- Follow hospital protocols for STI screening (some hospitals require it while others do not).

- All patients reporting sexual assault should be offered postexposure prophylaxis.
  - emergency contraception (after negative hCG test)
  - antibiotics and antiprotozoals (ceftriaxone, metronidazole, azithromycin and/or doxycycline)
  - HIV postexposure prophylaxis (PEP)
  - HPV vaccine

- Provide emotional support to patient.

- Provide patient with access to available resources for survivors of sexual assault, including hospital counselors and community sexual assault centers.

Legal Considerations

- Nurses should keep in mind that patients' medical records are legal documents that may be used in criminal or civil court proceedings.

- All interactions with patients should be carefully documented.

- Nurses who are asked to testify in court should confer with the hospital's legal team.

QUICK REVIEW QUESTIONS

8. A patient arrives at the ED stating they have been beaten and sexually assaulted. What is the nurse's priority?

   _____

9. What prophylactic measures should be offered to patients reporting sexual assault?

   _____

Gynecological Trauma

Pathophysiology

Patients presenting with complaints of genital pain or bleeding should undergo a thorough history and physical examination. External trauma can usually be identified easily; however, internal examination will be required to evaluate for deeper injury. Vulvar injuries may include lacerations and hematomas, while vaginal trauma may present with lacerations. Uterine and cervical injuries are generally associated with pregnancy; however, they can also be caused by vaginal or abdominal trauma. Undiagnosed vaginal trauma may result in secondary issues including dyspareunia, pelvis abscesses, and fistula formations.

HELPFUL HINT:

Patients may not be forthcoming with the details of gynecological trauma because of fear or embarrassment. The possibility of sexual assault or physical abuse must be considered and should be handled according to the appropriate protocols.

Physical Examination

- pain (vaginal, external, or visceral)

- vaginal bleeding

- external laceration, ecchymosis, or mutilation

- hematuria or dysuria

- foul-smelling vaginal discharge

- labial edema

- visible wound, penetration injury, or embedded object

Diagnostic Tests

- urinalysis for hematuria
- CT scan and pelvic/vaginal ultrasound to assess integrity of reproductive organs

Management

- pain management (analgesics, cold compresses)
- sutures for lacerations
- remove foreign object(s)

QUICK REVIEW QUESTIONS

10. What types of injuries should a nurse look for during assessment of a female patient with trauma to the genital region?

_____

11. A 22-year-old female patient seeks treatment in the ED after falling onto a metal hurdle during a track sporting event. In triage, the patient denies vaginal bleeding but complains of throbbing pain "down there." What interventions should the nurse initiate?

_____

ANSWER KEY

1. A young female patient may not disclose a history of sexual activity or potential pregnancy in the presence of a parent. The nurse should create an opportunity to ask these questions in a private setting such as a bathroom or exam room.

2. The nurse should determine if the patient takes blood thinners, and labs should be reviewed for PT/INR levels.

3. Symptoms of PID include cervical, uterine, or adnexal tenderness; vaginal discharge; abdominal or low back pain; right scapular pain (Fitz-Hugh–Curtis syndrome); postcoital bleeding; metrorrhagia; dyspareunia; pleuritic URQ pain; nausea and vomiting; and fever.

4. Chlamydia is treated with antibiotics.

5. A white, foul-smelling vaginal discharge with no other signs or symptoms is characteristic of bacterial vaginosis. The patient will likely be treated with a course of antibiotics such as metronidazole or clindamycin.

6. Ultrasound of the ovaries, usually transvaginal, is used to determine if there is an ovarian cyst and the status of the cyst (e.g., intact, ruptured, etc.).

7. Ovarian cysts may rupture or cause ovarian torsion, both of which present with severe, unilateral pelvic pain.

8. The nurse's priority is to assess the patient for serious or life-threatening injuries. Further interventions, including forensic exams and prophylaxis, will be provided based on the patient's wishes.

9. Patients reporting sexual assault should be offered emergency contraception, antibiotics and antiprotozoals, HIV postexposure prophylaxis, and the HPV vaccine.

10. The nurse should look for lacerations, hematomas, penetrating injuries, and embedded objects.

11. The patient likely sustained a straddle injury and is experiencing soft tissue swelling of the labia and external genitalia. A urine sample should be obtained and the patient prepped for a manual pelvic exam. Cold compresses can be provided to decrease swelling and provide localized pain relief.

7 OBSTETRICAL EMERGENCIES

BCEN OUTLINE: OBSTETRICAL EMERGENCIES

- Abruptio placenta
- Ectopic pregnancy
- **_Emergent delivery_**
- **_Hemorrhage (e.g., postpartum bleeding)_**
- Hyperemesis gravidarum
- Neonatal resuscitation
- Placenta previa
- Postpartum infection
- **_Preeclampsia, eclampsia, and HELLP syndrome_**
- Preterm labor
- Threatened/spontaneous abortion
- Obstetric trauma

Reproductive Anatomy and Physiology

- After an egg is fertilized with sperm, it develops into an **embryo**, which implants itself on the wall of the uterus.

- After approximately eight weeks, the embryo is described as a **fetus**.

- The fetus is surrounded by a fluid-filled membrane called the **amniotic sac**.

- The **placenta** is a blood-rich temporary organ attached to the wall of the uterus that provides nutrients and gas exchange for the fetus and eliminates waste.
- The placenta is attached to the fetus by the **umbilical cord**.

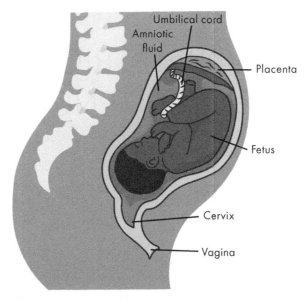

Figure 7.1. Fetus in Third Trimester

- **Full-term pregnancy** is 40 weeks and is divided into the first trimester (1 – 12 weeks), second trimester (13 – 26 weeks), and third trimester (27 – 40 weeks).
  - □ **Preterm labor** occurs between 20 and 37 weeks.
  - □ Post-term pregnancy occurs when the fetus has not been delivered by 42 weeks.
  - □ The likelihood of survival is very low for fetuses delivered before 24 weeks but increases with gestational age.
  - □ With access to appropriate neonatal care, around 90 percent of fetuses delivered at 27 weeks survive.
- Normal position for the fetus during delivery is head down. **Breech** position is when the fetus has its feet or buttocks downward.
- During pregnancy, the woman will experience physiological changes that may affect the delivery of medical care. These changes include:
  - □ increased blood volume (as much as 50 percent by the end of pregnancy)
  - □ increased heart rate (normal increase is around 15 beats per minute)
  - □ increased respiratory rate
  - □ increased oxygen demand and decreased lung capacity
  - □ increased clotting speed

HELPFUL HINT:

During pregnancy, the top of the uterus (**fundus**) may be as high as the xiphoid process. This limits movement of the diaphragm and chest wall, which may cause difficulty breathing.

□ displaced GI and respiratory organs

■ Normal **fetal heart rate** is 130 – 160 bpm.

Placental Disorders

Pathophysiology

Abruptio placentae (placental abruption) occurs when the placenta separates from the uterus after the twentieth week of gestation but before delivery. Abruption can lead to life-threatening conditions, including hemorrhage and DIC. Blood loss due to abruption can be difficult to quantify as blood may accumulate behind the placenta (**concealed abruption**) rather than exiting through the vagina.

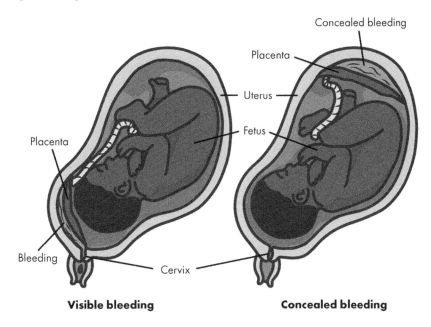

Figure 7.2. Abruptio Placentae

Placenta previa occurs when the placenta partially or completely covers the internal orifice of the cervix. A low lying placenta is located ≤ 2 cm from the cervix but does not cover it. Placenta previa is usually asymptomatic and is found on routine prenatal ultrasounds. The presence of previa makes the placenta susceptible to rupture or hemorrhage and necessitates a cesarean delivery.

Placenta previa is correlated with **placenta accreta**, particularly in women who have had multiple previous cesarean deliveries. In placenta accreta, the placenta attaches abnormally deeply into the myometrium. Because the placenta cannot detach from the uterus after delivery, placenta accreta can lead to hemorrhage and requires a hysterectomy.

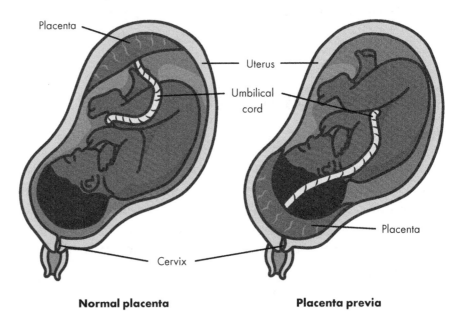

Normal placenta   **Placenta previa**

Figure 7.3. Placenta Previa

Risk Factors

- smoking
- cocaine use
- abruption:
  - hypertension
  - preeclampsia
  - fetal abnormalities
  - blunt trauma
- placenta previa:
  - age > 35
  - multifetal pregnancy
  - previous cesarean delivery
  - infertility treatment

Diagnosis

	Abruptio Placentae	**Placenta Previa**
Onset of Symptoms	**_sudden and intense bleeding with pain_**	asymptomatic or painless bleeding
Bleeding	bleeding may be vaginal or concealed	vaginal bleeding
Uterine Tone	firm	soft and relaxed
Imaging	transabdominal or transvaginal ultrasound	transabdominal or transvaginal ultrasound; no rectal or cervical exam until placenta placement is known

TABLE 7.1. Diagnosis of Abruptio Placentae and Placenta Previa

HELPFUL HINT:

Cervical exams and transvaginal ultrasounds should be done cautiously in patients with placenta previa because they may damage the placenta and lead to severe bleeding.

Management

- fetal heart rate monitoring
- monitor mother for signs of hemodynamic instability
- **_RhoGAM if mother is Rh negative_**
- IV fluids or blood products as needed
- patient admitted stat to OB

QUICK REVIEW QUESTIONS

2. What signs or symptoms indicate a significant separation of the placenta from the uterus?

_____

3. A patient presents to the ED in labor and says they have been diagnosed with placenta previa. What intervention should the nurse expect?

_____

Ectopic Pregnancy

Pathophysiology

In an **ectopic pregnancy**, the blastocyst implants in a location other than the uterus. In > 95% of cases, implantation occurs in the fallopian tubes (tubal pregnancy), but implantation can also occur in the ovaries, cervix, or abdominal cavity. Ectopic pregnancies are most often caused by tubal irregularities that are congenital or the result of infection or surgery. A tubal pregnancy may rupture the fallopian tube, causing a life-threatening hemorrhage.

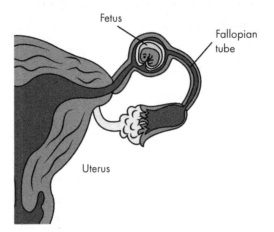

Figure 7.4. Ectopic Pregnancy (Tubal Pregnancy)

Risk Factors

- age > 35
- pelvic inflammatory disease
- STIs (chlamydia and gonorrhea)
- infertility or fertility treatments
- tubal surgery
- smoking

Physical Examination

- ***severe, unilateral pelvic pain***
- vaginal bleeding
- lower abdominal pain
- s/s of hemorrhage

Diagnostic Tests

- pregnancy confirmation with urine or serum hCG
- transvaginal ultrasound to locate pregnancy

Management

- RhoGAM if mother is Rh negative
- hemodynamically unstable patients: stabilize and prepare for surgery

- hemodynamically stable patients: OB referral for surgery or treatment with methotrexate

QUICK REVIEW QUESTIONS

4. A sexually active 19-year-old presents to the ED with vaginal bleeding and intermittent LLQ abdominal pain. Vital signs are stable, abdomen is tender, and the patient's uterus is soft and slightly enlarged. An ultrasound assessment confirms an ectopic pregnancy. What will be the most likely intervention for this patient?

_____

5. What are the signs and symptoms of a ruptured tubal ectopic pregnancy?

_____

Labor and Delivery ★

Pathophysiology

Labor and delivery occurs in 3 stages.

- Stage 1: onset of labor to full cervical dilation (12 – 16 hours)
- Stage 2: cervical dilation to expulsion of fetus (2 – 3 hours)
- Stage 3: delivery of placenta (10 – 12 minutes)

Delivery is **imminent** if the fetus is visible and/or the mother reports the urge to push with contractions. Alternatively, delivery can be considered imminent if the cervix is fully dilated (10 cm) and contractions are < 2 minutes apart.

Contractions and cervical dilation before the thirty-seventh week of gestation is **preterm labor.** If preterm labor begins between 34 and 37 weeks with no other complications, the patient should be transferred to the labor and delivery setting if delivery is not imminent. When preterm labor begins at < 34 weeks, the mother should be transferred to OB for treatment to delay delivery.

Risk Factors

- emergent delivery:
  - ☐ unrecognized pregnancy
  - ☐ unrecognized signs of labor
  - ☐ lack of prenatal care
  - ☐ trauma

HELPFUL HINT:

Umbilical cord prolapse occurs when the cord presents alongside (occult) or ahead of (overt) the presenting fetus during delivery. Exposure of the cord makes it vulnerable to compression or rupture, which disrupts blood flow to the fetus.

- preterm labor:
  - short cervical length
  - infections (e.g., bacterial vaginosis, UTI, STIs)
  - multifetal pregnancy
  - underweight or obese mother
  - diabetes

Physical Examination

- emergent delivery
  - ___ruptured amniotic membrane ("water broke")___
  - ___urge to push___
  - dilation of cervix
  - contractions

Diagnostic Tests

- pelvic exam: assess cervical dilation
- fetal Doppler to assess fetal heart rate
- transabdominal ultrasound: to identify presentation and number of fetus(es) and assess for possible complications

Management

- Assess patient to determine stage of labor and gestational age.
  - preterm labor or complications: OB consult stat
  - delivery not imminent: patient should be transferred to OB for delivery
  - delivery imminent and no complications: delivery will take place in the ED
- Monitor maternal blood pressure, heart rate, and contractions.
- Monitor fetal heart rate.
  - Administer RhoGAM if mother is Rh negative.
  - ___Administer betamethasone for imminent delivery of fetus < 34 weeks.___
  - Position mother is lithotomy position for delivery.
  - Clean perineum with antiseptic.
- Care of newborn postdelivery:
  - Wipe nose and mouth; suction airway if obstructed.
  - Dry and stimulate newborn.
  - Assign Apgar score.

HELPFUL HINT

Apgar scoring is 0 to 2 points for:
neonatal heart rate
respiratory effort
muscle tone
reflex irritability
color

- Care of mother postdelivery:
  - ☐ Deliver placenta.
  - ☐ Administer oxytocin IM or perform fundal massage.
  - ☐ Monitor for signs of hemorrhage.

Hemorrhage

Pathophysiology

Postpartum hemorrhage is bleeding that occurs any time after delivery up to 12 weeks postpartum and exceeds 1000 ml or that causes symptoms of hypovolemia. Primary hemorrhage occurs during the first 24 hours after delivery; secondary hemorrhage occurs between 24 hours and 12 weeks postpartum.

The etiology of hemorrhage varies.

- trauma: lacerations to uterus or vagina
- uterine atony: failure of the uterus to contract after delivery, often because of placental disorders
- subinvolution of the placental site: persistence of dilated arteries in placenta or uterus postpartum
- retained tissue
- coagulation disorders
- infection

Risk Factors

- placental disorders (accreta or previa)
- preeclampsia, eclampsia, or HELLP

HELPFUL HINT:

The causes of postpartum hemorrhage are known as the Four T's: tone, trauma, tissue, and thrombin.

- failure to progress in labor
- retained products of conception

Physical Examination

- vaginal bleeding
- s/s of hypovolemia

Management

- IV fluids and blood products as needed
- *tranexamic acid (to promote clotting)*
- uterine atony: uterine massage; oxytocin 20 – 40 IU/L 0.9% NaCl IV; ergot derivatives (contraindicated for preeclampsia and hypertension); vasopressors
- trauma: surgery to repair cause of bleed
- retained tissue: manual removal of placental tissue
- coagulopathy: replace clotting factors (platelets and/or FFP)

QUICK REVIEW QUESTIONS

9. A patient presents to the ED with heavy vaginal bleeding after a home birth. Her blood pressure is 110/65 mm Hg, her HR is 118, and her RR is 24. What priority intervention should the nurse prepare for?

    _____

10. What medication is often used to promote clotting during postpartum bleeding?

    _____

Hyperemesis Gravidarum

Pathophysiology

Hyperemesis gravidarum is severe nausea and vomiting that occur during pregnancy. While there is no definitive diagnostic line between hyperemesis and common "morning sickness," hyperemesis is generally defined as frequent vomiting that results in weight loss and ketonuria. Severe vomiting can lead to dehydration, hypovolemia, and electrolyte imbalances.

Hyperemesis usually presents around 6 weeks gestation and resolves around 16 to 20 weeks. However, for some women it may persist until delivery.

Risk Factors

- personal or family history of hyperemesis
- previous nausea and vomiting related to estrogen-based medications or motion sickness
- multifetal pregnancy
- young age
- hydatidiform mole

Physical Examination

- persistent vomiting (> 3 times per day)
- weight loss of > 5 pounds or > 5% of body weight
- s/s of hypovolemia

Diagnostic Tests

- elevated BUN
- elevated urine specific gravity
- serum electrolytes showing hypokalemia or other imbalances
- urinalysis positive for ketones
- elevated AST and ALT

Management

- IV fluids
  - □ initial infusion of lactated Ringer's followed by dextrose
  - □ urine output 100 ml/hour
- replace lost vitamins and minerals: IV thiamine, IV multivitamin, IV magnesium, calcium, or phosphorus as indicated by labs
- IV antiemetics

QUICK REVIEW QUESTIONS

11. How is hyperemesis gravidarum differentiated from morning sickness?

_____

12. What vitamins and minerals might a patient with severe hyperemesis gravidarum require?

_____

Neonatal Resuscitation

Pathophysiology

The transition to extrauterine life requires a complex series of changes in the cardiopulmonary system of a neonate. The alveoli in the neonate's lungs expand, usually beginning with the first breath, and the lungs are cleared of fluid. In addition, the clamping of the umbilical cord combined with the expansion of the lungs raises the neonate's blood pressure and pushes blood into the vasculature of the lungs.

A small number of neonates (around 10%) will require intervention to establish ventilation. Poor respiratory performance can have a number of causes:

- blocked airway
- lack of respiratory effort (usually the result of musculature or neurological deficits)
- persistent pulmonary hypertension in the newborn
- heart or lung defects
- preterm labor (lungs are not mature enough to clear and expand)

Physical Examination

- absence of spontaneous breath
- absence of vigorous cry
- airway obstruction (nares and/or trachea)
- cyanosis
- poor muscle tone

Management

- Stimulate the neonate by rubbing back, feet, and/or chest vigorously.
- Prevent heat loss by placing child in warmer.
- Clear airway of obstructions using bulb suction or wall suction (low suction).
- If stimulation and warming do not work, activate neonatal resuscitation code.
- Neonatal resuscitation is a specialized skill and requires supplemental education and certification. The ED nurse should be prepared to provide basic resuscitation of a neonate until the appropriate caregivers can arrive.

- Apply oxygen with positive pressure ventilation.
- ***If the neonate is apneic and the heart rate is < 60, initiate CPR.***

- Goals of neonate resuscitation:
  - spontaneous respiration
  - heart rate $\geq$ 100 bpm
  - SpO_2 85% to 95% by 10 minutes postdelivery

QUICK REVIEW QUESTIONS

13. A neonate is brought into the ED after an emergent delivery outside the hospital. The neonate's pulse is 45. What should the nurse do?

_____

14. A neonate delivered in the ED is receiving resuscitation measures. What assessment criteria would indicate that resuscitation measures have been successful?

_____

Postpartum Infection

Pathophysiology

Postpartum patients are frequently discharged soon after delivery and may develop **postpartum infections** at home that require further treatment. Possible sites of infection include the endometrium (**endometritis**), surgical incisions, breasts (mastitis), and urinary tract. The infection may spread and lead to septicemia, peritonitis, or sepsis.

HELPFUL HINT:

Endometritis is the most common postpartum infection requiring emergent care.

Risk Factors

- cesarean delivery
- vaginal infections
- manual rupture of membranes

Physical Examination

- fever of $\geq$ 100.4°F (38°C):
  - on more than 2 of the first 10 days postpartum
  - maintained over 24 hours after the end of the first day postpartum
- endometritis: uterine tenderness, midline lower abdominal pain
- surgical incision infection: erythema and inflammation at incision, purulent exudate
- mastitis: erythema and tenderness in breast

Diagnostic Tests

- labs show infection

Management

- endometritis and UTI: antibiotics, analgesics, antipyretics
- surgical incision: drain, irrigate, and debride wound
- mastitis: antibiotics, analgesics, antipyretics, empty breast of milk

QUICK REVIEW QUESTIONS

15. A postpartum patient returns to the ED 4 days following discharge from an uncomplicated vaginal delivery. She has a temperature of 101°F (38.3°C) and assessment shows erythema and discharge with an odor at her episiotomy site. What interventions should the nurse anticipate?

16. A patient with mastitis would present with what symptoms?

Preeclampsia and Eclampsia

Pathophysiology

Preeclampsia is a syndrome caused by abnormalities in the placental vasculature. The syndrome is characterized by hypertension in the mother paired with either proteinuria or end-organ dysfunction. Symptoms can appear after the twentieth week of pregnancy and most commonly appear after 34 weeks.

In most cases, preeclampsia will resolve after delivery, but symptoms can develop postpartum. Maternal **postpartum preeclampsia** generally occurs within 6 days after childbirth but can be delayed up to 6 weeks after delivery. It can occur even if there was no evidence of preeclampsia prior to delivery. Because preeclampsia is usually diagnosed during routine prenatal care, postpartum preeclampsia most commonly presents in the ED.

Preeclampsia is classified as being either with or without severe features. Preeclampsia with severe features can lead to life-threatening complications, including eclampsia, pulmonary edema, and abruptio placentae.

Eclampsia is the onset of tonic-clonic seizures in women with preeclampsia. Eclampsia can occur ante-, intra-, or postpartum. It is an emergent condition that requires immediate medical intervention.

Risk Factors

- age > 35
- personal or family history of preeclampsia
- obesity
- pregestational diabetes
- pregestational hypertension
- nulliparity or multifetal pregnancy
- chronic kidney disease

Physical Examination

- _hypertension: systolic BP > 140 mmHg or diastolic BP > 90 mmHg_
- facial edema
- rapid weight gain (> 5 pounds a week)
- severe preeclampsia: headache, epigastric pain, pitting edema
- eclampsia: tonic-clonic seizures

Diagnostic Tests

- _proteinuria diagnosed through urine sample_
  - 24-hour urine protein: ≥ 0.3 g
  - urine dipstick protein: ≥ 1+ (mild preeclampsia) to ≥ 3+ (severe preeclampsia)
  - serum creatinine: > 1.2 mg/dL indicates severe preeclampsia

Management

- definitive treatment: delivery of fetus
- management of symptoms
  - _antihypertensives_ (labetalol, hydralazine, or short-acting nifedipine)
  - _prophylactic magnesium_ (to prevent seizures)
- admit to OB

HELPFUL HINT:

Be aware of how an exam question on preeclampsia is worded. Do not confuse prepartum preeclampsia (which requires delivery of the fetus) with postpartum preeclampsia (which requires ICU monitoring and management).

★ HELLP Syndrome

Pathophysiology

HELLP syndrome is currently believed to be a form of preeclampsia, although the relationship between the two disorders is controversial and not well understood. Around 85% of women diagnosed with HELLP will also present with symptoms of preeclampsia (hypertension and proteinuria). HELLP is characterized by:

- _hemolysis (H)_
- _elevated liver enzymes (EL)_
- _low platelet count (LP)_

Physical Examination

- hypertension: systolic > 140 mmHg or diastolic > 90 mmHg
- RUQ abdominal pain
- nausea and vomiting
- severe headache or visual disturbances

Diagnostic Tests

- urine protein consistent with preeclampsia diagnosis
- schistocytes on blood smear
- platelets: ≤ 100,000 cells/μL
- total bilirubin: ≥ 1.2 mg/dL
- AST: > 70 units/L

Management

- antihypertensives (labetalol, hydralazine, or short-acting nifedipine)
- prophylactic magnesium (to prevent seizures)
- admit to OB

QUICK REVIEW QUESTIONS

19. What abnormal laboratory values confirm the diagnosis of HELLP?

20. What type of pain is associated with HELLP syndrome?

Threatened/Spontaneous Abortion

Pathophysiology

Spontaneous abortion (miscarriage) is the loss of a pregnancy before the twentieth week of gestation. (Death of the fetus after the twentieth week is commonly referred to as a **stillbirth**.) Spontaneous abortions are a common complication of early pregnancy. They can occur because of chromosomal or congenital abnormalities, material infection or disorders, or trauma.

Spontaneous abortions are classified by the location of the embryo/fetus and cervical dilation.

- **missed abortion**: occurs when the embryo/fetus is nonviable but has not been passed from the uterus and the cervix is closed

- **threatened abortion**: occurs when the patient has vaginal bleeding before 20 weeks and the cervix is closed; may progress to incomplete or complete abortion

- **inevitable abortion**: occurs when the patient has vaginal bleeding and the cervix is dilated but the embryo/fetus remains in the uterus; often accompanied by abdominal pain or cramps

- **incomplete abortion**: occurs when the patient has vaginal bleeding, the cervix is dilated, and the embryo/fetus is found in the cervical canal

- **complete abortion**: occurs when the embryo/fetus has been completely expelled from the uterus and cervix and the cervix is closed

- **septic abortion**: occurs when the abortion is accompanied by uterine infection; it is a life-threatening condition that requires immediate medical intervention

Risk Factors

- age > 35
- underweight or obese mother
- pregestational hypertension
- infection, particularly with fever
- endocrine disorders
- smoking
- cocaine or alcohol use

Physical Examination

- vaginal bleeding

- passage of fetal tissue

- radiating pelvic pain

- signs and symptoms of cessation of pregnancy (e.g., nausea, breast tenderness)

- s/s of infection with septic abortion

Diagnostic Tests

- fetal Doppler to assess for fetal cardiac activity

- transvaginal ultrasound to confirm pregnancy loss

Management

- RhoGAM if mother is Rh negative

- analgesics

- monitor patient for hemodynamic instability

- OB referral

- septic abortion: antibiotics and prep patient for surgery

QUICK REVIEW QUESTIONS

21. What is a septic abortion?

_____

22. A patient in the first trimester is admitted to the ED with complaints of abdominal cramping and spotting over the last 18 hours. During the assessment the nurse is palpating the breast for tenderness and the patient states that the tenderness is gone. Why is the lack of tenderness to the breast a concern for the nurse?

_____

Obstetrical Trauma

Pathophysiology

Trauma is the leading nonobstetric cause of death for pregnant people. Common causes of trauma include MVAs, falls, and intimate partner violence. Trauma is categorized as major if it involves the abdomen, includes high force, or results in vaginal bleeding or decreased fetal movement. Minor trauma does not involve the abdomen and may include no obvious signs and symptoms.

However, minor trauma can still be fatal for mother or fetus, so a thorough assessment should be done on any trauma patient who may be pregnant.

In the ED, the patient should be assessed and stabilized before the fetus is assessed. Pregnant patients presenting to the ED should be evaluated for any non–pregnancy-related issues and then referred to OB if necessary.

Physical Examination

- visible signs and symptoms of injury, including ecchymosis and lacerations
- vaginal bleeding
- tense abdomen
- decreased uterine tone
- presence of amniotic fluid due to membrane rupture

Diagnostic Tests

- transvaginal ultrasound to assess fetus, locate placenta, and assess for abruption
- FAST ultrasound to assess for hemorrhage if suspected

Management

- priority: assess mother's ABCs
- oxygen, respiratory intervention, or cardiac resuscitation as needed
- IV fluids or blood products as needed
- RhoGAM if mother is Rh negative
- betamethasone for imminent delivery of fetus < 34 weeks
- monitor fetal HR and uterine contractions
- OB consult for all obstetric trauma patients

QUICK REVIEW QUESTIONS

23. What steroid is administered to patients at high risk of preterm labor and why?

_____

24. A patient in the third trimester is admitted to the ED after a fall. The assessment shows no vaginal bleeding, but the patient's H/H is low. What should the nurse suspect?

_____

ANSWER KEY

1. The nurse should expect the patient's heart rate and respiratory rate to be increased. Some patients may also show a slight increase in BP resulting from increased cardiac output.

2. Significant separation of the placenta results in hemorrhage and rapid blood loss. Patients will show signs of hypovolemia, including heavy vaginal bleeding (unless abruption is concealed), hypotension, tachycardia, tachypnea, reduced urine output, and abnormal fetal heart rate.

3. The nurse should expect an immediate referral to OB for cesarian delivery.

4. Because the patient is stable, refer to OB for assessment. The pregnancy will be terminated using methotrexate or surgically.

5. A ruptured tubal ectopic pregnancy presents with vaginal bleeding and lower abdominal pain; the patient may have signs and symptoms of hemorrhage.

6. The patient will require fetal and patient monitoring, stat OB consult, and transfer to OB to delay delivery.

7. RhoGAM is administered to all Rh-negative mothers before delivery.

8. The Apgar score is 9: 1 for the appearance, 2 for the pulse, 2 for the grimace, 2 for the activity, and 2 for the respiratory effort.

9. The patient is showing early signs of hypovolemia (tachycardia and tachypnea accompanied by heavy blood loss). The nurse should monitor the patient for signs of hemodynamic instability and be prepared to deliver fluids or blood products as necessary.

10. Tranexamic acid is administered to promote clotting during postpartum bleeding.

11. Morning sickness is the common term for mild nausea and vomiting during early pregnancy. It does not usually affect fluid levels and can be managed with lifestyle changes. Hyperemesis gravidarum is defined as persistent nausea and vomiting in early pregnancy that leads to weight loss (> 5 pounds), dehydration, and possible hypovolemia and electrolyte imbalances.

12. Severe hyperemesis gravidarum may cause thiamine, folic acid, magnesium, calcium, and/or phosphorus deficiencies.

13. The nurse should call a neonatal code blue and initiate CPR.

14. The goal of resuscitation is for the neonate to have spontaneous respiration and a heart rate ≥ 100 bpm. The neonate's oxygen saturation should also be monitored and should reach 85% to 95% by 10 minutes postdelivery.

15. The patient most likely has a postpartum infection at the episiotomy site. The nurse should be prepared to drain and clean the wound and provide treatment for pain (ice packs or NSAIDs). The nurse may also be asked to order a culture and sensitivity of the discharge and administer broad-spectrum antibiotics.

16. A patient with mastitis would present with fever and erythema and tenderness in the breast.

17. The urinalysis of a patient with preeclampsia will show proteinuria.

18. The patient is presenting with signs and symptoms of preeclampsia. The nurse should be prepared to administer antihypertensives and magnesium and to begin maternal and fetal monitoring.

19. HELLP is characterized by hemolysis (H), elevated liver enzymes (EL), and a low platelet count (LP).

20. HELLP syndrome may present with RUQ abdominal pain.

21. A septic abortion is a spontaneous abortion occurring with a uterine infection.

22. A loss or lack of tenderness indicates hormone levels have decreased and a spontaneous abortion is in progress or is imminent.

23. Betamethasone is administered to patients at high risk of preterm labor because it speeds up fetal lung development.

24. The nurse should suspect occult bleeding. The patient will require an ultrasound to assess for an abruption or other sources of bleeding, and may need blood products. This patient will likely be admitted to OB.

8 MENTAL HEALTH EMERGENCIES

BCEN OUTLINE: MENTAL HEALTH EMERGENCIES

- *Aggressive and violent behavior*
- Anxiety disorders (e.g., PTSD, anxiety, panic attack)
- Mood disorders (e.g., bipolar, depression)
- *Homicidal and suicidal ideation*
- *Thought disorders (e.g., psychosis, schizophrenia)*
- Situational crisis (e.g., terminal diagnosis, job loss, relationship issues, unexpected death)
- Intentional overdose and ingestions*

*covered in chapter 12, "Medical Emergencies: Poisoning and Withdrawal"

Aggressive and Violent Behavior

Characteristics

Aggressive or violent behavior in patients may occur for many reasons, including:

- crisis or psychosis
- altered mental status
- influence of drugs or alcohol

- underlying organic processes
- traumatic brain injuries
- urosepsis, especially in patients > 65
- acute dementia or Alzheimer's disease

Management

- Management ranges from verbal de-escalation to mechanical restraint of the violent patient.
- **_De-escalation strategies_**:
  - verbal redirection
  - allowing the patient to express needs
  - allowing the patient to exercise
  - decreased environmental stimulation (quiet room time)
  - PRN medication administration (as requested by patient)
- Restraints may be used.
  - should be used conservatively
  - only for patients whose behavior cannot be controlled through less restrictive measures
  - require frequent assessment (every 5 – 15 minutes depending on organizational policy)
  - check vitals, assess pain, assess circulation and skin integrity of all restrained extremities, and address restroom needs
  - should be removed as soon as they are deemed unnecessary for patient and staff safety
- In patients with acute agitation, medications can be administered: **_olanzapine (Zyprexa), haloperidol (Haldol), or risperidone (Risperdal)_**

QUICK REVIEW QUESTIONS

1. A patient was placed in mechanical restraints after demonstrating violent and aggressive behavior toward nursing staff. It has been 15 minutes since the restraints were applied, and the nurse is preparing to assess the patient. What will the nurse include in her assessment?

   _____

2. What medications may be administered for patients with uncontrollable violent behavior?

   _____

Anxiety Disorders

Characteristics

Anxiety is feelings of fear, apprehension, and worry that can be characterized as mild, moderate, or severe (panic). Physical manifestations of anxiety include palpitations or chest pain, dyspnea, diaphoresis, and/or nausea.

Anxiety will impact other functions such as the respiratory, cardiac, and gastrointestinal systems. A key nursing consideration is to assess for organic causes for reported symptoms, as other life-threatening illnesses may present with similar symptoms.

Management

- Treatment of anxiety should be targeted at the level of anxiety the patient presents with (mild to panic).
- Non-pharmacological interventions include:
  - ☐ Place patient in calm environment.
  - ☐ Encourage rhythmic breathing.
  - ☐ Offer social support if possible.
- Pharmacological interventions (fast-acting anxiolytics) include:
  - ☐ _**benzodiazepines**_ (diazepam [Valium], lorazepam [Ativan])
  - ☐ antihistamines (hydroxyzine)

QUICK REVIEW QUESTIONS

3. A patient presents to the ED stating he was in a movie theater and suddenly began to feel fearful, apprehensive, and on edge. He is feeling mild chest pain and shortness of breath. What should the nurse ask in the assessment of this patient?

_____

4. What medications are usually administered to patients admitted to the ED with severe anxiety?

_____

Mood Disorders

Characteristics

Mood disorders can include mania and/or depression. **Depression** is a mood disorder characterized by feelings of sadness and hopelessness. Patients may also report feelings of suicidality. Depression can manifest as an exacerbation of bipolar disorder or as its own disease process. Depressive behaviors include:

- deep or intense feelings of sadness, worry, or anxiety
- decreased energy levels with associated decreased activity
- sleep and appetite disturbances
- suicidal ideation or focus on death

Bipolar disorder (previously called manic-depressive illness) is characterized by shifts in mood accompanied by manic behaviors or depressive behaviors. Manic behaviors include:

- feelings of elation
- high levels of energy and increased activity
- difficulty sleeping; may not sleep for several days
- increased rate of speech
- engaging in high-risk activities (e.g., excessive spending, risky sexual activity)

Management

HELPFUL HINT:

Organic causes of mania include neurological disorders (e.g., tumors), metabolic disorders (e.g., electrolyte imbalance), and exposure to drugs or toxins.

- Rule out possible medical causes for depression or mania (e.g., metabolic disorders).
- Assess for and treat conditions related to manic or depressive behaviors (e.g., dehydration, trauma injuries).
- Depression:
  - Screen for depression per protocols.
  - Evaluate for suicidal ideation (discussed in detail below).
  - Management of depression is long-term treatment with antidepressants and therapy.
- Bipolar disorder:
  - Treatment in ED addresses exacerbations (i.e., patients "in crisis").
  - Medications to treat symptoms of exacerbations include mood stabilizers, atypical antipsychotics, and antipsychotics.
  - Patients with extreme or long-term mania should be admitted to the hospital.

QUICK REVIEW QUESTIONS

5. What are some key considerations in the assessment of a patient with bipolar disorder on the third day of a manic episode?

_____

6. A nurse is performing an assessment of a patient with a chief complaint of fatigue. The patient tells the nurse that he has felt hopeless recently and has not slept well for the last 2 or 3 weeks. What follow-up questions should the nurse ask this patient?

Homicidal and Suicidal Ideation

Characteristics

Homicidal ideation is characterized by feelings of intent to harm other people, either groups or individuals.

Suicidal ideation is characterized by considering suicide, thoughts of attempting suicide, or planning suicide. Patients exhibiting suicidal ideation may have vague thoughts without a distinct plan, or they may have a specific plan and the means to carry it out.

A **situational crisis** is an acute change or event in a patient's life that may lead to feelings of anxiety, fear, depression, or other mental or emotional illness concerns. Examples of a situational crisis can include:

- divorce
- rape or sexual assault
- domestic violence or abuse
- loss of a job/retirement from a job
- loss of a family member
- any event that creates crisis from a patient's perspective

Nurses should understand that the crisis is as problematic as the patient perceives it to be. The key distinction is not the nature of the event, but the patient's response to the event. Patients may self-refer for situational crises, or the ED nurse may discover that the patient is experiencing a situational crisis during the course of the ED visit.

> **HELPFUL HINT:**
>
> The legal requirements for a **psychiatric emergency hold** vary by state. In most locations, patients can be involuntarily held for 48 to 72 hours if they are a danger to themselves or others.

Management

- Screen for depression and suicidal ideation.
  - ☐ Ask directly if the patient is considering suicide or has recently or in the past attempted suicide.
  - ☐ If the patient is having thoughts of suicide, do they have a concrete plan to carry it out?

□ Determine the presence of risk factors such as a history of substance abuse or chronic pain.

□ Assess the presence of social supports for the patient.

▪ *Interventions for patients with suicidal ideation*:

□ Secure a contract of safety that states they will remain safe while in the hospital and in the future.

□ Create a safe environment (e.g., removing dangerous items from the room).

□ Establish a 1:1 watch or line-of-sight supervision for the patient.

□ Have the patient evaluated by a psychiatrist before discharge.

▪ Homicidal ideation:

□ Assess level of intent.

□ Determine per local protocols if report to law enforcement is required.

QUICK REVIEW QUESTIONS

7. During triage, a patient expresses to the triage nurse that he wants to kill his boss. What should the nurse do next?

_____

8. How can the nurse address patient and staff safety when a patient reports thoughts of self-harm?

_____

★ Thought Disorders

Characteristics

HELPFUL HINT:

Underlying conditions that may cause symptoms of psychosis include DKA, hypoglycemia, stroke, sepsis, and electrolyte imbalances.

A patient experiencing an episode of **psychosis** will have delusions, hallucinations, paranoia, suicidal or homicidal ideation, and disturbances in thinking and perceptions. Psychosis can be the result of organic illnesses or an exacerbation of an existing or new-onset mental illness such as schizophrenia or bipolar disorder.

Schizophrenia is a chronic psychotic condition that is characterized by bouts of psychosis, hallucinations, and disorganized speech. Positive symptoms of schizophrenia are those not normally seen in healthy persons, and negative symptoms are disruptions of normal behaviors.

▪ Positive symptoms:

□ delusions and hallucinations

- □ disorganized speech
- □ odd or confusing behavior
- Negative symptoms:
  - □ social withdrawal
  - □ paranoia
  - □ flattened affect
  - □ poverty of speech

Management

- Rule out organic causes for behavior.
- Test for alcohol and recreational drugs.
- Patients with known history of schizophrenia should be tested to rule out lithium toxicity.
- Antipsychotics (e.g., risperidone or haloperidol) and/or benzodiazepines can be administered for acute exacerbations.

QUICK REVIEW QUESTIONS

9. A known schizophrenic patient presents to the ED after neighbors called the police concerned for her behavior. The patient appears unkempt, unclean, and not appropriately dressed for the weather. What key elements should the nurse assess this patient for?

   _____

10. What medications should the nurse expect to administer to a patient presenting with symptoms of psychosis and a history of schizophrenia?

    _____

ANSWER KEY

1. The nurse should assess the status of the patient, including orientation, vital signs, neurovascular status of the extremities restrained, and skin integrity at the restraint points.

2. Common medications used to manage uncontrollable violent behavior include benzodiazepines, olanzapine, haloperidol, or risperidone.

3. The nurse should obtain prior medical history to include cardiac and respiratory concerns and find out if the patient has a history of anxiety reactions in the past. The nurse should be prepared to address all life-threatening illnesses before addressing anxiety.

4. Severe anxiety is managed with benzodiazepines.

5. The nurse should do a physical assessment to include vital signs and sleep and eating habits to determine if the patient is adequately hydrated and fed. The nurse should determine if the patient has participated in any high-risk activities that may have either long-term or acute consequences to their health.

6. The nurse should use the statements from the patient to consider organic causes for the fatigue and difficulty sleeping but should also ask further questions regarding the patient's emotional and psychological state, including those about suicidal ideation and feelings of safety.

7. The nurse should determine if the patient is in possession of any weapons and follow organizational policy regarding notifying security and the emergency physician of the patient's intent.

8. The nurse should get a detailed accounting of the patient's plan for self-harm and determine if the patient is in possession of any objects or weapons that could cause harm to the patient or to staff. The patient's surroundings should be assessed for safety, with removal of any objects that could be used for harm. Suicide precautions should be initiated with procurement of a 1:1 safety companion assignment.

9. The nurse should perform a head-to-toe physical assessment to determine if any physical harm has come to the patient. The nurse should assess electrolyte balance, and determine if the patient is using recreational drugs or alcohol.

10. The nurse should expect to administer an antipsychotic or benzodiazepine.

9 MEDICAL EMERGENCIES: SHOCK

BCEN OUTLINE: MEDICAL EMERGENCIES

- *Allergic reactions and anaphylaxis*
- Hematologic disorders
- Electrolyte and fluid imbalance
- Endocrine disorders
- Immunocompromise (e.g., HIV/AIDS, oncology/ chemotherapy, transplant patient)
- Renal failure
- *Sepsis*
- *Hypovolemic and distributive shock*
- Substance use and abuse (e.g., alcohol and drug interactions, side effects, unintentional overdose)
- Withdrawal syndrome

Allergic Reactions and Anaphylaxis

ALLERGIC REACTIONS

Pathophysiology

An **allergic reaction** occurs when an irritant or allergen protein enters the body by inhalation, ingestion, or topical exposure. The allergen initiates a response from the immune system, which triggers acute inflammation and vasodilation.

Physical Examination

- topical dermatitis
- urticaria (hives)
- rhinorrhea and sneezing
- itchy skin, nose, mouth, or eyes
- circumoral tingling or pallor

Management

- pharmacological intervention based on location and severity of symptoms
- H1 antihistamines (diphenhydramine [Benadryl])
- H2 antihistamines (cimetidine) may be given with H1 antihistamines for severe symptoms
- PO or IV glucocorticoid (methylprednisolone, prednisone) for severe symptoms
- glucocorticoid or antihistamine nasal sprays for nasal congestion
- bronchodilator (albuterol) for respiratory symptoms
- topical antihistamines or steroids for skin symptoms

QUICK REVIEW QUESTIONS

1. A 6-year-old with a peanut allergy arrives at the ED with facial edema after eating a cookie at school. The patient shows no signs of increased work of breathing and has SpO_2 of 96%. What medications will likely be administered?

2. A patient arrives at the ED with diffuse poison ivy to the lower extremities, upper extremities, chest, and neck. The patient describes having taken 50 mg of loratadine (Claritin) by mouth prior to arrival. What other medications should the nurse anticipate administering?

ANAPHYLACTIC SHOCK
Pathophysiology

Anaphylaxis is triggered when a hypersensitive reaction to an allergen (e.g., foods, medications, insect sting, latex, radiocontrast dye, blood/blood products) causes an overwhelming inflammatory response. Symptoms appear minutes to a few hours after exposure to the allergen. If untreated or ineffectively treated, anaphylaxis will progress to anaphylactic shock, refractory hypotension, and possible death.

Anaphylactic shock is characterized by massive vasodilation, resulting in fluid loss into the extravascular space, hemoconcentration, and hypovolemia. Increased pulmonary vascular resistance may lead to pulmonary edema and respiratory arrest. Dysrhythmias (especially tachycardia) are common, and patients are at risk for MI.

Physical Examination

- urticaria, itching, and erythema
- pale skin
- nausea, vomiting, or diarrhea
- angioedema or tongue swelling
- laryngeal edema and difficulty swallowing
- bronchospasm and wheezing
- hypotension
- tachycardia
- alteration in LOC

Management

- first-line treatment
  - maintain airway
  - ***0.3 mg epinephrine 1:1,000 IM***
  - glucagon 5 – 15 mcg/min infusion if patient is on beta blocker
- second-line treatment
  - H1 blocker: diphenhydramine (25 – 50 mg IV/IM/PO)
  - H2 blocker: ranitidine (50 mg IV or 150 mg PO)
  - steroids: prednisone (50 mg PO) OR methylprednisolone (125 mg IV)
- shock management
  - airway management: oxygen therapy and bronchodilators (albuterol inhaler)
  - volume resuscitation: IV or IO colloid infusion with volume dependent on response (1 – 3 L rapid administration not uncommon)
  - circulatory management (decrease afterload and preload): epinephrine infusion (2 – 8 mcg/min), dopamine infusion (5 – 20 mcg/kg/min), or norepinephrine infusion (2 – 8 mcg/min)
- monitor for spontaneous or rebound/reemergence of anaphylaxis

HELPFUL HINT:

Doses of 1:10,000 – 1:100,000 IV epinephrine are used for cardiac arrest.

- patients who have self-administered an EpiPen monitored for at least 4 hours:
  - □ oxygen and IV fluids as needed
  - □ IV or IM epinephrine as needed

QUICK REVIEW QUESTIONS

3. A patient from an MVC is sent to radiology for a CT scan with contrast. Upon returning, the patient complains of dyspnea and dizziness and has hoarseness. What medication should the nurse anticipate giving?

    _____

4. What interventions should the nurse anticipate for a patient who has self-administered epinephrine for a bee sting allergy?

    _____

Sepsis and Septic Shock

Pathophysiology

Sepsis is a dysregulated inflammatory response to infection that can lead to organ system dysfunction. What starts as a localized response to infection leads to generalized inflammation, which in turn causes cellular damage across systems. Common organ-specific conditions seen during sepsis include:

- hypotension (due to massive vasodilation)
- pulmonary edema and ARDS
- AKI
- encephalopathy

Sepsis is a progressive process, and the guidelines for classifying its stages continue to evolve. Current Society of Critical Care Medicine guidelines define 3 stages of sepsis:

- **early sepsis:** infection + early indicators of organ dysfunction (e.g., increased RR or decreased SBP)
- **sepsis:** infection + signs of organ dysfunction (e.g., decreased PaO_2/FiO_2 ratio, increased creatine)
- <u>**septic shock:**</u> *sepsis + inability to maintain adequate MAP (MAP <65 mm Hg and lactate >2 mmol/L)*

  MODS is the most severe end of the sepsis spectrum. (Note that MODS is simply a description of organ dysfunction and can have noninfectious causes.) Commonly used indicators of organ dysfunction are given below.

- **neurologic**: confusion, lethargy, disorientation, delirium, coma, seizure
- **cardiovascular**: tachycardia, dysrhythmias, elevated troponin level, hypotension requiring fluid resuscitation and vasopressor support, decreased SVR, abnormal CVP (low or high)
- **pulmonary**: tachypnea, dyspnea, hypoxemia, ARDS
- **renal**: oliguria, decreased GRF, elevated creatinine, critical-level electrolyte imbalances
- **endocrine**: hypoglycemia or hyperglycemia, adrenal insufficiency
- **hepatic**: decreased albumin, jaundice, elevated liver function tests
- **hematologic**: thrombocytopenia, coagulopathy, increased D-dimer levels
- **metabolic**: metabolic acidosis, elevated lactate levels

Older sepsis guidelines also include **systemic inflammatory response syndrome (SIRS)** as part of the sepsis continuum. SIRS is defined as 2 or more of the following:

- HR > 90 bpm
- temperature >100.5°F (38.0°C) OR <96.8°F (36.0°C)
- RR >20 OR $PaCO_2$ <32 (respiratory alkalosis)
- WBC >12,000 OR WBC <4,000 OR a shift of bands to the left >10%

Patients with SIRS and a suspected or confirmed infection are considered to have sepsis. Noninfectious causes of SIRS include pancreatitis, burns, thromboembolism, and trauma.

Management

- stat lab work:
  - □ 2 sets of blood cultures: 2 separate sites; obtain before initiating antibiotic therapy
  - □ CBC with differential, lactate levels
- *implement sepsis bundle (per facility guidelines): broad-spectrum antibiotics, IV fluids, and vasopressors as indicated*
- identify causative agent: antibiotic/antiviral/antifungal therapy ASAP
- first-line treatment: IV fluid challenges
  - □ initiated when lactate level >4 mmol/L
  - □ 30 mL/kg to start to support BP
- second-line treatment: vasopressors to maintain MAP ≥65
- ionotropic therapy if cardiac dysfunction: dobutamine infusion
- PRBCs if Hgb <7.0

HELPFUL HINT:

Lactate may be considered a marker of tissue perfusion. Elevated lactate levels sustained >6 hours lead to increased mortality. Lactate >4.0 mmol/L is associated with a >28% mortality rate.

- focused reassessment exam after initial fluid resuscitation:
    - assess tissue perfusion and volume status
    - lactate level should decrease by 10% with each fluid bolus

Hypovolemic Shock

Pathophysiology

Hypovolemic shock is characterized by a profound reduction in circulating volume, leading to impaired tissue perfusion. External causes of hypovolemic shock include hemorrhage, burns, GI/renal losses, or excessive diaphoresis. Hypovolemic shock can also be caused by fluid pooling in the intravascular compartment (third-spacing). Shock caused by bleeding is categorized as **hemorrhagic shock**; all other causes of hypovolemic shock are **nonhemorrhagic**.

HELPFUL HINT:

SVR remains high during hypovolemic state: do NOT give vasopressors.

Physical Examination

- tachycardia
- hypotension
- *narrowing pulse pressure (decrease in SBP, increase in DBP)*
- tachypnea
- oliguria
- dizziness, confusion, and weakness
- nausea
- cool, clammy skin

Management

- determine and treat cause (assessment performed concurrently with fluid resuscitation)
- secure airway and obtain 2 large-bore IV access sites
- rapidly replace volume:
    - 0.9% NaCl or lactated Ringer's (crystalloid fluids)
    - fluid warmer if giving more than 2 L/hr

- maintenance treatment when HR returns to baseline to meet target parameters:
  - MAP ≥ 65
  - CVP 6 – 10 mm Hg
  - urine output ≥ 0.5 mL/kg/hr
- management of hemorrhagic shock:
  - manage bleeding
  - *hemorrhagic shock Class I and II (blood loss <1500 mL, BP normal): crystalloid fluids*
  - *hemorrhagic shock Class III and IV (blood loss >1500 mL, decreased BP): crystalloids and PRBC units*
  - *FFP, cryoprecipitate, and/or platelets (because PRBCs do not contain plasma or platelets)*
  - indications for massive transfusion resuscitation: traumatic injuries; liver transplants; OB emergencies; ruptured aortic or thoracic aneurisms; Hgb <7.0 (generally transfused at higher level for MI, lactic acidosis, severe hypoxemia, or continued active bleeding)
  - ensure Hgb >7.0 and coagulation profile/platelets normalized before moving to maintenance treatment
- blood administration risks:
  - hypothermia: use blood warmer if possible
  - hemolytic and nonhemolytic transfusion reactions
  - hypocalcemia and hypomagnesemia
  - coagulopathy: requires platelets and plasma therapy

HELPFUL HINT:

Cold blood increases hemoglobin's affinity for oxygen and decreases tissue uptake, creates platelet dysfunction, and deforms RBCs

QUICK REVIEW QUESTIONS

7. What are the classic hemodynamic changes found in hypovolemic shock?

_____

8. A patient is admitted to the ED with arterial bleeding from lacerations to the forearm. Crystalloid fluids have been administered. The patient's BP is 80/52 and the physician orders 4 units of PRBCs to be transfused immediately. What other orders should the nurse expect?

_____

ANSWER KEY

1. The patient with an allergic reaction will be administered H1 antihistamines; they may also be administered glucocorticoids or H2 antihistamines.

2. Loratadine is an H1 blocker. H2 blockers, glucocorticoids, and topical antihistamines will also help reduce the allergic response to poison ivy.

3. The nurse should expect to administer epinephrine 1:1,000 IM 0.01 mg/kg.

4. The nurse should assess the patient and monitor their airway. Interventions may include supplemental O_2, IV fluids, and preparation for further IV or IM doses of epinephrine as needed.

5. Septic shock is defined as the presence of sepsis and the inability to maintain MAP ≥65 mm Hg without use of vasopressors.

6. The nurse should anticipate administering a vasopressor such as norepinephrine.

7. Patients in hypovolemic shock will be tachycardic and hypotensive with a narrowing pulse pressure (dropping SBP with increasing or maintaining DBP).

8. Patients who have experienced massive hemorrhage require administration of clotting factors, such as FFP and platelets, to promote coagulation.

10 MEDICAL EMERGENCIES: RENAL DISORDERS

Renal System Assessment and Interventions

- Kidney function is assessed by measuring the rate of filtration and buildup of metabolic waste in the blood.

- The **glomerular filtration rate (GFR)** is the approximate volume of fluid filtered from the glomeruli per minute.

- **Creatinine clearance (CrCl)** is the volume of plasma cleared of creatinine per minute. (Normal rate is 90 – 140 mL/min for men and 80 – 125 mL/min for women.)

- **Blood urea nitrogen (BUN) and serum creatinine** tests assess the levels of metabolic waste products that are normally cleared by the kidneys.
- During renal hypoperfusion, urea may be reabsorbed in the proximal tubules because of compensating increases in the reabsorption of sodium and water. Creatinine is not reabsorbed, so an increased **BUN-to-creatinine ratio** indicates hypoperfusion.

TABLE 10.1. Kidney Function Tests

Test	Description	Normal Range
Serum Tests		
BUN	byproduct of ammonia metabolism; filtered by the kidneys; high levels can indicate insufficient kidney function	7 – 20 mg/dL
Creatinine	product of muscle metabolism; filtered by the kidneys; high levels can indicate insufficient kidney function	0.6 – 1.2 mg/dL
BUN-to-creatinine ratio	increased ratio indicates dehydration, AKI, or GI bleeding; decreased ratio indicates renal damage	10:1 – 20:1
GFR	volume of fluid filtered by the renal glomerular capillaries per unit of time; decreased GFR indicates decreased renal function	men: 100 – 130 mL/min/1.73 m^2 women: 90 – 120 mL/min/1.73 m^2 GFR <60 mL/min/1.73 m^2 is common in adults >70 years
Potassium (K$^+$)	helps with muscle contraction and regulates water and acid-base balance	3.5 – 5.2 mEq/L
Sodium (Na$^+$)	maintains fluid balance and plays a major role in muscle and nerve function	135 – 145 mEq/L
Calcium (Ca^{2+})	plays an important role in skeletal function and structure, nerve function, muscle contraction, and cell communication	8.5 – 10.3 mg/dL

Test	Description	Normal Range
Serum Tests		
Chloride (Cl⁻)	plays a major role in muscle and nerve function	98 – 107 mEq/L
Magnesium (Mg²⁺)	regulates muscle, nerve, and cardiac function	1.8 – 2.5 mg/dL
Urinalysis		
Leukocytes	presence of WBCs in urine indicates infection	negative
Nitrate	presence in urine indicates infection by gram-negative bacteria	negative
Protein	presence in urine may indicate diabetic neuropathy, nephritis, or eclampsia	negative
pH	decreased (acidic) pH may indicate systemic acidosis or diabetes mellitus; increased (alkali) pH may indicate systemic alkalosis or UTI	4.5 – 8
Blood	presence in urine may indicate infection, renal calculi, a neoplasm, or coagulation disorders	negative
Specific gravity	concentration of urine; decreased concentration may indicate diabetes insipidus or pyelonephritis; increased concentration may indicate dehydration or syndrome of inappropriate antidiuretic hormone secretion (SIADH)	1.010 – 1.025
Urine osmolality	concentration of urine; more accurate than specific gravity	300 – 900 mOsm/kg
Ketones	produced during fat metabolism; presence in urine may indicate diabetes, hyperglycemia, starvation, alcoholism, or eclampsia	negative

- **Renal replacement therapies** are considered when the GFR is <30 mL/min.
- During **intermittent hemodialysis**, blood is pumped through an external dialyzer.
  - standard method of dialysis for hemodynamically stable patients
  - heparin administered to prevent microemboli formation
  - complications usually related to shifts in fluid volume; include hypotension, angina, dyspnea, and dysrhythmias
- **Continuous renal replacement therapy (CRRT)** uses an extracorporeal blood pump to continuously move blood through a hemofilter. It is used in patients who cannot tolerate changes in water and electrolyte levels during intermittent hemodialysis.
- During **peritoneal dialysis**, the dialysate fluid is infused into the peritoneal cavity and allowed to remain there for several hours. It is the preferred method for hemodynamically unstable patients who cannot tolerate hemodialysis.
- **Dialysis disequilibrium syndrome (DDS)** is a set of neurological symptoms that occur during dialysis, due to cerebral edema. Signs and symptoms include headache, blurred vision, and altered LOC or mental status.

QUICK REVIEW QUESTIONS

1. What conditions can cause an increased BUN-to-creatinine ratio?

   _____

2. Why is intermittent hemodialysis contraindicated for patients with TBI or increased ICP?

   _____

Electrolyte and Fluid Imbalance

Electrolytes are positively or negatively charged ions located in both the intracellular fluid (ICF) and the extracellular fluid (ECF). These ions are necessary for the maintenance of homeostasis, cellular excitability, and the transmission of neural impulses.

TABLE 10.2. Electrolyte Imbalances

Imbalance	Clinical Manifestation	Treatment and Management	Etiology
Sodium (normal: 135 – 145 mEq/L)			
Hyponatremia	tachycardia hypotension weakness dizziness headache abdominal cramping cerebral edema increased ICP **_seizure_**	sodium replacement, ≤ 12 mEq/L/24 hr in a 24-hour period PO sodium replacement as tolerated isotonic IV solutions (lactated Ringers or 0.9% normal saline) restrict fluid intake, and monitor fluid I/O	dilutional depletion of Na⁺ CHF diarrhea diaphoresis use of thiazides
Hypernatremia	hypotension tachycardia polydipsia lethargy or irritability edema warm, flushed skin hyperreflexia seizures	restrict dietary sodium increase PO fluid or free-water intake diuretics D5W or other hypotonic IV solutions	sodium overload volume depletion impaired thirst renal or GI loss inability to replace fluid losses
Potassium (normal: 3.5 – 5 mEq/L)			
Hypokalemia	dysrhythmias: • **_flat or inverted T waves_** • **_prominent U waves_** • ST depression • prolonged PR interval	potassium replacement PO or IV IV administration ≤ 20 mEq/hr stop infusion if urine output < 30 mL/hr	acid-base shifts alkalosis true depletion or deficits IV dextrose use diarrhea

continued on next page

TABLE 10.2. Electrolyte Imbalances (continued)

Imbalance	Clinical Manifestation	Treatment and Management	Etiology
Potassium (normal: 3.5 – 5 mEq/L)			
Hypokalemia (continued)	hypotension altered mental status leg cramps or muscle cramps hypoactive reflexes flaccid muscles	cardiac monitoring necessary presents with hypercalcemia	alcoholism Cushing's syndrome medications: steroids, diuretics, amphotericin, insulin
Hyperkalemia	dysrhythmias or cardiac arrest: • ***tall, peaked T waves*** • prolonged PR interval • wide QRS complex • absent P waves • ST depression • abdominal cramping and diarrhea • anxiety	***calcium gluconate*** ***IV insulin and D50*** ***loop diuretics*** ***sodium polystyrene sulfonate (Kayexalate)*** sodium bicarbonate beta 2 agonists (albuterol) hypertonic IV solution (3% normal saline) ECG and continued cardiac monitoring restrict PO intake of potassium-containing foods may require dialysis	increased intake of salt substitutes or potassium-sparing medications hemolysis, burns, crushing injury, or rhabdomyolysis decreased urine output

Imbalance	Clinical Manifestation	Treatment and Management	Etiology
Magnesium (normal: 1.3 – 2.1 mEq/L)			
Hypomagnesemia	dysrhythmias: • **_torsades de pointes_** • flat or inverted T waves • ST depression • prolonged PR interval • widened QRS complex hypertension seizures hyperreflexia	magnesium sulfate IV, 1 – 2 g over 60 minutes monitor for seizures, dys-rhythmias, and magnesium toxicity	excessive loss from GI tract or kidneys diuretic use alcoholism
Hypermagnesemia	bradycardia (more common) or tachy-cardia **_respiratory depression lethargy/ decreased LOC_** dysrhythmias or cardiac arrest: • prolonged PR interval • wide QRS complex • peaked T waves	**_calcium gluconate loop diuretics_** isotonic IV solutions (lactated Ringers or 0.9% normal saline) may require dialysis	increased intake renal dysfunction hepatitis Addison's disease
Calcium (normal: 4.5 – 5.5 mEq/L)			
Hypocalcemia	dysrhythmias or cardiac arrest: • prolonged QT interval • flattened ST segment	PO or IV calcium replacement calcium gluconate dilute IV solution with D5W only, never with normal saline	low serum proteins decreased intake renal failure hypoparathyroid-ism vitamin D defi-ciency

continued on next page

TABLE 10.2. Electrolyte Imbalances (continued)

Imbalance	Clinical Manifestation	Treatment and Management	Etiology
Calcium (normal: 4.5 – 5.5 mEq/L)			
Hypocalcemia (continued)	hypotension third-space fluid shift decreased clotting time laryngeal spasm or bronchospasm seizures ***Chvostek sign*** ***Trousseau sign*** hyperactive deep-tendon reflexes	vitamin D supplements seizure precautions	pancreatitis medications: calcitonin, steroids, loop diuretics
Hypercalcemia	anxiety cognitive dysfunction constipation nausea/vomiting shortened QT interval muscle weakness	loop diuretics isotonic IV solutions (0.9% normal saline) glucocorticoids and calcitonin	malignancies hyperthyroidism and hyperparathyroidism Paget's disease medications: lithium, androgens, tamoxifen, excessive vitamin D, excessive thyroid replacement therapy
Phosphate (normal: 1.8 – 2.3 mEq/L)			
Hypophosphatemia	respiratory distress or failure tissue hypoxia chest pain seizures decreased LOC increased susceptibility to infection nystagmus	PO or IV phosphate replacement seizure precautions	increased renal excretion

Imbalance	Clinical Manifestation	Treatment and Management	Etiology
Phosphate (normal: 1.8 – 2.3 mEq/L)			
Hyperphosphatemia	tachycardia hyperreflexia soft-tissue calcifications	saline and loop diuretics phosphate binders (e.g., aluminum hydroxide) limit dietary intake of phosphates dialysis may be appropriate	decreased renal excretion

QUICK REVIEW QUESTIONS

3. A nurse is reviewing the ECG of a patient who came into the ER for a racing heart rate. The T waves are tall and peaked. What abnormal labs would be expected to cause this?

   _____

4. Lab values reveal that a patient's sodium level is 157 mEq/L. What precautions should be initiated?

   _____

5. A patient receiving enteral feedings has had severe diarrhea. The patient becomes irritable and is twitching. Vital signs are BP 92/53 mm Hg, HR 108 bpm, RR 20 breaths per minute, and oral temperature 100.9°F (38.3°C). What condition should the nurse suspect?

   _____

Acute Kidney Injury

Acute kidney injury (AKI), previously called acute renal failure, is an acute decrease in kidney function characterized by increased serum creatinine (**azotemia**) with or without decreased urine output. Changes in kidney function may result in multiple systemic conditions that require intervention. These conditions include:

- fluid imbalance (hypo- or hypervolemia)
- electrolyte imbalance
- acid-base imbalance
- hematological abnormalities (e.g., anemia, low platelet count)

AKI has a diverse etiology and is characterized as prerenal, intrarenal, or postrenal, based on the cause of injury.

PRERENAL DISEASE

Pathophysiology

Prerenal disease is renal hypoperfusion caused by hemodynamic compromise (e.g., hypovolemia, systemic vasodilation) or renal ischemia. Prerenal disease presents with no damage to renal tubules and can usually be reversed by treating the underlying condition.

HELPFUL HINT:

NSAIDs, ARBs, and ACE inhibitors can cause or worsen prerenal disease and ATN.

Diagnostic Tests

- *increased creatinine and BUN*
- *elevated BUN-to-creatinine ratio (>20:1)*
- low urine Na⁺ (<20 mEq/L)
- increased urine osmolality and specific gravity
- normal finding on urine microscopy (no casts)
- serum creatinine returns to normal value after fluid repletion

Management

- *treat underlying cause to maintain MAP >65 mm Hg*
  - □ fluids to rehydrate
  - □ vasopressors as needed to manage vasodilation

> **QUICK REVIEW QUESTION**
>
> 6. A patient with sepsis has received 3 L of normal saline over the past 24 hours and currently has maintenance fluids at 125 mL/hr. The nurse notes that urine output is at 250 mL for the past 4 hours. The last serum creatinine is 1.8 mg/dL, and BUN is 38 mg/dL. What interventions should the nurse anticipate?

INTRARENAL DISEASE

Pathophysiology

Intrarenal (or intrinsic) disease is caused by damage to the kidneys. The most common intrarenal condition in critical care settings is **acute tubular necrosis (ATN)**, the destruction of the renal tubular epithelium. ATN may be ischemic (usually caused by severe prerenal disease) or nephrotoxic. Common nephrotoxic substances include contrast dyes, NSAIDs, ARBs, ACE inhibitors, and aminoglycosides. ATN may also occur secondary to rhabdomyolysis or after cardiovascular surgery.

Intrarenal disease and recovery occurs in 4 phases.

1. The **onset phase** occurs immediately after the triggering event but before cell injury. Patients may have reduced urine output but few other symptoms.

2. During the **oliguric phase** (1 – 2 weeks), urine output is reduced to <400 mL/day, and creatinine and BUN serum levels will increase. In rare cases, patients may become **anuric** (urine output <100 mL/day). The inability of the kidneys to excrete urine may cause fluid overload, electrolyte imbalances (particularly hyperkalemia), and metabolic acidosis.

3. The **diuretic phase** (1 – 2 weeks) begins when the underlying cause of AKI has been corrected and GFR begins to increase. This phase is characterized by increased urine output (>3 L/day). Patients should be monitored for hypovolemia and electrolyte depletion.

4. The **recovery phase** may last up to a year as kidney function slowly returns.

Diagnostic Tests

- ***increased creatinine and BUN***
- ***BUN-to-creatinine ratio <20:1***
- oliguric phase
    - increased urine osmolality and specific gravity
    - urine Na^+ <10 mEq/L
- diuretic phase
    - decreased urine osmolality and specific gravity
    - urine Na^+ <40 mEq/L
- casts seen through urine microscopy
- serum creatinine does not respond to fluid repletion

Management

- treat underlying cause
- discontinue or minimize use of nephrotoxic medications
- fluid volume management
    - IV fluids for hypovolemia
    - loop diuretics for hypervolemia (if not anuric)
    - daily weights and strict monitoring of fluid I/O

- correct electrolyte imbalances and monitor for related complications (including cardiac monitoring)
- sodium bicarbonate for metabolic acidosis
- ***indications for urgent dialysis in patients with AKI:***
  - □ severe or symptomatic hyperkalemia
  - □ severe metabolic acidosis
  - □ volume overload
  - □ pulmonary edema
  - □ uremia

QUICK REVIEW QUESTION

7. A patient is admitted with intrarenal disease related to the use of imaging contrast dye. The patient's I/O are being monitored closely, with outputs of approximately 500 mL per shift charted. The patient's assessment is as follows: BP 165/92, HR 85 bpm, 3+ pitting edema, auscultation of crackles in the bases of lungs, and SpO_2 92%. What condition should the nurse suspect, and what intervention will be required?

POSTRENAL DISEASE
Pathophysiology

Postrenal conditions are characterized by the blocked drainage of urine, usually because of prostatic hypertrophy or renal calculi. Treatment addresses the underlying cause of obstruction.

Diagnostic Tests

- oliguria
- increased serum creatinine and BUN
- normal BUN-to-creatinine ratio
- possible pain or hematuria

QUICK REVIEW QUESTION

8. What lab values can be used to differentiate between pre- and postrenal failure?

Chronic Kidney Disease

Pathophysiology

Chronic kidney disease (CKD) is long-term (>3 months) kidney damage or dysfunction caused by destruction of nephrons. Like AKI, the etiology of CKD can be categorized as pre-, intra-, or postrenal. Common causes of CKD include:

- decreased perfusion due to heart failure or cirrhosis
- hypertensive nephrosclerosis
- diabetic nephropathy
- renal artery stenosis (usually due to atherosclerosis)
- glomular or tubulointerstitial disease
- chronic urinary obstruction

The kidneys initially compensate by hyperfiltration in individual nephrons, so patients are initially asymptomatic and present only with abnormal creatinine or BUN values. As the kidneys' ability to remove excess fluid and metabolic waste is further impaired, patients show signs and symptoms related to hypervolemia and decreased GFR. Related conditions that may require acute care include pulmonary edema and electrolyte imbalances.

Diagnostic Tests

- decreased GFR
  - Stage 1: >90 mL/min
  - Stage 2: 60 – 89 mL/min
  - Stage 3: 30 – 59 mL/min
  - Stage 4: 15 – 29 mL/min
  - Stage 5: <15 mL/min (**end-stage renal disease [ESRD]**)
- increased serum creatinine and BUN
- increased K^+ and decreased Ca^{2+}
- decreased HgB
- increased serum bicarbonate

Management

- reverse initial cause of kidney injury
- sodium restriction and diuretics for hypervolemia
- sodium bicarbonate for acidosis
- ACE inhibitors or ARBs for hypertension

- erythropoietin for anemia
- renal replacement therapy (hemodialysis or peritoneal dialysis)

QUICK REVIEW QUESTION

9. Why would diuretics be prescribed for a patient with CKD?

_____

ANSWER KEY

1. Common causes of an increased BUN-to-creatinine ratio include dehydration, AKI, and GI bleeding.

2. The rapid removal of urea from the blood can lower plasma osmolality, which results in fluid shift to the intracellular space. For patients at risk for ICP, the resulting cerebral edema can cause neurological deterioration.

3. Hyperkalemia or hypermagnesemia may cause tachycardia and tall, peaked T waves.

4. Seizure and fall precautions should be initiated for patients with hypernatremia.

5. The patient's history and symptoms suggest hypernatremia, likely due to the dehydration associated with diarrhea and possibly insufficient free water administered with the enteral feedings.

6. The patient is likely experiencing sepsis-induced prerenal disease. The nurse should ensure optimal perfusion through continued fluid replacement and titrating vasopressors to keep MAP >65 mm Hg. The physician should be notified if the patient does not respond with improving urine output.

7. These symptoms may indicate pulmonary edema. The nurse should immediately inform the physician and prepare the patient for hemodialysis.

8. In prerenal disease, the BUN-to-creatinine ratio will be >20:1. In postrenal disease, the ratio will be normal (10:1 – 20:1).

9. Diuretics are prescribed to manage conditions related to hypervolemia in patients with CKD, including PE and hypertension. Diuretics may also be used to lower K^+ levels (loop diuretics).

11 MEDICAL EMERGENCIES: ENDOCRINE DISORDERS

Endocrine System Anatomy and Physiology

- The endocrine system is made up of **glands** that regulate numerous processes throughout the body by secreting chemical messengers called **hormones**.

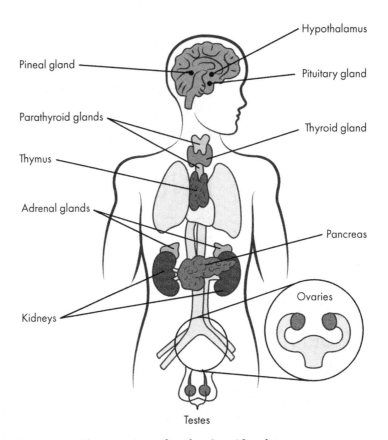

Figure 11.1. The Location of Endocrine Glands

Gland	Regulates	Hormones Produced
TABLE 11.1. Endocrine Glands and Their Functions		
Hypothalamus	pituitary function and metabolic processes including body temperature, hunger, thirst, and circadian rhythms	thyrotropin-releasing hormone (TRH), dopamine, growth-hormone-releasing hormone (GHRH), gonadotropin-releasing hormone (GnRH), oxytocin, vasopressin
Pituitary gland	growth, blood pressure, reabsorption of water by the kidneys, temperature, pain relief, and some reproductive functions related to pregnancy and childbirth	human growth hormone (HGH), thyroid-stimulating hormone (TSH), prolactin (PRL), luteinizing hormone (LH), follicle-stimulating hormone (FSH), oxytocin, antidiuretic hormone (ADH)
Pineal gland	circadian rhythms (the sleep-wake cycle)	melatonin
Thyroid gland	energy use and protein synthesis	thyroxine (T_4), triiodothyronine (T_3), calcitonin

Gland	Regulates	Hormones Produced
Parathyroid	calcium and phosphate levels	parathyroid hormone (PTH)
Adrenal glands	"fight or flight" response and regulation of salt and blood volume	epinephrine, norepinephrine, cortisol, androgens
Pancreas	blood glucose levels and metabolism	insulin, glucagon, somatostatin
Testes	maturation of sex organs and secondary sex characteristics	androgens (e.g., testosterone)
Ovaries	maturation of sex organs, secondary sex characteristics, pregnancy, childbirth, and lactation	progesterone, estrogens
Placenta	gestation and childbirth	progesterone, estrogens, human chorionic gonadotropin, human placental lactogen (hPL)

QUICK REVIEW QUESTION

1. Which endocrine gland regulates blood glucose levels?

_____

Adrenal Insufficiency

Pathophysiology

Adrenal insufficiency is an endocrine disorder characterized by a decrease in circulating corticosteroids (both glucocorticoids and mineralocorticoids). **Primary adrenal insufficiency** (Addison's disease) is caused by the inability of the adrenal glands to produce corticosteroids. **Secondary adrenal insufficiency** is caused by low production of **adrenocorticotropic hormone (ACTH)** in the pituitary gland. (ACTH stimulates corticosteroid production.)

The condition can be chronic or acute. The most common cause of **chronic adrenal insufficiency** is autoimmune conditions that damage the adrenal cortex.

Acute adrenal insufficiency (adrenal crisis) causes distributive shock and is a medical emergency that requires immediate care. It usually occurs when infection or trauma exacerbate chronic adrenal insufficiency, but may occur following damage to the adrenal or pituitary glands. Rarely, it may be caused by withdrawal from long-term glucocorticoid use.

The information below describes the diagnosis and management of adrenal crisis.

Physical Examination

- shock (e.g., hypotension, tachycardia, oliguria)
- abdominal pain/tenderness
- nausea, vomiting, or diarrhea
- fever
- hyperpigmentation (from chronic adrenal insufficiency)

Diagnostic Tests

- *low cortisol* or aldosterone levels
- ACTH stimulation test shows low cortisol level
- *low serum Na+*
- *high serum K+*
- *low blood glucose*
- elevated renin

Treatment and Management

- IV fluid resuscitation
- *empiric administration of IV glucocorticoids* (usually hydrocortisone or dexamethasone)
- replacement of mineralocorticoids may be required (e.g., fludrocortisone)
- management of hypoglycemia and electrolyte imbalances as needed

QUICK REVIEW QUESTIONS

2. What abnormalities should the nurse expect to see in the labs for a patient in acute adrenal crisis?

   _____

3. A 19-year-old patient who has recently stopped a course of prednisone for asthma exacerbation arrives at the ED with BP of 78/40 mm Hg, HR of 135 bpm, fatigue, and extreme thirst. What medication does the nurse anticipate giving this patient?

   _____

Diabetes Mellitus

Diabetes mellitus (DM) is a metabolic disorder affecting insulin production and insulin resistance. It is classified as type 1 or type 2.

HELPFUL HINT:

Fever caused by infection may precipitate an adrenal crisis, or the fever itself may be caused by low corticosteroid levels.

- **type 1**: an acute-onset autoimmune disease most prominent in children, teens, and adults <30. Beta cells in the pancreas are destroyed and are unable to produce sufficient amounts of insulin, causing blood sugar to rise. Patients with type 1 diabetes require regular insulin injections.
- **type 2**: a gradual-onset disease most prominent in adults >30. Individuals develop insulin resistance, which prevents the cellular uptake of glucose and causes blood sugar to rise. Patients with type 2 diabetes may manage the condition through lifestyle changes or may require antidiabetic medications.

Physical Examination

- polyuria, polyphagia, and polydipsia
- fatigue and weakness
- altered mental status

Diagnostic Tests

- fasting blood glucose ≥126 mg/dL
- 2-hour plasma glucose ≥200 mg/dL (75 g OGTT)
- A1C ≥6.5%

Management

- treat hypo- or hyperglycemia as indicated
- manage related conditions (e.g., peripheral neuropathy, diabetic retinopathy)
- for patients with diabetes but presenting with unrelated complaints:
  - □ regular glucose monitoring with moderate glycemic controls (140 – 180 mg/dL)
  - □ dosing of insulin or oral hypoglycemics may change in light of presenting complaint
  - □ IV fluids with dextrose for NPO patients

QUICK REVIEW QUESTION

4. A patient with a history of type 1 diabetes arrives at the ED after sustaining a shoulder dislocation and is put on NPO status in anticipation of surgical intervention. The nurse should anticipate an IV infusion of what fluid to maintain a therapeutic blood glucose level?

Hyperglycemia

Pathophysiology

Diabetic ketoacidosis (DKA) occurs when the body does not produce insulin. The elevated glucose levels increase the serum osmolality, resulting in osmotic diuresis that causes polyuria, with significant water loss. Simultaneously, the body also begins to break down fat cells for fuel, producing a buildup of serum ketones, resulting in acidosis. As acidosis worsens, potassium is shifted out of cells, resulting in an initial presentation with hyperkalemia. However, continued osmotic diuresis eventually leads to hypokalemia in most patients.

Hyperosmolar hyperglycemic state (HHS), also called **hyperglycemic hyperosmolar nonketotic syndrome (HHNK)**, is a slow-onset, high-mortality complication of type 2 DM. It occurs when the pancreas produces insufficient insulin. As with DKA, blood glucose levels become high, resulting in osmotic diuresis and hypovolemia. With decreased kidney perfusion and oliguria from dehydration, less glucose is removed and serum hyperosmolality increases. Serum potassium may be elevated, but total body potassium will be depleted due to osmotic diuresis. In HHS, insulin production is sufficient to prevent ketoacidosis, differentiating it from DKA.

HELPFUL HINT:

HHS is often mistaken for a neurological event as intracerebral dehydration may cause profound CNS symptoms, including coma.

Diagnosis

TABLE 11.2. DKA and HHS	
DKA	**HHS**
Etiology	
• undiagnosed/ineffectively managed type 1 DM • destabilized type 2 DM (less common) • acute illness (e.g., MI, pancreatitis) • medications (e.g., steroids, epinephrine, thiazide diuretics, atypical antipsychotics) • stress of critical illness • endocrine disorders (e.g., hyperthyroidism, Cushing's syndrome)	• most common in older adult patients with obesity, type 2 DM, and underlying cardiovascular disease • patients who control diabetes through diet only • TPN • use of steroids or thiazides • pancreatitis • serious illness or infection (e.g., MI, pneumonia)

DKA	HHS
Physical Examination	
• rapid onset • polyuria (early); oliguria (late) • signs and symptoms of hypovolemia • **_Kussmaul respirations and fruity breath odor_** • polyphagia and polydipsia • nausea, vomiting • abdominal pain • malaise and weakness • decreased LOC	• slow onset • polyuria • signs and symptoms of hypovolemia • rapid, extremely shallow breaths • polydipsia • mild nausea or vomiting • weight loss • diplopia • malaise and weakness • **_stupor or coma_**
Diagnostic Findings	

• **_elevated blood glucose (>250 mg/dL)_**
• **_metabolic acidosis_**
  • pH <7.3
  • HCO_3- <18 mEq/L
  • anion gap >10
• **_increased serum ketones_**
• low serum Na^+ and Ca^{++}
• increased serum K^+
• elevated BUN and creatinine
• fluid deficit (negative 50 – 100 mL/kg common)
	• **_elevated blood glucose (>600 mg/ dL)_**
	• **_high serum osmolality (>350 mOsm/kg)_**
	• no diagnostic findings of acidosis (i.e., normal pH and serum HCO_3)
	• serum K^+ normal or high
	• elevated BUN and creatinine
	• **_fluid deficit may be as high as 150 mL/kg total body weight_**

HELPFUL HINT:

For fluid resuscitation in DKA, think "Oh, oh, ease off": isOtonic, hypOtonic, hypErtonic.

Management

- **_IV fluid protocols_**
  - first hour: 1 – 3 L of isotonic fluids (lactated Ringer's or 0.9% normal saline)
  - second hour: 1 L of hypotonic fluids (0.45% normal saline)
  - when blood glucose reaches 250 mg/dL: 1 L of hypertonic fluids with dextrose (D5 in half-normal saline).
- IV K^+ replacement if K^+ <5.3 mEq/L
- **_continuous IV insulin_** (0.1 units/kg/hr)
  - initiate only when K^+ >3.3 mEq/L
  - slow blood glucose reduction (decrease by 50 – 75 mg/dL/hr)

QUICK REVIEW QUESTIONS

5. What diagnostic findings differentiate HHS from DKA?

    _____

6. What is the IV fluid protocol for patients with severe hyperglycemia?

    _____

Hypoglycemia
Pathophysiology

Hypoglycemia is the sudden fall of blood glucose below normal levels. The decreased glucose levels result in neurological dysfunction. In addition, the adrenal medulla is triggered to release adrenaline (also called epinephrine) to restore normal glucose levels, leading to increased sympathetic nervous system activity.

Risk Factors

- use of insulin (IV or subcutaneous)
- interruption of oral, enteral, or parenteral feedings
- adrenal insufficiency
- infection
- pancreatitis
- vomiting
- drinking excess alcohol, or liver disease

Physical Examination

- cardiovascular
  - □ tachycardia
  - □ diaphoresis
  - □ irritability, restlessness
  - □ cool skin
- neurological
  - □ lethargy
  - □ weakness
  - □ slurred speech or blurred vision
  - □ anxiety or confusion
  - □ seizure (at blood glucose 20 – 40 mg/dL)
  - □ coma (at blood glucose <20 mg/dL)

HELPFUL HINT:

Beta blockers may hide cardiovascular symptoms in patients with hypoglycemia.

Diagnostic Tests

- *serum glucose <70 mg/dL*

Treatment and Management

- overall treatment goal: maintain blood glucose level >70 mg/dL
  - blood glucose 60 – 70 mg/dL: 4 oz of juice if oral intake is not contraindicated
  - blood glucose 40 – 60 mg/dL: D50 via IV push (12.5 g = 0.5 ampule)
  - blood glucose <40 mg/dL: D50 via IV push (25 g = 1.0 ampule)
- refractory hypoglycemia
  - continuous infusion of D10 (dextrose 10% solution) via peripheral IV
  - continuous infusion of D20 (dextrose 20% solution) via central line
- longer-acting carbohydrates (oral intake, tube feeding, or TPN) after patient is stabilized
- seizure prophylaxis
- identify and treat underlying cause

QUICK REVIEW QUESTIONS

7. What serum glucose level is generally defined as hypoglycemic?

_____

8. What hormone is released from the adrenal gland to restore glucose levels in hypoglycemia?

_____

Hyperthyroidism

Pathophysiology

Hyperthyroidism (thyrotoxicosis) occurs when the thyroid produces an excess of the thyroid hormones triiodothyronine (T3) and/or thyroxine (T4). Chronic hyperthyroidism presents with a characteristic set of symptoms, including anxiety, weakness, palpitations, tremor, and weight loss.

Thyroid storm is a severe form of thyrotoxicosis usually seen in patients with hyperthyroidism after a precipitating event (e.g., trauma, infection). Thyroid storm has a high mortality rate and requires immediate treatment.

The information below describes the diagnosis and management of thyroid storm.

Physical Examination

- tachycardia (>140 bmp)
- hypotension
- hyperpyrexia
- altered mental status (agitation, confusion)
- decreased LOC (progressing to coma)

Diagnostic Tests

- _**elevated T4 and/or T3**_
- low TSH

Management

- _**pharmacological suppression of thyroid hormones**_ (e.g., thionamides, iodine, and glucocorticoids)
- beta blockers (for cardiac symptoms)
- respiratory support as needed
- aggressive cooling measures (e.g., ice packs)

QUICK REVIEW QUESTIONS

9. A patient is admitted to with new onset of thyroid storm. Which physiological system should be a main focus of symptom management?

   _____

10. What medications should the nurse expect to administer to a patient in thyrotoxic crisis?

    _____

Hypothyroidism

Pathophysiology

Hypothyroidism is characterized by low levels of the hormones T3 and T4. **Primary hypothyroid** disease results from damage to the thyroid. **Secondary hypothyroidism** is the result of a hypothalamic-pituitary disease. Symptoms of chronic hypothyroidism are related to slowing of metabolic process and include fatigue, bradycardia, cold intolerance, weight gain, and localized non-pitting edema (myxedema).

Myxedema coma is severe hypothyroidism usually seen in patients with chronic hypothyroidism after a precipitating event (e.g., MI, infection). It is a medical emergency that requires immediate treatment.

The information below describes the diagnosis and management of myxedema coma.

Physical Examination

- decreased LOC (confusion and lethargy progressing to coma)
- hypothermia
- bradycardia
- hypotension

Diagnostic Tests

- low serum T4
- low serum Na$^+$
- ABGs show respiratory acidosis

Management

- empiric administration of IV levothyroxine (T4) and liothyronine (T3)
- glucocorticoids (usually hydrocortisone)
- fluids and vasopressors
- passive rewarming

QUICK REVIEW QUESTIONS

11. What diagnostic findings should the nurse expect for a patient severe hypothyroidism?

_____

12. Why would a patient with suspected myxedema coma be administered glucocorticoids?

_____

ANSWER KEY

1. The pancreas controls blood glucose levels by producing and releasing insulin and glucagon.

2. Patients with acute adrenal crisis will have decreased serum cortisol; labs may also show hyperkalemia, hyponatremia, or hypoglycemia.

3. The patient will be administered IV corticosteroids.

4. The nurse will administer D5W or other dextrose-containing IV fluids.

5. The preferred diagnostic indicator is serum osmolality: patients with HHS will have a higher serum osmolality (>350 mOsm/kg) than with DKA. HHS also presents with higher blood glucose (>600 mg/dL) than DKA, and patients may have a higher fluid deficit (as high as 150 mL/kg of body weight). Because no ketoacidosis is present with HHS, there will be no significant serum ketones or findings associated with acidosis.

6. The IV fluid protocol for patients with severe hyperglycemia is:

   • first hour: 1 – 3 L of isotonic fluids

   • second hour: 1 L of hypotonic fluids

   • when blood glucose reaches 250 mg/dL: 1 L of hypertonic fluids with dextrose

7. Hypoglycemia is a blood glucose <70 mg/dL.

8. Adrenaline (epinephrine) increases blood glucose levels and increases cardiac output.

9. Patients with thyroid storm typically have severe cardiac disturbances and need supportive care to maintain hemodynamic stability. The patient should be placed on cardiac telemetry and the nurse should be prepared for emergent cardioversion and treatment with beta blockers.

10. Patients in thyrotoxic crisis may be administered beta blockers, thionamide, iodine, glucocorticoid, and/or antipyretics.

11. The nurse should expect to see low serum T4 and low serum Na⁺.

12. Myxedema coma is often concomitant with secondary adrenal insufficiency. Because adrenal crisis requires immediate treatment with glucocorticoids, they are often administered to patients with myxedema coma until adrenal insufficiency has been ruled out.

12 MEDICAL EMERGENCIES: POISONING AND WITHDRAWAL

BCEN OUTLINE: MEDICAL EMERGENCIES

- Allergic reactions and anaphylaxis
- Hematologic disorders
- Electrolyte and fluid imbalance
- Endocrine disorders
- Immunocompromise (e.g., HIV/AIDS, oncology/chemotherapy, transplant patient)
- Renal failure
- Sepsis
- Hypovolemic and distributive shock
- ***Substance use and abuse (e.g., alcohol and drug interactions, side effects, unintentional overdose)***
- ***Withdrawal syndrome***

Poisoning and Intoxication

TOXIDROMES ★

Toxidromes are groups of signs and symptoms present in patients who have large amounts of toxins or poisons in the body. General signs and symptoms are given below, but these may vary based on the specific drug (or combination of drugs) ingested.

TABLE 12.1. Signs and Symptoms of Toxidromes

Toxidrome	HR	BP	RR	Temp	Bowel Sounds	Pupils	Skin	Mental Status
Anticholinergic antihistamines, antipsychotics, tricyclic antidepressants (TCA), scopolamine, atropine, some medications used for COPD and asthma	↑	↑	—	↑	↓	↑	dry	agitated and delirious
Cholinergic anticholinesterase, insecticides and pesticides, nerve agents (e.g., sarin)	—	—	—	—	↑	↓	moist	—
Hallucinogenic LSD, psilocybin ("magic mushrooms"), mescaline, DMT, salvia divinorum, dextromethorphan (DXM), PCP	↑	↑	↑	—	↑	↑	—	disoriented
Sympathomimetic cocaine, amphetamines, methamphetamines, hallucinogenic amphetamines (MDMA, MDA), khat and related substances (methcathinone, "bath salts"), cold medications, diet supplements containing ephedrine	↑	↑	↑	↑	↑	↑	moist	agitated and delirious

Toxidrome	HR	BP	RR	Temp	Bowel Sounds	Pupils	Skin	Mental Status
Sedative-hypnotic benzodiazepines, barbiturates, antipsychotics, zolpidem (Ambien), clonidine, GHB	↓	↓	↓	↓	↓	—	dry	lethargic and confused

QUICK REVIEW QUESTION

1. What symptoms should the nurse expect to see in a patient who has intentionally consumed a bottle of atropine eye drop solution in an attempt to self-harm?

ACETAMINOPHEN POISONING

Pathophysiology

During **acetaminophen (Tylenol)** poisoning, toxic metabolites accumulate in the liver causing hepatotoxicity from mitochondrial dysfunction and cellular destruction. Gastritis symptoms usually appear within hours; symptoms of hepatotoxicity may not appear for 48 hours. Hepatoxicity rapidly advances to acute liver failure often complicated by encephalopathy, pulmonary edema, pancreatitis, and AKI.

Time and amount of drug are important considerations in acetaminophen overdose treatment. Plasma acetaminophen levels can be measured 4 – 24 hours after ingestion to predict risk of hepatotoxicity using the **Rumack-Matthew nomogram.**

Management

- *__antidote: N-acetylcysteine (Mucomyst)__* (best response occurs when it is administered within 24 hours of ingestion)
  - N-acetylcysteine dosing (IV): IV 150 mg/kg over 1 hour; 50 mg/kg over next 4 hours; 100 mg/kg over next 16 hours
  - N-acetylcysteine dosing (PO): 140 mg/kg loading dose; 70 mg/kg every 4 hours
- activated charcoal (within 4 hours of ingestion)

BENZODIAZEPINE POISONING

Benzodiazepine poisoning causes a depression of spinal reflexes and the reticular activating system by enhancing the neurotransmitter GABA. Generally, respiratory arrest occurs with ingestion of benzodiazepines. Cardiopulmonary arrest is seen in rapid diazepam injections or when benzodiazepines are used with other depressant drugs. Onset of symptoms are seen in 30 – 120 minutes (specific to the benzodiazepine used).

Benzodiazepines have a very high therapeutic index, and the majority of benzodiazepine overdose cases do not require respiratory intervention or the use of an antagonist.

Physical Examination

- classis presentation: CNS depression with normal vital signs
- lethargy
- slurred speech and ataxia
- pinpoint pupils (midline fixated and unresponsive to light)

Management

- priority: management of airway and breathing
- antidote: flumazenil (Romazicon)
  - 0.2 mg IVP every 1 – 6 minutes or IV infusion 0.3 – 0.4 mg/hr
  - monitor for re-sedation after flumazenil administration

CARDIOVASCULAR MEDICATION POISONING

- **Beta blockers** block beta-adrenergic receptors in the heart (beta$_1$) and blood vessels (beta$_2$), resulting in lowered BP and HR and decreased cardiac output. They are prescribed to treat a wide range of conditions, and most overdoses are unintentional.

□ Symptoms of toxicity will be seen 1 – 2 hours after ingestion and usually are most pronounced around 20 hours post-ingestion.

□ General signs and symptoms: bradycardia, hypotension, hypoglycemia, altered mental state.

- **Calcium channel blockers (CCBs)** restrict the flow of calcium into cells in vascular and cardiac tissues and result in vasodilation, decreased contractility, and decreased conduction velocity in the cardiac nodes.

- Management of beta blocker and CCB overdose:

□ CCB toxicity causes severe hemodynamic instability with hypotension and dysrhythmias.

□ Patients may present with tachycardia or bradycardia, depending on the type and quantity of medication taken.

□ Activated charcoal (within 2 hours of ingestion); whole bowel irrigation for timed-release medication

□ *First-line treatment: IV fluids and atropine*

□ *Additional treatments: IV glucagon, IV calcium, vasopressors, IV insulin and dextrose*

QUICK REVIEW QUESTION

4. A 58-year-old is brought to the ED after ingesting 25 enteric-coated diltiazem pills 3 hours earlier. He is administered 0.5 mg atropine and intubated. Fluid resuscitation is started with 3 L 0.9% NaCl. What other medications should the nurse expect to administer if the patient's hemodynamic status does not improve?

Acute Opioid Intoxication

Pathophysiology

Opioids depress the CNS and lower the perception of pain by stimulating dopamine release. Opioid overdose causes an excessive depressive effect on the portion of the brain that regulates RR and can be fatal. Opioid overdose can be a complication of substance abuse, unintentional or intentional overdose, or therapeutic drug error.

Physical Examination

- opioid overdose triad: pinpoint pupils, respiratory depression, decreased LOC

- hypotension

- wheezing or dyspnea

- nausea or vomiting
- seizure

Management

HELPFUL HINT:

Co-ingestion of CNS depressants—such as alcohol, opioids, and benzodiazepines— significantly increases the risk of respiratory complications.

- priority: airway management and supplemental oxygen
- *antidote: naloxone (Narcan)*, an opioid antagonist administered IV, IM, or intranasally.
  - □ indicated for patients with agonal breathing, RR < 12 bpm, or SpO_2 <90% to restore respiratory status
  - □ BVM before and after administration for patients with low respiration rates
  - □ standard dose: IV 0.4 mg titrated until adequate ventilation is achieved
  - □ patients who are opioid dependent: a slow dose of naloxone (0.1 – 0.4 mg every 1 – 3 minutes) to prevent withdrawal symptoms
  - □ monitor closely: effects of naloxone may wear off, resulting in the reappearance of overdose symptoms

QUICK REVIEW QUESTION

5. A patient is brought to the ED after taking an unknown number of Vicodin pills. The patient is drowsy but responsive to verbal stimulation, has a RR of 13 breaths per minutes, and SpO_2 is 92% on room oxygen. What interventions should the nurse expect?

SYMPATHOMIMETIC DRUG INTOXICATION
Pathophysiology

HELPFUL HINT:

Cocaine-associated chest pain is caused by cocaine-induced vasoconstriction which may lead to myocardial ischemia.

Sympathomimetic drugs mimic CNS agonists and stimulate the CNS. The resulting vasoconstriction in coronary arteries may lead to myocardial injury or dysrhythmias. These drugs also increase levels of neurotransmitters (e.g., serotonin, dopamine), leading to feelings of euphoria, agitation, aggression, or psychosis.

Sympathomimetic drugs include:

- amphetamines (both prescription drugs (e.g., methylphenidate [Ritalin]) and street drugs (e.g., crystal methamphetamine [crystal meth])
- hallucinatory amphetamines (MDMA)
- cocaine

- khat
- synthetic cathinones ("bath salts")

Physical Examination

- tachycardia
- hypertension
- hyperthermia
- agitation
- psychosis

Management

- cardiac and pulse ox monitoring
- *benzodiazepines for sedation and to reduce hypertension*
- *cooling measures*
- protective measures for patient and staff when managing aggressive patients
- activated charcoal or whole bowel irrigation for "body packers" (people who swallow large amounts of drugs for transport)

QUICK REVIEW QUESTION

6. A patient presents to the ED with chest pains that started after intranasal cocaine use. ECG and troponin labs rule out myocardial injury. What medication should the nurse expect to administer to manage the patient's symptoms?

Acute Substance Withdrawal

ALCOHOL WITHDRAWAL

Pathophysiology

Alcohol is a central nervous system depressant that directly binds to gamma-aminobutyric acid (GABA) receptors and inhibits glutamate-induced excitation. Chronic alcohol use alters the sensitivity of these receptors; when alcohol use is stopped, the result is hyperactivity in the central nervous system.

Symptoms develop 6 to 24 hours after last consuming alcohol. **Delirium tremens (DTs)** is type of severe alcohol characterized by hallucinations and hyperthermia. Symptoms occur 2 to 4 days after stopping alcohol intake.

Chronic alcohol use inhibits the absorption of nutrients, including thiamine and folic acid. Consequently, patients admitted with symptoms of alcohol withdrawal are also at risk for disorders related to vitamin deficiency, including Wernicke's encephalopathy and megaloblastic anemia.

Alcohol withdrawal can be fatal and requires medical management.

Physical Examination

- tachycardia
- anxiety and irritation
- tachypnea
- diaphoresis
- seizures
- _DTs: hallucinations, hyperthermia_

Assessment

The **Clinical Institute Withdrawal Assessment (CIWA)** is a ten-item scale used to objectively assess withdrawal symptoms and ensure withdrawing patients are given the correct amount of medication. Patients are given a score of 0 to 7 for each symptom, based on its severity, except orientation, which is scored from 0 to 4.

- nausea and emesis
- paroxysmal sweats
- level of anxiety
- level of agitation
- tremors
- headache symptoms
- auditory disturbances
- visual disturbances
- tactile disturbances
- orientation

The numerical values for the sections are totaled and the number is used to guide the use of withdrawal medication.

- < 10: very mild withdrawal
- 10 to 15: mild withdrawal
- 16 to 20: modest withdrawal
- > 20: severe withdrawal

Management

- IV fluids and electrolytes as needed

- treat for vitamin deficiencies and malnutrition with glucose, thiamine, folate, parenteral multivitamins

- benzodiazepines for agitation

- lorazepam for seizures

- *for severe drug-resistant DTs: drug "cocktail" that includes lorazepam, diazepam, and midazolam (Versed) or propofol*

QUICK REVIEW QUESTIONS

7. A 45-year-old man is admitted to the ED with vomiting, profuse sweating, and complaint of a headache. Assessment shows a HR of 130 bpm and blood pressure of 130/102 mm Hg. The nurse checks the patient's chart and notes that the patient has a history of alcohol abuse. What should the nurse prepare to do next?

8. What medication is most commonly used to treat alcohol withdrawal–induced seizure activity?

OPIOID WITHDRAWAL

Pathophysiology

Opioids are synthetically and naturally occurring substances that bind to opioid receptors in the brain, depressing the central nervous system. Chronic use of opioids increases excitability of noradrenergic neurons, and withdrawal leads to hypersensitivity of the central nervous system. Opioid withdrawal is rarely fatal, but death can occur, usually as a result of hemodynamic instability or electrolyte imbalances.

Assessment

The **Clinical Opiate Withdrawal Scale (COWS)** is an 11-item scale to help objectively assess withdrawal symptoms and ensure that patients are given the correct amount of medication.

Patients are given a score based on the severity of each symptom.

- resting heart rate

- sweating

- restlessness

- pupil size

- bone or joint aches

HELPFUL HINT:

Commonly used opioids include codeine, fentanyl, heroin, hydrocodone, hydromorphone, meperidine, methadone, morphine, and oxycodone.

- rhinorrhea or lacrimation
- GI upset
- tremor
- yawning
- anxiety or irritability
- piloerection

The numerical values for the sections are totaled and the amount is used to guide the use of withdrawal medication.

- 5 – 12: mild withdrawal
- 13 – 24: moderate withdrawal
- 25 – 36: moderate to severe withdrawal
- > 36: severe withdrawal

Management

- supportive care for symptoms: *__alpha-2 adrenergic agonists (clonidine or lofexidine)__* benzodiazepines, antiemetics, antidiarrheals, IV fluids as needed
- medically supervised withdrawal
  - opioid replacement therapy: methadone or buprenorphine relieve symptoms without producing intoxication
  - opioid antagonists: naltrexone and naloxone block the effects of opioids

---

QUICK REVIEW QUESTIONS

9. What medication is commonly administered to patients in opioid withdrawal to manage symptoms?

_____

10. The nurse assesses a patient using COWS and calculates a result of 32. What conditions should the nurse monitor for?

_____

ANSWER KEY

1. Symptoms of anticholinergic overdose include increased BP and HR, hyperthermia, flushing, blurred vision, dry skin, agitation or delirium, urinary retention, and decreased bowel sounds.

2. Acetaminophen is hepatotoxic, but symptoms of liver failure will not appear for 24 to 72 hours. The earlier the patient is administered the antidote, the less likely he is to develop liver failure.

3. The nurse should expect to monitor the patient's airway and breathing and be prepared to provide respiratory support if the patient shows signs of respiratory depression.

4. Second-line treatments for calcium channel blocker overdose include IV calcium, IV glucagon, IV insulin and dextrose, and vasopressors.

5. The patient is currently stable, so the nurse should expect to monitor the patient and frequently reassess his respiratory status.

6. Benzodiazepines are administered to patients with cocaine intoxication to reduce cardiovascular symptoms.

7. The nurse should anticipate assessing the patient using the CIWA scale and administering medications per the ED's protocol.

8. Lorazepam is used to treat alcohol withdrawal–induced seizure activity.

9. Alpha-2 adrenergic agonists (clonidine or lofexidine) are given to patients in opioid withdrawal to manage anxiety, nausea, diarrhea, and cramping.

10. Patients with severe diarrhea or vomiting due to opioid withdrawal are at risk of electrolyte imbalances and hemodynamic instability.

13 MEDICAL EMERGENCIES: HEMATOLOGY AND IMMUNOLOGY

BCEN OUTLINE: MEDICAL EMERGENCIES

- Allergic reactions and anaphylaxis
- _Hematologic disorders_
- Electrolyte and fluid imbalance
- Endocrine disorders
- _Immunocompromise (e.g., HIV/AIDS, oncology/ chemotherapy, transplant patient)_
- Renal failure
- Sepsis
- Hypovolemic and distributive shock
- Substance use and abuse (e.g., alcohol and drug interactions, side effects, unintentional overdose)
- Withdrawal syndrome

Hematological Anatomy and Assessment

- **Plasma,** the liquid part of blood, includes albumin (which maintains osmotic pressure), serum globulins, and clotting factors.

- **Red blood cells (RBCs** or **erythrocytes)** transport oxygen (and, to a lesser extent, CO_2).
  - □ High RBC counts may indicate chronic hypoxia, dehydration, bone marrow overproduction, or kidney disease.

- □ Low RBC counts indicate anemia caused by disease processes that result in underproduction or destruction of RBCs.
- □ **Erythropoiesis**—the production of RBCs—is triggered by the release of erythropoietin from the kidneys. RBCs grow to maturity within the bone marrow.
- □ RBCs are broken down in the liver and spleen through **phagocytosis**; waste products are excreted as bilirubin and biliverdin in bile.
- ■ White blood cells (WBCs or leukocytes) fight infection.
  - □ High WBC counts occur during infections, physiological distress, and steroid use.
  - □ Low WBC counts occur during bone marrow suppression and chemotherapy.
- ■ A **WBC differential** includes the percentage or absolute number of different types of WBCs.
  - □ **Left shift** refers to an increased presence of band neutrophils in the peripheral blood. This shift may be due to inflammation, infection, steroids, or stress.
  - □ Viral infections show a decreased overall WBC count and high lymphocytes.
  - □ Malignancies show a high count of one type of WBC or high counts of numerous immature WBCs.

TABLE 13.1. CBC With Differential

Test	Description	Normal Range
Complete Blood Count (CBC)		
White blood cells (WBCs)	cells that fight infection; a high WBC count can indicate inflammation or infection	4,500 – 10,000 cells/µL
Red blood cells (RBCs)	cells that carry oxygen throughout the body and filter carbon dioxide	men: 5 – 6 million cells/µL women: 4 – 5 million cells/µL
Hemoglobin (HgB)	protein that binds oxygen in the blood	men: 13.8 – 17.2 g/dL women: 12.1 – 15.1 g/dL
Hematocrit (Hct)	percentage of the blood composed of red blood cells	men: 41% – 50% women: 36% – 44%
Mean corpuscular volume (MCV)	average size of RBCs	80 – 95 fL

Test	Description	Normal Range
Complete Blood Count (CBC)		
Mean corpuscular hemoglobin (MCH)	average amount of HgB in RBCs	27.5 – 33.2 pg
Mean corpuscular hemoglobin concentration (MCHC)	average concentration of HgB in RBCs	334 – 355 g/L
Platelets	blood components that play a role in clotting	150,000 – 450,000 platelets/μL
WBC Differential		
Neutrophils	first responders that quickly migrate to the site of infection to destroy bacterial invaders	2,000 – 7,000/μL (40% – 60%)
Band neutrophils	immature neutrophils (also called bands)	<700/μL (<5%)
Lymphocytes	B cells, T cells, and natural killer cells; all 3 types develop from common lymphoid progenitors	1,000 – 3,000/μL (20% – 40%)
Monocytes	cells that engulf and destroy microbes and cancer cells	200 – 1,000/μL (2% – 8%)
Eosinophils	cells that attack parasites and regulate inflammation	20 – 500/μL (1% – 4%)
Basophils	cells responsible for inflammatory reactions, including allergies	20 – 100/μL (0% – 2%)

- **Hemostasis** is the process of stopping blood loss from a damaged blood vessel.

- Blood loss is stopped through **coagulation**, the process of turning liquid blood into a semisolid **clot** composed of platelets and red blood cells held together by the protein **fibrin**.

- The process of coagulation is a complex cascade of reactions involving proteins called **clotting factors**.
  - □ Platelet aggregation is initiated by the exposure to **von Willebrand factor (vW)** and **tissue factor (TF)**.
  - □ During coagulation, the protein **fibrinogen** (factor I) is converted to fibrin by the enzyme **thrombin** (factor IIa).
  - □ **Prothrombin** (factor II) is a precursor to thrombin.

- The **intrinsic pathway** is activated via damage within a blood vessel.
  - □ This pathway is monitored by measuring the activated partial thromboplastin time (aPTT).

- □ Heparin disrupts the intrinsic pathway.
- ■ The **extrinsic pathway** is activated by damage outside the vasculature.
  - □ This pathway is monitored by measuring the prothrombin time (PT).
  - □ Warfarin disrupts the extrinsic pathway.
- ■ Both pathways activate clotting factor X and produce a fibrin clot.

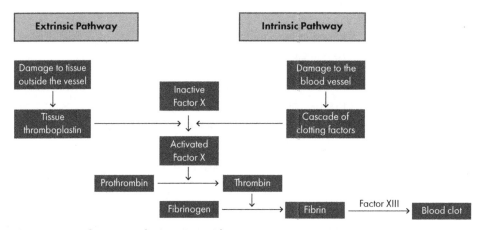

Figure 13.1. The Coagulation Cascade

- ■ Laboratory tests can be used to measure coagulation time and levels of clotting factors.

TABLE 13.2 Coagulation Studies

Test	Description	Normal Range
Prothrombin time (PT)	how long it takes blood to clot	10 – 13 seconds
International normalized ratio (INR)	standardized PT for patients taking Warfarin	healthy adults: < 1.1 patients receiving anticoagulants: 2.0 – 3.0
Partial thromboplastin time (PTT)	the body's ability to form blood clots	60 – 70 seconds
Activated partial thromboplastin time (aPTT)	the body's ability to form blood clots using an activator to speed up the clotting process	20 – 35 seconds
D-dimer	protein fragment produced during fibrinolysis	negative
Fibrin split products (FSP) or fibrin degradation products (FDP)	components produced during fibrinolysis	< 10 mg/L

Test	Description	Normal Range
Fibrinogen	amount of fibrinogen (clotting factor I)	200 – 400 mg/dL
Plasminogen	substrate involved in fibrinolysis	10 – 16 mg/dL

QUICK REVIEW QUESTION

1. Congenital hypofibrinogenemia is an inherited condition characterized by low circulating levels of fibrinogen (< 150 mg/dL). What abnormal laboratory values should a nurse expect in a patient with severe hypofibrinogenemia?

Disseminated Intravascular Coagulation (DIC)

Pathophysiology

Disseminated intravascular coagulopathy (DIC) is a coagulation disorder with simultaneous intervals of clotting and bleeding. DIC occurs when injury exposes blood to TF, causing a rapid increase in circulating thrombin and fibrin. Microclots cascade throughout the vascular system, causing hypoxia and ischemia in multiple organs. The use of platelets in clot formation results in thrombocytopenia, decreased fibrinogen, and overall increased clotting time. Subsequent fibrinolysis of the clots leads to elevated D-dimer and FSP.

Acute (or decompensated) DIC occurs when the presence of large amounts of TF cause rapid depletion of platelets and clotting factors, resulting in severe bleeding. **Chronic (or compensated) DIC** is the result of long-term exposure to TF. The body is able to compensate for lost platelets and clotting factors, but the risk of thromboembolic complications is high.

Risk Factors

- sepsis
- trauma
- cancers (especially leukemia and brain tumors)
- blood transfusion reaction
- recent procedure or surgery with anesthesia
- obstetrical complications (e.g., preeclampsia)
- cardiac arrest

Physical Examination

- bleeding (e.g., spontaneous hemorrhage, petechiae)
- thromboembolic event (e.g., PE, DVT)

Diagnostic Tests and Findings

- acute DIC
  - *decreased platelets (moderate to severe)*
  - *prolonged PT and PTT*
  - *decreased fibrinogen*
  - *severely elevated D-dimer and FSP*
- chronic DIC
  - decreased platelets (mild)
  - normal or slightly prolonged PT and PTT
  - normal or slightly decreased fibrinogen
  - elevated D-dimer and FSP

Management

- identify and treat underlying cause
- IV fluid resuscitation
- vasopressors
- transfusion of blood products (FFP, PRBCs, platelets, or cryoprecipitate)
- heparin for chronic DIC

QUICK REVIEW QUESTIONS

2. How is acute DIC differentiated from chronic DIC?

3. What findings would confirm a diagnosis of acute DIC in a patient recovering from postpartum hemorrhage?

HELPFUL HINT:

Hemarthrosis, bleeding into the joints, is one of the most common presentations of hemophilia.

Hemophilia

Pathophysiology

Hemophilia is a recessive, X-chromosome-linked bleeding disorder characterized by the lack of coagulation factor VIII (hemophilia A), factor IX (hemophilia B), or factor XI (hemophilia C). The deficiency in coagulation factors causes abnormal bleeding after an injury or medical procedures, and spontaneous bleeding can occur in patients with severe hemophilia. Hemophilia is usually diagnosed in infancy or childhood, but mild forms may not be diagnosed until the patient experiences injury or surgery later in life.

Physical Examination

- excessive bleeding

Diagnostic Tests

- prolonged aPTT
- normal platelet count and PT
- decreased activity level for factors VIII, IX, or XI

Management

- *first line: factor VIII for hemophilia A or factor IX for hemophilia B*
- standard treatment protocols for bleeding/hemorrhage

QUICK REVIEW QUESTIONS

4. What abnormalities should the nurse expect to see on labs for a patient with hemophilia?

_____

5. An 8-year-old boy with a known history of hemophilia A arrives at the ED after sustaining a closed radial ulna fracture when he fell off a swing at school. What intervention should the nurse anticipate performing first?

_____

Sickle Cell Disease

Pathophysiology

Sickle cell disease is an inherited form of hemolytic anemia that causes deformities in the shape of the RBCs. When oxygen levels in the venous circulation are low, the RBCs dehydrate and form a sickle shape. This process can be exacerbated by exposure to cold temperatures or high altitudes. Sickle cell disease is a chronic disease that can lead to complications that require emergency care.

- Sickle cell crisis *(also called vaso-occlusive pain): sickle-shaped cells clump together and restrict blood flow, causing localized ischemia, inflammation, and severe pain.*

HELPFUL HINT:

In the United States, most diagnoses of sickle cell trait are made following newborn screenings.

- **Acute chest syndrome (ACS):** *vaso-occlusion in the lungs (often after an infection) that results in chest pain and respiratory distress.*
- **Aplastic crisis:** anemia that occurs after an infection, usually by human parvovirus; rapid decline of hemoglobin caused by the inability of the bone marrow to produce new cells.
- **Splenic sequestration:** pooling of RBCs in the spleen; can lead to anemia and hypovolemia.
- **Infection:** the leading cause of death for children with sickle cell disease; common infections include bacteremia, pneumonia, and osteomyelitis.
- **Acute infarctions:** blood clots caused by clumped sickle-shaped cells; can lead to hypoxia and infarction (MI, stroke, PE, DVT, etc.).
- **Priapism:** a common complication for men with sickle cell disease.

Management

- treatment based on patient's signs and symptoms
- transfusion of packed RBCs for ACS, splenic sequestration, and symptomatic anemia
- ACS: IV fluids, analgesics, oxygen, low-molecular-weight heparin, hydroxyurea
- sickle cell crisis: analgesics (usually IV opioids)
- standard treatment protocols for other complications (e.g., DVT, priapism, infection)

QUICK REVIEW QUESTIONS

6. A 26-year-old male with a history of sickle cell disease arrives at the ED with fever, jaundice, and priapism. What symptom is most urgent to address?

_____

7. What symptoms would a nurse expect to see in patients with sickle cell crisis?

_____

Thrombocytopenia

- **Thrombocytopenia** is an abnormally low platelet level that can lead to severe bleeding or thrombosis. It can generally be classified by the number of platelets:
  - mild: 100,000 – 150,000/μL
  - moderate: 50,000 – 100,000/μL
  - severe: < 50,000/μL

- Thrombocytopenia has a diverse etiology. It is commonly seen in patients with cancer, bone marrow disorders, sepsis, chronic liver disease, and autoimmune diseases.

- **Heparin-induced thrombocytopenia (HIT)** is acute-onset thrombocytopenia in patients receiving heparin therapy.
  - Causes platelet activation, significantly increasing risk of thrombosis.
  - Thrombocytopenia and thrombosis occur 5 – 10 days after exposure to heparin (particularly unfractionated heparin).
  - If HIT is suspected, immediately discontinue heparin and administer anticoagulants.

- **Idiopathic thrombocytopenic purpura (ITP, immune thrombocytopenia)** is an autoimmune disorder that causes the destruction of platelets.
  - S/s include mild bleeding (e.g., petechiae, purpura); severe GI bleeding and hematuria are more rare.
  - Treatment includes corticosteroids and IVIG.

HELPFUL HINT:

Heparin is neutralized with protamine sulfate. Warfarin is neutralized with Vitamin K.

QUICK REVIEW QUESTIONS

8. What laboratory result would be classified as severe thrombocytopenia?

_____

9. What are the likely medical interventions for a patient with ITP who presents with lower GI bleeding and a platelet count of 35,000/μL?

_____

Immunocompromise

Pathophysiology

Immune deficiencies can be primary disorders (i.e., inherited) or secondary to disease, medications, or malnutrition. Immune deficiencies commonly seen in emergency care are discussed below.

- **Leukopenia** is the general term for a WBC < 4000/μL. It can occur as the result of impaired production or rapid use of WBCs.

- **Acquired immunodeficiency syndrome (AIDS)** is the end-stage progression of HIV. Patients with AIDS have a depletion of T lymphocytes and are susceptible to opportunistic and sometimes emergent infections.

- **Leukemia,** cancer of the WBCs, occurs in the bone marrow and disrupts the production and function of WBCs. In the absence of functioning WBCs, the patient becomes immunocompromised. The types of leukemia are differentiated by which WBCs are affected (lymphocytes or myeloid cells).

- **Chemotherapy** is conducted with a class of cytotoxic medications that destroy cancer cells by disrupting cell mitosis and DNA replication. A side effect of chemotherapy is severe **neutropenia** (a decrease in circulating neutrophils).

- Poorly managed **diabetes mellitus**, and associated hyperglycemia, increases the risk of infection. Patients with diabetes are more prone to infections, particularly skin infections.

Management

- treat patient's complaints and symptoms, usually fever and infection
- specialized care to prevent opportunistic infections
  - □ appropriate precautions for patient, providers, and visitors
  - □ maintain patient skin integrity
  - □ ensure adequate nutrition and hydration
  - □ prophylactic antibiotics

QUICK REVIEW QUESTION

10. A patient receiving chemotherapy presents with onset of cough and fever. A CBC reveals a WBC count of 20,000/µL and a left shift. Blood cultures are drawn, with results pending, and the patient's lactic acid level is 2.9 mmol/L. Chest X-ray shows bilateral pulmonary infiltrates. What diagnosis does the nurse anticipate?

ANSWER KEY

1. Fibrinogen (clotting factor I) is a substrate necessary for coagulation. Patients with very low fibrinogen levels are at risk for severe bleeding and will have prolonged PTs, INRs, PTTs, and aPTTs.

2. Acute DIC is characterized by severe bleeding; chronic DIC is associated with high risk of thrombosis.

3. Diagnostic findings that would confirm a diagnosis of DIC include thrombocytopenia, prolonged clotting times (PT and PTT), decreased fibrinogen, and increased levels of fibrinolysis products (D-dimer and FSP).

4. Labs for patients with hemophilia will show prolonged aPTT and decreased activity level for factors VIII, IX, or XI.

5. Factor VIII transfusion should be initiated immediately if not previously started by the parent or school nurse.

6. Priapism can lead to permanent impotence, sexual dysfunction, and tissue necrosis. This symptom requires immediate treatment to restore blood flow.

7. Sickle cell crisis presents with localized ischemia, inflammation, and severe pain.

8. Severe thrombocytopenia is defined as platelets $<50,000/\mu L$.

9. The patient will require platelet transfusion, corticosteroids, and IVIG.

10. The nurse should suspect septic pneumonia. Chemotherapy immunocompromises patients, making them more susceptible to infection.

14 MUSCULOSKELETAL EMERGENCIES

BCEN OUTLINE: MUSCULOSKELETAL EMERGENCIES

- Amputation
- *Compartment syndrome*
- Ligament tendon injuries (e.g., sprains, strains, ruptures)
- *Fractures (e.g., open, closed, fat embolus)*
- Dislocations
- Inflammatory conditions (e.g., costochondritis)
- Osteomyelitis

Amputation

Pathophysiology

An **amputation** occurs when a body part is separated from the body by surgical or traumatic means. Traumatic amputations typically occur in the extremities and may include fingers, toes, hands, feet, arms, or legs. Amputations are categorized as complete or incomplete (partial).

- **Complete amputations** occur when the body part is entirely separated from the body.

- **Incomplete** or **partial amputations** occur when the body part is non-functional but still technically connected by a tendon, ligament, or other tissue.

Severe hemorrhaging may be absent in some amputations due to the tendency for severed blood vessels to spasm and retract. Partial amputations or those with significant tissue damage (such as crush injuries) will likely result in more blood loss than cleanly severed body parts.

Replantation (surgical reattachment of the amputated body part) may be considered based on the patient and type of injury. Indicators for a high chance of successful replantation include:

- pediatric patients
- patients with amputated digits, wrists, or forearms
- patients with sharp amputation (instead of blunt)
- <6 hours since amputation (longer for digits or for cooled tissue)

Management

- direct pressure and pressure dressing for bleeding
- IV fluids and blood products as needed
- preserve detached limb
    - wrap in sterile gauze and moisten with normal saline
    - place in tightly sealed bag and place bag on ice
- gently replace attached tissue and maintain normal positioning
- cleanse area with sterile saline solution and cover with thick material
- analgesics, antibiotics, and tetanus immunization as needed

---

QUICK REVIEW QUESTION

1. A 32-year-old patient is brought to the ED with a partially severed LLE after a snowmobile accident. Bleeding was controlled by EMS via a tourniquet and the patient is being prepared for surgery. What can the nurse do in the interim to promote limb preservation?

★ # Compartment Syndrome

Pathophysiology

Compartment syndrome is the result of increased intracompartmental pressure, usually as a result of a fracture or crush injury. When the increased pressure in the closed compartment exceeds the pressure of perfusion, blood circulation is impaired, resulting in ischemia of the nerves and muscle tissue. Oxygen deficiency and the buildup of waste produce nerve irritation, resulting in pain and a decrease in sensation. With progression of ischemia, muscles become necrotic, which can lead to rhabdomyolysis, hyperkalemia, and infection if left untreated.

Lower legs and arms are the most common areas; compartment syndrome can also occur in the abdomen.

Risk Factors

- extremity fractures (most common)
- crush injuries, severe contusions, or burns
- sepsis
- casting or compression bandage
- blood clots
- prolonged periods of unconsciousness
- after abdominal surgery or repair of vascular injury

Physical Examination

- *the 5 P's*
  - ☐ pain (not proportional to injury and does not respond to opioid medications)
  - ☐ paresthesia
  - ☐ pallor
  - ☐ paralysis
  - ☐ pulselessness
- decreased urine output
- hypotension
- tissue tight on palpation
- edema with tight, shiny skin

Diagnostic Tests

- **intracompartmental pressure > 30 mm Hg**
- delta pressure (DBP – compartment pressure) < 30 mm Hg

Treatment and Management

- remove casts or dressings to relieve pressure
- IV fluids: maintain urine output > 30 cc/hr
- intracompartmental pressure > 30 mm Hg: prepare patient for fasciotomy
- intracompartmental pressure 10 – 30 mm Hg: monitor pressure and hemodynamic status
- analgesics

QUICK REVIEW QUESTION

2. A patient with a femur break and subsequent setting and casting returns to the ER 2 days later with numb toes and increased pain. The cast is opened to reveal tight, shiny skin. What pressure measurement would warrant an emergent fasciotomy?

Ligament Tendon Injuries

Pathophysiology

Sprains, strains, and rupture are very common injuries and share similar signs and symptoms.

- **Sprains** are the tearing or stretching of ligaments.
- **Strains** are the separation of muscle or tendon from bone.
- A **rupture** occurs when a tendon is torn or separates from muscle. Common locations of tendon ruptures include the Achilles tendon, the bicep tendons, and the patellar tendon.

Risk Factors

- overextension with severe stress applied (e.g., pivoting on knee, falling on wrist)
- falling
- throwing objects when running or jumping
- heavy lifting
- awkward position when lifting

Physical Examination

- localized pain and edema
- decreased ROM
- hear or feel a pop on incident

Diagnostic Tests

- X-ray to rule out fracture

Management

- mild sprains or strains typically treated at home
- _**RICE: rest, ice, compression, and elevation**_

- analgesics as needed
- immobilization for severe injury

QUICK REVIEW QUESTION

3. A parent brings their 8-year-old child to the ED for foot and ankle pain after a misstep during dance class. An X-ray rules out a fracture. What nursing interventions would be expected?

Fractures

Pathophysiology

A **fracture** is any break in a bone. **Open fractures** include a break in the skin; with a **closed fracture**, the skin is intact. Fractures to the hand, wrist, arm, lower leg, foot, and ankle can often be managed in an acute care setting with reduction and splinting/casting. Complications such as hemorrhage, neurological damage, or compartment syndrome may require additional consultations or hospital admission.

Further classifications of fractures are made based on the configuration of the fracture.

- **Non-displaced**: Broken area of the bone remains in alignment; this is the optimal condition for reduction and healing.

- **Displaced**: Broken areas of bone are not aligned. It may require manual or surgical reduction including hardware for fixation.

- **Transverse**: A horizontal break in a straight line across the bone occurs from a force perpendicular to the break.

- **Oblique**: A diagonal break occurs from a force higher or lower than the break.

- **Spiral**: A torsion or twisting break around the circumference of the bone is common in sports injuries.

- **Comminuted**: The break is fragmented into 3 or more pieces. This is more common in people older than 65 and those with brittle bones.

- **Compression**: The break is crushed or compressed, creating a wide, flattened appearance. It frequently occurs with crush injuries.

- **Segmental**: Two or more areas of the bone are fractured, creating a segmented area of "floating" bone.

- **Greenstick**: In this type of incomplete break, the bone is not completely separated and bends to one side; it is common in children.

HELPFUL HINT:

A **supracondylar fracture** of the humerus puts the patient at risk of neurovascular injury and requires hospital admission for assessment and monitoring. This type of fracture is most common in children who fall on outstretched arms.

- **Avulsed**: A "chip" fracture displaces small segments of bone from the main bone at the area of tendon/ligament attachment. It results from tension/pulling of the tendons/ligaments away from the bone.

- **Torus/buckle fracture**: This is an incomplete fracture with bulging of the cortex, common in children.

- **Impacted**: The ends of the bone are impacted or "jammed" into each other from forceful impact.

- **Salter-Harris**: This is a growth plate fracture, classified as I – V

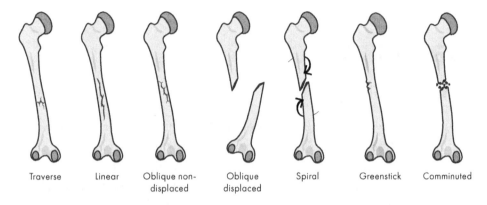

Figure 14.1. Types of Fractures

Fractures of the pelvis or femur require complex stabilization and place patients at high risk of complications, including internal hemorrhage, organ perforation, hematoma formation, and lipid embolisms.

Fat embolism syndrome (FES) is caused by fat in the pulmonary circulatory system that can occur after long bone or pelvic fractures. _**A cardinal cutaneous sign of fat emboli is reddish-brown non-palpable petechiae that appear over the upper body (particularly in the axilla region) 24 – 36 hours after the trauma event.**_ Other symptoms include hypoxemia, dyspnea, altered mental status/decreased LOC, and fever.

Physical Examination

- pain and tenderness increasing with movement
- swelling
- visual or palpated deformity
- crepitus
- abnormal movement or decreased ROM
- inability to bear weight
- contusions or bleeding

Diagnostic Tests

- X-ray

Management

- analgesics
- cleanse open wounds and cover with sterile dressing
- reduce (manual or surgical as indicated)
- immobilize
  - □ stabilize at the joints above and below the injury
  - □ position the splinted limb as close to anatomically normal as possible
  - □ do not reposition the limb if there is resistance or evidence of further injury
  - □ reassess pulses, motor function, and sensation after the splint is in place
- pelvic or femur fracture:
  - □ pelvic binder/traction splint
  - □ ***be prepared to administer blood products as needed***
- IV fluids and respirator support for FES

QUICK REVIEW QUESTIONS

4. A 16-year-old was admitted to the ED following a fall on outstretched hand (FOOSH) while skateboarding. The patient denies hitting their head and complains of nausea and pain increasing with movement. The physical assessment findings are tenderness, slight deformity, lateral and medial bruising, and progressive swelling to the affected (left) hand. Radial pulse is strong and palpable and capillary refill time is brisk. No pallor of the extremity is present. What should the nurse do next?

5. A 28-year-old patient has been receiving care in the ED for a closed femur fracture caused by an MVC. After being hemodynamically stable with a GCS of 15 for twenty-four hours post-injury, the patient is now unable to follow commands. His vital signs are: HR 122 bpm, RR 30, temperature 101°F (38.5°C). What condition should the nurse suspect, and how will it be diagnosed?

Dislocations

Pathophysiology

Dislocations involve bones being separated or "disrupted" from the joint they are a part of. Most dislocations are caused by sudden, abnormal force placed on the joint. Common causes of dislocations include falls, motor vehicle collisions, and athletics; common sites include shoulders, fingers, hips, and knees.

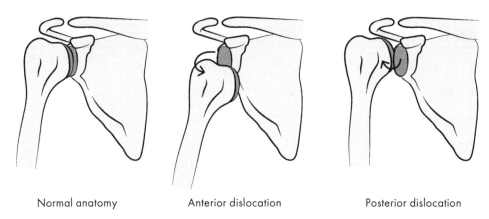

Normal anatomy   Anterior dislocation   Posterior dislocation

Figure 14.2. Shoulder Dislocation

Dislocations usually result in damage to ligaments and tendons and may damage muscles and blood vessels. Significant damage may still have occurred even if the joint was restored (sometimes done by the patient or bystanders).

Physical Examination

- intense, localized pain at the joint
- deformity of joint
- loss of function or range of motion
- absent pulses distal to injury (with blood vessel damage or constriction)

Diagnostic Tests

- X-ray

Management

- assess distal pulses, motor function, and sensation
- reduce as splint as soon as possible to prevent neurovascular injury

QUICK REVIEW QUESTION

6. A 73-year-old patient is being treated for right hip pain. Upon assessment, the right leg appears to be several inches shorter than the left. What diagnostic test should be ordered?

HELPFUL HINT:

Patellar dislocation is most often caused by a sudden twisting motion with the foot planted. It often self-reduces.

Knee dislocation involves dislocation of the tibia relative to the femur. It is caused by high-energy impact and is usually associated with major damage to tendons and vasculature

Inflammatory Conditions

ARTHRITIS

Pathophysiology

Arthritis is inflammation in the joints caused by autoimmune conditions or accumulation of chemical byproducts in the connective tissues. Inflammation causes a thickening of the synovial membrane and leads to irreversible damage to the joint capsule and cartilage from scarring. Both acute and chronic conditions result in pain, erythema, swelling, stiffness.

Common types of arthritis include:

- rheumatoid arthritis: progressive, symmetric inflammation of joints (most common in hands)
- psoriatic arthritis: arthritis accompanied by psoriasis
- osteoarthritis: progressive, usually presents in one to a few joints (most common form of arthritis)
- ankylosing spondylitis: arthritis of the spine
- gout: arthritis caused by buildup of uric acid in joints

Physical Examination

- erythema
- pain, edema, stiffness, deformity, and loss of function in joints
- fever or chills
- muscle pain and stiffness

Management

- treatment based on disease type, age, health, history, and severity of disease
- treat underlying disease
- topical or oral analgesics (NSAIDs)
- corticosteroids

QUICK REVIEW QUESTION

7. A 75-year-old woman arrives at the ED complaining of severe pain in both hands. She has limited income and has not sought prior treatment. She states the pain has increased recently, she is progressively losing function of her hands, and her knees have recently started hurting as well. On assessment the nurse finds the joints in both hands to be reddened, swollen, and disfigured, and the patient's knees slightly swollen. What condition should the patient's symptoms lead the nurse to suspect?

COSTOCHONDRITIS

Pathophysiology

HELPFUL HINT:

Idiopathic costochondritis is more common in women, particularly children and teenagers.

Costochondritis is the inflammation of the costal cartilage, which joins the ribs to the sternum. ***It usually affects the fourth, fifth, and sixth ribs.*** The inflammation causes the chest wall to be tender and painful upon palpation. There is no known definite cause, and the condition will generally resolve without treatment.

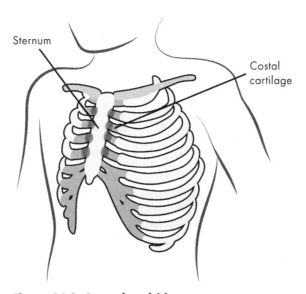

Figure 14.3. Costochondritis

Physical Examination

- sharp pain at chest wall; radiating to abdomen or back
- tenderness on palpation of rib joints
- rib pain increases with deep breathing and movement of the trunk
- can cause dyspnea or anxiety

Management

- application of heat or ice
- anti-inflammatories
- steroid injection with local anesthetic if anti-inflammatory is ineffective
- rest and avoidance of sports and exercise

QUICK REVIEW QUESTION

8. What clinical findings would lead the nurse to suspect costochondritis in a 13-year-old girl with a complaint of chest pain?

Osteomyelitis

Pathophysiology

Osteomyelitis is an infection in the bone that can occur directly (after a traumatic bone injury) or indirectly (via the vascular system or other infected tissues). In children, osteomyelitis is most commonly found in the long bones of the upper and lower extremities, while in adults it is most common in the spine.

Physical Examination

- may be asymptomatic
- fever or chills
- pain at site of infection
- s/s of local infection (warmth, exudate)

Diagnostic Tests

- MRI or CT scan
- positive blood culture or culture of bone biopsy

Treatment and Management

- surgical debridement
- *IV antibiotics*

HELPFUL HINT:

Spreading infection from open wounds (e.g., fractures) is the most common cause of osteomyelitis.

CONTINUE

ANSWER KEY

1. The limb should be maintained in as normal a position as possible and the affected area gently cleansed with sterile saline solution and covered with thick, non-adhering gauze.

2. An intracompartmental pressure >30 mm Hg or a delta pressure <30 mm Hg would likely require a fasciotomy.

3. The nurse should expect to wrap, ice, and elevate the foot and to treat pain with analgesics.

4. The nurse should prepare the patient for X-ray and administer analgesics.

5. The patient has signs and symptoms of FES. FES is a clinical diagnosis, so the nurse should assess for other symptoms (e.g., petechial rash) and anticipate a CXR to rule out a PE.

6. An X-ray of the hip joint should be done to determine whether the injury is a dislocation or a break.

7. The nurse should suspect the patient has rheumatoid arthritis. The patient exhibits several physical findings relating to this disease: it is progressive, affects bilateral joints, and causes disfigurement.

8. Chest pain with tenderness on palpation of the fourth, fifth, and sixth ribs is the classic sign of costochondritis.

9. The nurse should expect an MRI and bone biopsy to confirm a diagnosis of osteomyelitis.

15 WOUND EMERGENCIES

Wound Assessment and Management

- **Skin** is composed of 3 layers.
  - The **epidermis** is the outermost layer of the skin. This waterproof layer contains no blood vessels and acts mainly to protect the body.
  - Under the epidermis lies the **dermis**, which consists of dense connective tissue that allows skin to stretch and flex. The dermis is home to blood vessels, glands, and **hair follicles**.
  - The **hypodermis** is a layer of fat below the dermis that stores energy (in the form of fat) and acts as a cushion for the body. The hypodermis is sometimes called the **subcutaneous layer**.

→

CONTINUE

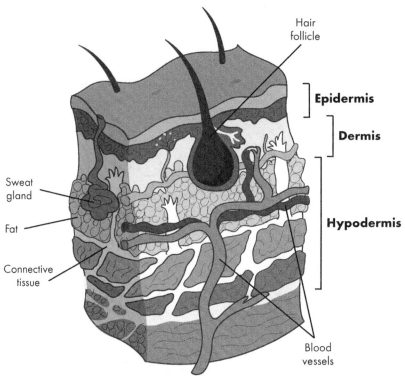

Hair follicle

Epidermis

Dermis

Hypodermis

Sweat gland

Fat

Connective tissue

Blood vessels

Figure 15.1. Anatomy of the Skin

General guidelines for wound care are outlined below.

1. History and physical examination of wound:
   □ Should be done after patient is stable.
   □ Get vaccination history: Tetanus vaccination (DTaP, DT, Tdap, or Td) is required if patient has not been vaccinated within the last 5 years. Tetanus immunoglobulin (Tig) is required for unvaccinated patients with high risk of wound infection.
   □ Include neurovascular assessment and examination of anatomy of wound.
   □ X-rays as needed.

2. Local anesthesia:
   □ Local anesthesia (injected or topical) should be administered before the wound is cleaned and closed.
   □ Common anesthetics include lidocaine (duration 1 – 2 hours), bupivacaine (duration 4 – 8 hours), and procaine (duration 15 – 45 minutes).
   □ Epinephrine may be added to anesthetic agents to increase duration of effect.

3. Wound cleaning:
   □ Irrigate with sterile water or normal saline to flush debris from wound.

HELPFUL HINT:

Anesthesia agents with epinephrine should never be used on the digits or in the ears, nose, or penis.

□ Remove foreign bodies.

□ Debride nonviable tissue.

4. Wound closure:

Methods of primary closure include sutures, staples, wound tape, and glue.

□ Glue should not be used in high-tension areas (e.g., joints) or on mucous membranes.

□ Staples should only be used in areas where scars will not be visible.

□ Wound tape may be used for superficial wounds but may fall off when exposed to moisture.

■ Topical antibiotics may be applied after wound closure for wounds at high risk for infection.

5. Wound dressing:

□ gauze and non-adherent pads: used for dry, closed wounds

□ wet-to-dry dressings: innermost layer is wet and keeps wound bed moist

□ transparent film: securement for IVs, moisture-retentive

□ calcium alginate dressing: absorbs wound exudate

□ hydrogel: promotes moisture within wound bed

□ foam dressing: provides cushioning over bony prominences

TABLE 15.1. Types of Wound Closure

Type	Description
Primary	• closure within 4 to 8 hours of wound occurrence • used with minimal risk, clean or clean-contaminated wounds • tissue integrity is maintained, and there is no tension created with closure
Secondary	• wound is left to heal on its own • used when wounds are contaminated, have edges that cannot be approximated, have penetration to an organ, or have a high risk for infection • may take longer to heal, and healing may become halted at the full thickness stage
Tertiary	• wound is left intentionally open to allow for improved healing • used when infection or edema is present

QUICK REVIEW QUESTIONS

1. The ED nurse is performing a skin assessment on an 86-year-old nursing home resident admitted for hypotension and bradycardia. The nurse notes a reddened but blanchable area on the hip. What dressing is the most appropriate?

2. A 65-year-old patient arrives at the ED after stepping on a nail outside. The nail has punctured through the shoe, and the wound is bleeding. What question about vaccination should the nurse ask during the history?

Specific Wounds

TABLE 15.2. Diagnosis and Management of Trauma Wounds	
Wound	**Management**
Avulsion full thickness injury in which skin is separated from the body by an external force tearing or pulling the tissue; exposed ligaments, tendons, muscle fibers, and bone may be visible **Degloving injury** an avulsion where the skin is completely separated from the underlying structures	• control bleeding • local or topical anesthetic • debride wound (remove detached tissues as needed) • irrigate wound with saline solution (avoid application of soap, hydrogen peroxide, or alcohol directly on wound) • cover wound with an absorbent, non-adhering bandage or dressing • ice, analgesics, and antibiotics as needed
Laceration a tear of the soft tissue; external lacerations that involve full thickness of the skin layers into the subcutaneous tissue are at high risk for infection due to bacteria or debris from the object causing the injury	• control bleeding • local anesthetic • irrigate with normal saline • prepare for closure (suturing, stapling, Dermabond adhesive, or Steri Strips as appropriate) • dress wound • ice, analgesics, and antibiotics as needed • degloving injury: realign tissue and cover with sterile dressing

Injection injury	
injection of substances (e.g., paint, grease, industrial chemicals) through an almost unseen point of entry via high-pressure equipment; can result in tissue necrosis, compartment syndrome, or infection	• debride, irrigate, and dress wound • prophylactic antibiotics • surgical consult ASAP • monitor for compartment syndrome

Wound	Management
Missile injury damage from a projectile (e.g., bullet); injury is dependent on the type, trajectory, and velocity of the bullet and on the characteristics of the tissue or organs involved	• remove clothing • primary survey for entry/exit wounds; secondary survey to diagnose all injuries • imaging: CT angiogram, eFAST, X-ray, or MRI • IV fluids or blood products as needed • pressure/tourniquet to bleeding injuries • analgesics • surgical consult
Puncture wounds caused by an object entering through soft tissue, resulting in hemorrhage and damage to the skin and underlying tissues; the penetrating object also deposits organisms or foreign bodies into the deeper tissue, increasing the risk for infection	• irrigate wound with saline solution • topical anesthetic or ice • cover using clean, moist dressing or nonstick/non-adherent dressing • antibiotics

HELPFUL HINT:

Unresolved infection of a wound may indicate a retained foreign body and requires further medical attention.

QUICK REVIEW QUESTIONS

3. Following treatment in the ED last week for a puncture injury from a tool, a patient returns stating increased pain and oozing at the site. What should the nurse prepare the patient for?

_____

4. A construction worker is brought to the ED with an injection injury of industrial lubricant from a high-powered injector. The injury is to the left lower extremity, the pain has increased to 10/10, and the patient is losing feeling in the toes. What medical emergency may be occurring?

_____

5. A patient is treated in the ED following a bicycle accident. The patient has a large area of road rash along the right outer leg and across both palms. The wounds present with scant bleeding and serous drainage mixed with copious amounts of →

CONTINUE

dirt and debris. Fractures and vascular injury have been ruled out, and full range of motion is intact. What should the nurse anticipate for wound care for this patient?

Wound Infections

Pathophysiology

Trauma wounds are at high risk for infection because they are contaminated by debris and microorganisms. Surgical site infections may also require emergency care, particularly if the patient had a preexisting infection or there was spillage from the GI tract during surgery. If not treated properly wound infections prevent proper healing and may lead to complications including cellulitis, endocarditis, septicemia, and osteomyelitis.

HELPFUL HINT:

Wound infection is more likely to occur in patients with diabetes, malnutrition, decreased mobility, impaired circulation, or depressed immune systems.

Physical Examination

- fever
- pain, erythema, and edema around wound
- purulent exudate from wound

Diagnostic Tests

- CBC with differential and cultures to identify infectious organism

Management

- wound care, including drainage, debridement, and appropriate dressings
- incision and drainage of abscesses
- topical antibiotics for non-purulent, local infections
- oral antibiotics for purulent local infections
- IV antibiotics for systemic infections or high-risk patients

QUICK REVIEW QUESTION

6. A 34-year-old patient presents to the ED with a 4-day-old knife wound on her right palm that occurred while slicing vegetables. Her palm is red and swollen, and the nurse notes purulent discharge from the wound. The patient's vital signs are normal. What intervention should the nurse anticipate?

ANSWER KEY

1. The skin is intact, so the nurse should apply a foam dressing to further protect the bony prominence and document characteristics of the pressure injury in the chart.

2. The nurse should ask the patient if she has had a tetanus booster vaccine in the last 5 years.

3. The patient requires X-ray or CT imaging to check for retained foreign body.

4. The patient has s/s of compartment syndrome.

5. The nurse should irrigate with saline solution or assist the patient in cleansing with mild soap and water; apply topical antibiotic ointment if ordered; cover the wounds with nonstick or moist dressings; and apply ice over the dressing.

6. The patient has a local wound infection with no systemic symptoms. The nurse should expect to irrigate and dress the wound, and the patient will likely be prescribed oral antibiotics.

16 MAXILLOFACIAL EMERGENCIES

BCEN OUTLINE: MAXILLOFACIAL EMERGENCIES

- Abscess (e.g., peritonsillar, dental)
- *Epistaxis*
- Facial nerve disorders (e.g., Bell's palsy, trigeminal neuralgia)
- *Maxillofacial infections (e.g., Ludwig's angina, otitis, sinusitis, mastoiditis)*
- Acute vestibular dysfunction (e.g., labrinthitis, Ménière's disease)
- *Maxillofacial trauma*

Abscess

Pathophysiology

Peritonsillar abscess is an acute medical emergency that compromises the airway. Purulent exudate accumulates between the tonsillar capsule and the pharyngeal constrictor muscle causing cellulitis and edema. This is a life-threatening condition that can quickly advance to mediastinitis, intracranial abscess, necrotizing fasciitis, streptococcal toxic shock syndrome, and empyema if the infection is not aggressively managed.

Risk Factors

- most common in teenagers and young adults ages 20 – 40
- acute tonsillitis

- smoking
- poor oral hygiene

Physical Examination

HELPFUL HINT:

Dental abscesses may be periodontal or periapical (at the apex of the tooth). They present with intense localized pain, fever, and halitosis. Management includes antibiotics, analgesics, and antipyretics. Incision and drainage may be required for fluctuance.

- visible abscess on soft palate
- severe sore throat
- enlarged lymph nodes
- fever
- trismus
- drooling
- dysphagia
- halitosis

Management

- maintain airway
- analgesics, antibiotics, and/or corticosteroids
- incision and drainage or needle aspiration

QUICK REVIEW QUESTIONS

1. An 18-year-old patient arrives at the ED with a complaint of sore throat, drooling, and severe halitosis that the nurse can detect from several feet away. In the triage setting, what can the nurse immediately assess for to determine the level of acuity for this patient?

   _____

2. What age group is most at risk for peritonsillar abscess?

   _____

★ # Epistaxis

Pathophysiology

Epistaxis is hemorrhage or bleeding in the nasal passages caused by rupture of vasodilated vessels in the mucous membranes. Rupture can occur in one or more vessels and more commonly presents unilaterally. Emergency treatment should be considered if bleeding cannot be self-controlled or compromises the airway.

Epistaxis may originate anteriorly or posteriorly. **Anterior bleeding** compromises the majority of epistaxis cases and is usually self-limiting. _Posterior bleeding is less common but requires more aggressive treatment._ Risk factors for posterior bleeding include hypertension, use of anticoagulants, and recent nasal surgery.

HELPFUL HINT:

Do not have patients with epistaxis tilt their head backward because it can direct blood to the airway.

Physical Examination

- visible frank bleeding from nares
- nasal speculum used to visualize source of bleeding

Diagnostic Tests

- facial X-ray for injury

Management

- _manage airway_
- position patient sitting upright and leaning forward to prevent aspiration
- anterior epistaxis
  - continuous pressure to midline septum by pinching with fingers for up to 15 minutes
  - nasal decongestant spray (oxymetazoline) for vasoconstriction
  - electrical or chemical (silver nitrate) cautery
  - nasal packing if bleeding continues
- posterior epistaxis
  - nasal packing (balloon catheter)
  - hospital admission

QUICK REVIEW QUESTION

3. A patient with acute epistaxis has continued bleeding after application of silver nitrate and anterior packing. What intervention should the nurse anticipate next?

Facial Nerve Disorders

BELL'S PALSY

Pathophysiology

Bell's palsy is a unilateral facial paralysis or weakness caused by inflammation of the facial nerve (seventh cranial nerve). Onset is sudden and facial droop is similar in appearance to droop present with a cerebrovascular accident. In most cases the weakness will resolve over weeks to months; occasionally, it may recur. Bell's palsy typically occurs in younger adults and children. Cause is unknown but may be related to viral infections, autoimmune disease, or vascular ischemia.

Risk Factors

- pregnancy
- diabetes
- viral infection (herpes simplex virus, herpes zoster, flu)

Physical Examination

- mild to total unilateral paralysis of facial muscles
- characteristic facial droop
- painful sensations on affected side
- difficulty speaking
- dysphagia

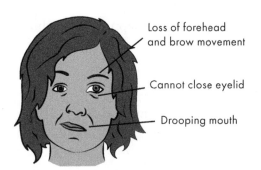

Loss of forehead and brow movement

Cannot close eyelid

Drooping mouth

Figure 16.1. Bell's Palsy

Management

- ***initial diagnostics to rule out CVA***
- corticosteroids
- antivirals if indicated
- patch on affected eye if diminished blink reflex to limit risk for corneal abrasion
- oral glycerin swabs for dry mouth
- Yankauer suction for excess saliva

QUICK REVIEW QUESTIONS

4. When Bell's palsy is suspected, what other serious ailment should be ruled out?

_____

5. A patient with Bell's palsy has a reddened eye and is unable to blink effectively. What can be provided to prevent eye damage?

_____

TRIGEMINAL NEURALGIA

Pathophysiology

Trigeminal neuralgia—or tic douloureux—is a condition of the trigeminal nerve (fifth cranial nerve) that causes unilateral stabbing, shooting pain and burning sensations along the nerve branches. Paroxysms can affect any or all of the three nerve branches: ophthalmic, maxillary, and mandibular. The cause is unknown, but pressure and compression of the vascular vessels near the trigeminal nerve root is suspected.

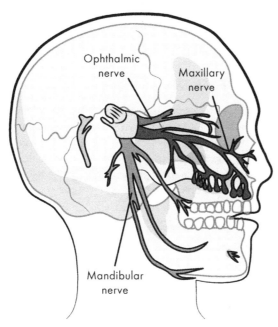

Figure 16.2. The Trigeminal Nerve

Trigeminal neuralgia is chronic, and the slightest touch or stimulation may precipitate a painful episode. Painful spasms both start and end abruptly. The initial attacks may be short; however, it can progress to longer and more frequent attacks.

Risk Factors

- age-related anatomical changes of the cerebral artery and veins: most common in ages 50 – 60
- more common in women

- multiple sclerosis
- facial trauma

Physical Examination

- *__characteristic unilateral pain along branches of the fifth cranial nerve__*
- abrupt onset and ending of pain lasting several minutes to several days
- facial muscle contractions causing eye to close and mouth to twitch on affected side

Diagnostic Tests

- MRI or CT to rule out neurovascular injury or lesion

Treatment and Management

- initial diagnostics to rule out CVA
- first-line medications: carbamazepine or oxcarbazepine
- second-line medications: gabapentin, lamotrigine, baclofen
- surgical decompression if pain does not respond to medications

---

QUICK REVIEW QUESTIONS

6. A 50-year-old female patient arrives at the ED with a complaint of excruciating pain when anything touches her face and when eating, brushing her teeth, and putting on makeup. Her symptoms have evolved over the past few weeks. Her medical history includes possible multiple sclerosis. She could not tolerate being touched for the physical assessment and made it partway through the neurological exam. What treatment should the nurse anticipate?

    _____

7. A patient with trigeminal neuralgia comes to the ED for excruciating pain that has lasted several days. The physician orders 50 mcg of fentanyl to treat pain. What should the nurse question about this order?

    _____

★ Maxillofacial Infections

- **Acute otitis media** is inflammation of the middle ear that usually results from inflammation in the mucous membranes. It is one of the most common reasons for ED visits in children.
  - Diagnosis: otalgia; otorrhea; tugging on ear; perforated, opaque, bulging, or erythematous tympanic membrane

□ Management: *usually heals spontaneously*; oral antibiotics if membrane is intact; antibiotic drops in affected ear if membrane is ruptured; analgesics

■ **Ludwig's angina** is a gangrenous cellulitis in the soft tissue of the neck and the floor of the mouth, generally following dental abscess. *Edema in the neck and mouth places the patient at high risk for airway obstruction.*

□ Diagnosis: tongue enlargement and protrusion; sublingual pain and tenderness; compromised breathing; difficulty swallowing; drooling; labs and s/s consistent with infection

□ Management: manage airway; IV antibiotics; incision and drainage

■ **Mastoiditis** is a bacterial infection of the mastoid air cells within the mastoid bone. It typically occurs secondary to acute otitis media.

□ Diagnosis: otitis media; tympanic membrane rupture; papilledema; erythema and edema over mastoid process

□ Management: antibiotics; analgesics

■ **Sinusitis** is inflammation and edema of the membranes lining the sinus cavities.

□ Diagnosis: facial pressure and pain; headache; nasal congestion and blockage; green or yellow nasal discharge

□ Management: decongestant\antihistamine; analgesics; antibiotics; corticosteroids; humidified air, warm compress, or saline nasal drops

HELPFUL HINT:

Otitis media is the second most common reason for ED visits in children < 1 year old. (Fever is the most common.)

QUICK REVIEW QUESTIONS

8. What are the typical signs and symptoms of sinusitis?

_____

9. A 2-year-old is brought to the ED for a severe earache. The physician orders antibiotic drops for the ears. The parent asks why oral antibiotics are not ordered. What should the nurse explain?

_____

10. A male patient is admitted to the ED one week after oral surgery with pain and swelling to the left side of his face and neck, which has progressed through the day. He states he has had difficulty swallowing and is drooling. He rates the pain 7/10 and vital signs reveal a temperature of 100.0°F (37.8°C) and pulse of 114 bpm. The oral cavity is tender and painful upon palpation. What diagnosis is appropriate for these signs and symptoms, and what test can be ordered to confirm?

_____

⟶
CONTINUE

Acute Vestibular Dysfunction

LABYRINTHITIS

Pathophysiology

Labyrinthitis occurs in the inner ear when the vestibulocochlear nerve (eighth cranial nerve) becomes inflamed as the result of either bacterial or viral infection. The inflammation affects hearing, balance, and spatial navigation. Onset is characterized as acute, sudden, and painless. The initial episode is most severe, with subsequent episodes showing less intensity. Labyrinthitis symptoms can extend from several weeks to several months.

Physical Examination

- dizziness and vertigo
- nausea and vomiting
- loss of balance
- tinnitus or hearing loss

Diagnostic Tests

- imaging/labs to rule out neurological condition, Ménière's disease

Management

- antibiotics or antivirals
- corticosteroids
- supportive care for symptoms: antihistamines, antiemetics, benzodiazepines

> **QUICK REVIEW QUESTION**
>
> 11. A 40-year-old female is diagnosed with labyrinthitis in the ED after all other potential neurological causes for sudden onset of vertigo, nausea, and tinnitus have been ruled out. While the nurse is preparing the patient for discharge, the patient asks if she can return to work tomorrow. What should the nurse anticipate discussing with the patient about the course of this disease?

MÉNIÈRE'S DISEASE

Pathophysiology

Ménière's disease is the result of chronic excess fluid in the inner ear. Fluid accumulation is the result of malabsorption in the endolymphatic sac or

HELPFUL HINT:

Tumarkin's otolithic crisis (drop attacks) occur in the late stages of Ménière's disease. They occur when a sudden loss of balance causes the patient to fall. The patient remains conscious and usually recovers quickly.

blockage of the endolymphatic duct. The excess fluid causes the endolymphatic space to enlarge, increasing inner ear pressure and possibly rupturing the inner membrane (not to be confused with rupture of the tympanic membrane in the middle ear as seen with otitis media).

While typically only one ear is affected, it does occur bilaterally in about 20% of cases. Onset may be minor with subtle symptoms, with subsequent episodes manifesting with more severe symptoms. Attacks can occur frequently, up to several times per week, or infrequently, several months or years apart. Attacks typically last anywhere from 20 minutes to 24 hours.

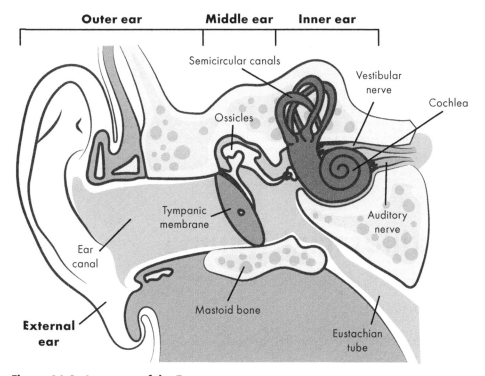

Figure 16.3. Anatomy of the Ear

Physical Examination

- *__classic triad of symptoms: fluctuations in hearing/hearing loss, tinnitus, vertigo__*

- pre-attack (aura): loss of balance, dizziness, pressure in ear, hearing loss or tinnitus, headache

- mid-attack: sudden severe vertigo, anxiety, GI symptoms, blurred vision, nystagmus, palpitations

- post-attack: extreme exhaustion and need for sleep

- late-stage disease: permanent hearing loss and increases in balance/ visual disturbances

Diagnostic Tests

- imaging/labs to rule out neurological condition, labyrinthitis

Management

- intratympanic gentamicin and steroids (injected by ENT)
- diuretics (non-potassium-sparing) and reduced sodium diet
- supportive care for symptoms: antihistamines, antiemetics, benzodiazepines

QUICK REVIEW QUESTION

12. A 43-year-old female patient arrives at the ED with a complaint of vertigo and tinnitus lasting >20 minutes. Patient states that the onset was sudden and occurred while she was shopping. Patient states she has had vertigo in the past but never this severe. She denies cold and flu symptoms. Vital signs: temperature of 98.6°F (37.0°C), pulse of 88 bpm, RR 16 BPM, BP 112/74 mm Hg, O$_2$ sat 99% on room air. What key information leads the nurse to suspect Ménière's disease versus labyrinthitis?

Maxillofacial Trauma

 ## MAXILLOFACIAL FRACTURES

Pathophysiology

Maxillofacial fractures occur from both blunt and penetrating traumas. Emergency management focuses on maintaining a patent airway and stabilizing the patient for surgical intervention. Most fractures will involve the integrity of surrounding tissues, requiring complex repair to muscular, vascular, and dermal structures as well as the reduction and fixation of the affected bone.

Types of maxillofacial fractures:

- nasal: most common of all facial fractures and least likely to need specialist consultation
- orbital rim and blowout fractures: fractures of orbital floor or lateral and medial orbital walls; occur from direct blow to the orbit such as from a baseball or fist
- mandibular: fractures of the lower jaw; may be singular or multiple
- maxillary: fractures of the upper jaw
- Le Fort I: horizontal fracture; separates teeth from upper structures—"floating palate"

- Le Fort II: pyramidal fracture; teeth are the base of the pyramid, fracture passes diagonally along the lateral wall of the maxillary sinuses, apex of pyramid is the nasofrontal junction—"floating maxilla"

- Le Fort III: craniofacial disjunction transverse fracture line passes through the nasofrontal junction, maxillofrontal suture, orbital wall, zygomatic arch, and zygomaticofrontal suture—"floating face"

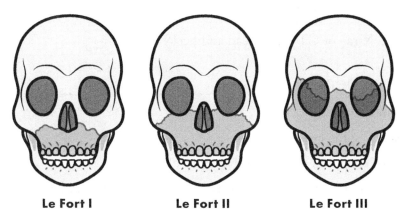

Le Fort I   **Le Fort II**   **Le Fort III**

Figure 16.4. Types of Maxillary Fractures

- Zygomaticomaxillary complex (tripod) fracture: simultaneous fracture of the lateral and inferior orbital rim, the zygomatic arch, and lateral maxillary sinus wall; occurs from direct blow to the lateral cheek

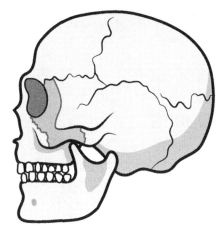

Figure 16.5. Zygomaticomaxillary Complex (Tripod) Fracture

Physical Examination

- visible facial injury or deformity

- pain, tenderness, or paresthesia over affected area

- epistaxis

- ecchymosis

- ocular: diplopia, restricted extraocular movements, decreased vision, enophthalmos, periorbital hematoma or edema, subconjunctival hemorrhage
- dental/oral: visible dental fractures or avulsions, impaired mastication, malocclusion, trismus, rhinorrhea of cerebrospinal fluid

Diagnostic Tests

- facial X-ray or CT scan (head and neck)

Management

HELPFUL HINT:

Cervical spine injuries are seen in around 15 percent of unconscious patients with maxillofacial fractures.

- maintain airway
- cervical spine precautions
- treatment based on type and severity of injury
- goal of all treatments is to preserve function and minimize disfigurement

QUICK REVIEW QUESTIONS

13. What diagnostic test needs to be performed stat on a patient with a suspected mandibular fracture that presents with dental avulsions?

14. While transferring an unconscious patient with a suspected Le Fort III fracture, what precautions should be taken?

SOFT TISSUE INJURIES
Pathophysiology

Penetrative and blunt trauma injuries to the maxillofacial region will cause soft tissue injuries that may obstruct the airway.

Physical Examination

- visible entry wound or foreign object
- bleeding
- contusions, hematoma, or tissue edema
- nasal drainage (rule out cerebrospinal fluid)

Management

- priority: maintain airway
- immobilize spine and neck as warranted
- IV fluids as needed for hemorrhage
- apply direct pressure for hemorrhage
- clean or irrigate wounds, then dress
- analgesics
- remove foreign object(s) when it is safe to do so; surgery to remove objects may be required

QUICK REVIEW QUESTION

15. A patient is brought to the ED via ambulance following a hunting accident. A friend states that the patient had lowered the butt of the shotgun to the ground and it accidently fired buckshot into the right side of the patient's neck, chin, and cheek. The patient's neck, face, eye, and mouth exhibit severe swelling and bleeding at entry points, and the patient is unable to speak and has labored breathing. What are the priority steps for the nurse to stabilize this patient?

ANSWER KEY

1. The nurse can use a penlight to assess the tonsillar tissue and soft palate for presence of a peritonsillar abscess. Peritonsillar abscess is an emergent finding and requires rapid evaluation by a medical provider.

2. Teenagers and adults ages 20 – 40 are most at risk for peritonsillar abscess.

3. Bleeding through anterior packing suggests posterior epistaxis. The nurse should anticipate posterior packing using a catheter.

4. Bell's palsy signs and symptoms are similar to CVA, so the patient should be worked up for a stroke.

5. The patient should be provided an eye patch.

6. Based on signs and symptoms, the patient is suffering from trigeminal neuralgia. The nurse should anticipate administration of carbamazepine or oxcarbazepine.

7. Trigeminal neuralgia originates from nerve pain and does not typically respond to analgesics.

8. Symptoms of sinusitis include facial pressure and pain, headache, nasal congestion and blockage, and green or yellow nasal discharge.

9. Oral antibiotics are not ordered if the ear membrane is ruptured as it is able to drain, so drops are more effective in this case.

10. Signs and symptoms are consistent with early onset of Ludwig's angina. A CT scan to evaluate the soft tissue would be appropriate.

11. Labyrinthitis runs a course of several weeks to several months. The nurse should educate the patient that bedrest is essential and that use of prescribed medications will manage symptoms. It is likely that additional episodes will occur, although they may be less severe than the onset of disease.

12. Ménière's disease presents with sudden vertigo and tinnitus with no fever or cold/flu symptoms. A history of less severe episodes of vertigo is consistent with progressive chronic disease.

13. The patient should receive a chest X-ray to assess for aspiration of avulsed teeth and bone fragments.

14. Spinal precautions should be taken with a patient with a suspected Le Fort III fracture.

15. This is a traumatic injury with the risk of death. The nurse should start with the ABCs: stabilizing the airway is priority. Prepare for intubation before the airway is lost and administer oxygen or bag patient until airway is secured. Suction oral cavity and start large-bore IVs and fluids for blood loss. Apply direct pressure or pressure bandages to bleeding wounds and administer IV pain medication and sedative. Once the patient is stable, evaluation and removal of buckshot can follow.

17 OCULAR EMERGENCIES

Ocular Anatomy and Assessment

The eye is a delicate organ supported by 6 extraocular muscles attached to the **sclera**, a white protective layer composed of tough, fibrous connective tissue. The sclera extends from the cornea to the **optic nerve**.

- Covering the sclera and inner eyelids, the **conjunctiva**:
  - lubricates eye tissues
  - protects the eye from debris and injury
- The **central retinal artery** and **central retinal vein** run parallel to the optic nerve.
- Light passes through the **cornea**, the clear tissue that covers and protects the front of the eye.

- Light is then filtered by the **iris**, which contracts and dilates to control how much light passes through the pupil.
- The **lens** sits directly behind the pupil.
  - Light passing through the lens is concentrated through a process called **accommodation.**
  - Accommodation helps the eye to focus on objects based on their distance.
- The **retina** is light-sensitive specialized tissue that lines the back of the eye.
  - Sensory cells in the retina send electronic signals to the brain, translating the light received into an image.
- **Vitreous humor**, a jellylike substance, fills the eye.

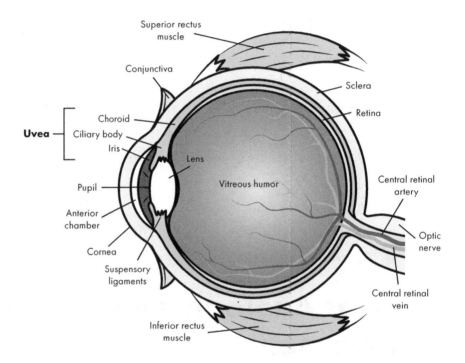

Figure 17.1. Anatomy of the Eye

- **Visual acuity** should be measured during triage.
  - Methods of assessment include a Snellen chart, an E chart (used for patients who cannot read), and an Allen card (used for children).
  - If the patient is unable to read the chart, measure the distance at which they can see motion and determine if they can perceive light.
  - Measure visual acuity both with and without the patient's corrective lenses.
- The most common method of measuring intraocular pressure in the ED is a **Tono-Pen**. Topical anesthetic should be applied to the cornea before use.

- **Fluorescein staining** is used to diagnose damage to the cornea. The stain is applied to the eye and will gather in areas of epithelial damage.

- A **fundoscopic exam** is used to examine the posterior chamber of the eye. Pupil-dilating drops may be administered to allow for ease of inspection of the retina.

- A **slit lamp** is used to examine the anterior chamber of the eye. A vertical slit of light is shone on the eye while a microscope is used to identify damage to the retina, cataracts, corneal injury, and retinal vessel blockages.

- A **Seidel test** uses fluorescein staining and a slit lamp to test for ocular leaks after orbital injury.

QUICK REVIEW QUESTION

1. A patient is admitted to the ED after an MVC. The patient is reporting loss of eyesight in the left eye, and there is significant bruising around the orbital socket. The provider orders a Seidel test. The nurse knows that this test assesses for what indication?

Abrasions

Pathophysiology

A **corneal abrasion** is a scratch or abrasive friction on the outer surface of the epithelium (the cornea's outer layer). Symptoms, severity, and outcome are variable based on the layers of the cornea involved and the size of the area affected. Corneal abrasions typically heal within 24 – 72 hours without complications, but in some cases may progress to infection, keratitis, or ulceration.

Corneal lacerations extend into the deeper layers of the cornea and are more symptomatic and painful than corneal abrasions. Lacerations are considered partial thickness (closed globe) and do not penetrate the globe structure of the eye.

Physical Examination

- painful pressure or burning sensation
- sensation of foreign body or grit
- lacrimation or discharge
- erythema or edema
- decrease in visual acuity: may be described as blurred, dull, or foggy

Diagnostic Tests

- fluorescein staining
- slit lamp or Woods lamp exam to identify the degree of injury or illness

Management

- irrigate to remove foreign body, if present
- topical anesthetic, NSAIDs, and antibiotics
- ophthalmic lubricating solution
- lacerations may require surgery

QUICK REVIEW QUESTIONS

2. A patient arrives in the ED complaining of a burning sensation in both eyes with increased tearing. The patient states he had "day surgery" for tooth extraction about 8 hours ago and noticed the pain shortly after being discharged. The nurse identifies that the pain is bilateral, making the presence of a foreign body unlikely. What diagnostics should the nurse anticipate for this patient?

3. A patient with a closed globe injury is observed holding a facecloth over the affected eye "for comfort" but has removed the protective eye shield to do so. What complication of introducing external pressure to this eye does the nurse need to monitor for?

Burns

Pathophysiology

Ocular burns are classified as chemical (subdivided as alkali- or acid-based) or radiant energy (thermal or ultraviolet). Chemical burns occur through splash, spray, or direct touch. Alkali burns penetrate deep into the eye, causing liquefactive necrosis, while acidic burns cause a coagulated necrosis closer to the surface of the injury. Radiant energy burns occur from exposure to intense heat, explosions, hot cooking oils, electrical arc, lasers, and direct gaze into ultraviolet light.

The outcome varies based on the agent of exposure, time length of exposure, and ocular structures involved, but usually involves some degree of vision loss. Ocular burns tend to occur bilaterally and often in combination with other injuries such as dermal burns, penetrating objects, and compromised airways.

Physical Examination

- extreme pain or burning sensation
- erythema and edema
- copious lacrimation
- decrease in visual acuity
- history of chemical or radiant energy exposure

Management

- maintain airway and assess for concurrent injury
- irrigate for minimum of 30 minutes with isotonic solution
    - assess pH level after irrigation; if > 7.4, continue with additional irrigation
    - topical anesthetics may be added to irrigant solution
    - Morgan Lens: as needed assist with irrigation
- topical corticosteroids, antibiotics, and cycloplegics
- occlusive dressing as needed
- obtain chemical safety data sheet and consider consultation with regional poison control center

HELPFUL HINT:

Irrigation should be deferred if globe rupture is suspected.

QUICK REVIEW QUESTIONS

4. A 38-year-old male patient arrives at the ED clutching his face after an automobile battery exploded, splashing acidic liquid into his eyes. Irrigation with 1 L normal saline is initiated immediately. How will the nurse assess if the irrigation has been effective or if additional irrigation may be needed?

5. A 14-year-old is brought into the ED after playing with a welding arc without proper eye protection. The patient is visibly in pain and unable to open the eyes. What can be used to facilitate the assessment?

Foreign Bodies

Pathophysiology

Ocular foreign bodies are any substance or object that does not belong in the eye. Size, shape, substance, impact velocity, and location will greatly impact severity of symptoms and ultimate outcome.

Foreign bodies are described based upon their location.

- extraocular (lid, sclera, conjunctiva, and cornea)
- intraocular (anterior chamber, iris, lens, vitreous, retina, and intraorbital)

Physical Examination

- visible foreign object
- sensation of foreign body or grit
- painful pressure or burning sensation
- penetrating injury: bleeding
- lacrimation or discharge
- erythema or edema
- blepharospasm
- photosensitivity or decrease in visual acuity

Diagnostic Tests

- fluorescein staining
- slit lamp or Woods lamp exam to identify the degree of injury or illness

Management

- irrigate with normal saline or eye wash solution
- evert upper lid to confirm absence/presence of foreign body
- Morgan Lens for extraocular foreign bodies, or if sensation of foreign body is present but foreign body is not visible
- remove foreign body using cotton-tipped applicator, metal spud, or 25-gauge needle (extraocular only)
- topical anesthetic, NSAIDs, and antibiotics
- ophthalmic lubricating solution
- patch if foreign body is retained (pending ophthalmology referral)
- immediate ophthalmology referral for all intraocular foreign bodies

HELPFUL HINT:

Ophthalmic corticosteroids are used cautiously and only by ophthalmologists as they can worsen underlying infections in the eye.

QUICK REVIEW QUESTIONS

6. A patient in a small community hospital is diagnosed with a retained foreign body to the left lens with vitreous leakage present. The patient will require transfer to a larger hospital for emergent ophthalmology consult. How will the nurse prepare this patient for transport?

7. A 45-year-old construction worker arrives at the ED from the work site with extreme eye irritation in one eye. Assessment does not reveal an obvious cause of the irritation. What can be used to assist with checking for a foreign body?

Increased Intraocular Pressure

Pathophysiology

Glaucoma is a group of eye diseases that cause an increase in **intraocular pressure (IOP)**, resulting in compression of the optic nerve. The compression causes degeneration of the optic nerve fibers and apoptosis of the retinal ganglion cells, resulting in permanent vision loss.

Types of glaucoma include:

- primary open-angle glaucoma
- normal tension (low-pressure) glaucoma
- secondary glaucoma related to diabetes or cataracts
- angle-closure glaucoma

Most glaucomas are chronic and develop slowly and painlessly over time. The emergency nurse should be familiar with the visual impact of these chronic glaucomas, as the patient may have a deficit of peripheral vision that can impact communication methods.

Acute angle-closure glaucoma is a medical emergency that occurs when IOP increases rapidly to 30 mm Hg or higher (normal pressure is 8 – 21 mm Hg). Permanent vision loss from compression of the optic nerve can occur in as little as several hours if not rapidly treated. Additionally, scarring of the trabecular meshwork can lead to chronic forms of glaucoma, and cataracts can develop as latent complications. Acute onset commonly occurs in conjunction with pupil dilation, such as when transitioning from light to dark environments.

The information below relates to acute angle-closure glaucoma.

Risk Factors

- family history
- being of Asian descent
- more common in women
- age > 60
- hyperopic vision
- shallow anterior chamber
- thickened lens

Physical Examination

- abrupt onset of pain
- visual changes: described as blurry, cloudy, or halos of light
- headache
- nausea and vomiting
- erythema

Diagnostic Tests

- corneal edema with clouding
- fixed pupil, mid-dilated (5 – 6 mm)
- Tono-Pen: increased intraocular pressure
- fundoscopic exam: pale, cupped optic disc
- slit lamp exam: shallow anterior chamber

Management

- first-line pharmacological treatment:
  - topical miotic ophthalmic drops (pilocarpine)
  - topical beta-blockers (timolol)
  - topical alpha-adrenergic agents (apraclonidine)
- IV administration of acetazolamide or mannitol
- immediate ophthalmology referral and consult

QUICK REVIEW QUESTIONS

8. Two patients arrive at the ED separately, each complaining of acute onset of eye pain. The first patient, a 35-year-old Asian male, describes pain in his left eye as burning, with onset occurring while he was outside in his yard. Clear tearing and erythema are present. The second patient is a 65-year-old Caucasian female who describes her pain as deep and sharp with onset occurring as she was leaving a matinee show at a movie theater. Which patient does the nurse recognize as needing emergent medical evaluation?

9. A patient in the ED diagnosed with elevated intraocular pressure has received topical pilocarpine, timolol, and apraclonidine. The physician evaluates the patient and finds that the pressure has not reduced as expected. What is the next action the nurse should anticipate?

Ocular Infections

- **Conjunctivitis** (pink eye) is the inflammation of the thin connective tissue that covers the outer surface of the sclera (bulbar conjunctiva) and lines the inner layers of the eyelids (palpebral conjunctiva).
  - Diagnosis: burning or itching sensation; increased lacrimation (clear or yellow); erythema of sclera and inner eyelids; edema of palpebra; typically no decrease in visual acuity
  - Management: warm or cool compress for comfort; topical antibiotics if indicated; topical steroid if severe periorbital edema is present; ophthalmic lubricating solution

- **Uveitis** is the inflammation of any of the structures in the uvea, including the iris (iritis or anterior uveitis), the ciliary body (intermediate uveitis), or the choroid (choroiditis or posterior uveitis).
  - Diagnosis: pain described as global aching or tenderness; cilliary spasm; conjunctival erythema; photophobia; vision changes; vitreous floaters; keratitis; Tono-Pen (increased intraocular pressure)
  - Management: topical mydriatic ophthalmic drops to dilate the pupil; topical corticosteroids; referral to ophthalmology within 24 hours

QUICK REVIEW QUESTIONS

10. A 35-year-old female with a known history of HIV is diagnosed in the ED with iritis following an acute onset of erythema, tenderness, and photophobia. Clinically, the left pupil is small and irregular in shape. The patient asks the nurse when her eye will "return to normal." What patient education should the nurse anticipate delivering?

11. What treatment would be expected for a patient presenting with uveitis?

Retinal Artery Occlusion

Pathophysiology

Retinal artery occlusion (sometimes referred to as an ocular stroke) occurs when there is a blockage of vascular flow through the retinal arteries, resulting in a lack of oxygen delivery to the nerve cells in the retina. Blockage may occur from thrombi or emboli.

Risk Factors

- heart or vascular disease
- artificial heart valves
- A-fib
- diabetes
- hypertension
- sickle cell disease
- pregnancy
- use of oral contraceptives
- IV substance abuse

Physical Examination

- unilateral, sudden, painless loss of vision

Diagnostic Tests

- Tono-Pen (increased intraocular pressure)
- dilated fundoscopic exam
  - □ red fovea (cherry-red spot)
  - □ optic disc pallor and edema

Management

- topical beta blockers
- IV acetazolamide
- IV mannitol
- IV methylprednisolone
- ocular massage
- immediate referral to ophthalmology

QUICK REVIEW QUESTIONS

12. A patient present to the ED after experiencing a sudden loss of sight in the right eye while outside gardening 60 minutes before arrival. The nurse obtains the following medication list from the patient: metformin 500 mg twice daily, chewable aspirin 81 mg daily, warfarin (Coumadin) 5 mg daily, diltiazem (Cardizem) 60 mg three times daily, cetirizine (Zyrtec) 10 mg daily, and metoprolol (Lopressor) 25 mg twice daily. What risk factors for retinal arterial occlusion can the nurse identify based upon the diagnosis and medication history?

Retinal Detachment

Pathophysiology

Retinal detachment occurs when the pigmented epithelial layer of the retina separates from the choroid layer (visualize how thin layers of an onion peel can separate from each other) because of tension, trauma, or fluid accumulation between the layers. Vision loss results from lack of available oxygen and deterioration of photoreceptor cells.

Risk Factors

- age > 65
- history of cataract surgery
- trauma
- high myopia (nearsightedness)
- diabetes
- Marfan's syndrome
- uveitis inflammation
- hypertension
- neovascular ("wet") macular degeneration

Physical Examination

- painless onset of visual changes
- loss of vision is not immediate (unlike retinal artery occlusions)
- reduction in peripheral vision and curtain-like shadow over visual field
- sudden or gradual increase of multiple floaters (wispy spider web-like formations that "float" across the visual field

Diagnostic Findings

- fundoscopic exam to assess for Schafer's sign, vitreous hemorrhage, and scleral depression
- ocular ultrasound

Management

- stabilize patient and treat underlying injuries
- bedrest and quiet environment
- immediate referral to ophthalmology

QUICK REVIEW QUESTION

14. A 25-year-old female patient arrives at the ED with complaint of "a curtain" shading her peripheral vision and "hazy strings" floating across her visual field. Onset was yesterday but is becoming progressively worse. Medical history is nonsignificant except for tonsillectomy at age 8. The nurse conducts a visual acuity test and the patient states results are consistent with her baseline sight of 20/100 without glasses. Explain how this patient may be at risk for retinal detachment.

Ocular Trauma
GLOBE RUPTURE
Pathophysiology

HELPFUL HINT:

Common sources of ocular trauma include occupational injuries, MVCs, and falls (especially children and the elderly).

A **global rupture** (open globe) occurs from a full thickness laceration or tearing of the cornea and sclera. Rupture may occur as the result of blunt trauma, penetrating injury (entry wound without exit), or a perforating injury (entry and exit wounds present). Rupture can also occur post-trauma due to a rapid rise in intraocular pressure.

Physical Examination

- eccentric or teardrop-shaped pupil
- sunken eye appearance and loss of volume
- gross deformity or misshapen eye
- ocular pain
- subconjunctival hemorrhage
- decreased visual acuity

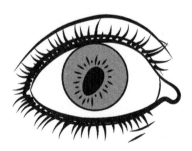

Figure 17.2. Teardrop Pupil

- edema, erythema, or ecchymosis
- tenting of the sclera or cornea at the site of globe puncture

Diagnostic Findings

- Seidel test positive (indicating leakage of aqueous humor)

Management

- maintain bedrest; elevate head of bed 30 degrees
- manage IOP
- shield both eyes (to prevent eye movement)
- keep patient NPO and prep for surgery
- Do NOT:
  - irrigate
  - remove foreign body or penetrating objects
  - measure intraocular pressure
  - use pressure or absorbent dressings

QUICK REVIEW QUESTION

15. A 22-year-old male patient arrives at the ED after sustaining injury to his left eye during a bar fight. The eye is edematous, there is visual prolapse of the uvea, and vitreous extrusion is present. The patient exhibits signs of pain and is unable to tolerate visual acuity testing at this time. What nursing interventions does the nurse anticipate?

HYPHEMA
Pathophysiology

Hyphema is a collection of blood inside the anterior chamber between the cornea and iris. Blood accumulates as a result of a traumatic tear in the vascular structure of the iris or pupil, and it may rise to a level that fully occludes all vision.

Hyphema bleeding differs in appearance from bleeding that is seen with a subconjunctival hemorrhage. Hyphema is dependent; the blood rises in a horizontal fashion in front of the iris as it accumulates, similar to how water levels rise in a closed chamber.

→
CONTINUE

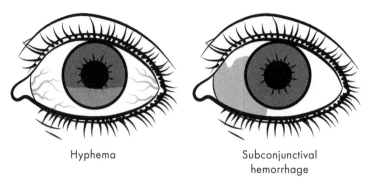

Hyphema

Subconjunctival hemorrhage

Figure 17.3. Hyphema versus Subconjunctival Hemorrhage

A **subconjuctival hemorrhage** is painless and occurs from rupture of localized surface vessels in the sclera. A subconjuctival hemorrhage is irregularly shaped, covers the white portion of the eye, and does not result in visual deficit or loss.

Physical Examination

- visible accumulation of blood

- decreased visual acuity

- pain and headache

Management

- maintain bedrest; elevate head of bed ≥ 45 degrees

- manage IOP

- low-risk patients: rest and monitoring

- high-risk patients: pharmacological management (topical corticosteroids, cycloplegics, beta blockers, or alpha-adrenergic agents [clonidine])

QUICK REVIEW QUESTION

16. A patient is admitted to the ED with severe inflammation around the right eye. He stated he was hit with a baseball and complains of severe pain, pressure, sensitivity to light, and blurred vision. As the nurse's assessment progresses she notes blood filling the area over the iris under the cornea. What treatment should the nurse anticipate?

Ulcerations and Keratitis

Pathophysiology

Ulcerative keratitis is characterized by crescent-shaped inflammation of the epithelial layer that progresses to necrosis of the corneal stroma. Ulcers may occur from infectious or noninfectious causes, and they form scar tissue when healing. Without treatment, ulcers may infiltrate deeper structures of the eye, causing secondary uveitis, prolapse of the iris or cilliary body, hypopyon, and endophthalmitis/panophthalmitis.

Risk Factors

- traumatic injury
- diabetes
- immunodeficiency
- systemic side effects of some medications (e.g., amiodarone, flouro-quinilones, antimetabolites/neoplastic agents, tamoxifen, NSAIDs, thorazine)
- side effects of topical medications (allergic ulcerative keratitis)
- use of contact lenses

Physical Examination

- painful pressure, severe pain, or burning sensation
- increased lacrimation
- erythema and edema
- white or cloudy spot on cornea
- sensation of foreign body or grit
- decrease in visual acuity: may be described as blurred, dull, or foggy

Diagnostic Findings

- culture and sensitivity

Management

- empiric administration of broad-spectrum antibiotics
- warm compress
- topical cycloplegics

QUICK REVIEW QUESTIONS

17. What is a distinguishing characteristic of ulcerative keratitis?

_____

→

CONTINUE

18. A patient was seen in the ED and diagnosed with a corneal abrasion. The patient returns 6 days later stating that pain has become significantly worse and that the front of his eye appears white in color, impacting his central vision. The patient admits to not completing the course of prescribed antibiotic ophthalmic drops and reinserting his contact lenses the following day. The contact lens remains in the affected eye as the patient was unable to remove it before returning to the ED. How would the nurse explain to the patient how the corneal abrasion progressed to ulcerative keratitis?

_____

ANSWER KEY

1. A Seidel test assesses for ocular leaks after an orbital injury.

2. A slit lamp or Woods lamp exam and fluorescein staining will assess for corneal abrasion.

3. This patient is at risk for developing an open globe rupture. External pressure can elicit an increase in intraocular pressure, causing strain at the weakest point of the sclera at the insertion point of the extraocular muscles.

4. Assess pH level with litmus paper or pH indicator strips. Touch the paper or test strip to the conjunctival fornix; if results are > 7.4, additional irrigation is warranted.

5. The eyes may be flushed with an irrigant combined with a topical anesthetic (e.g., 1% lidocaine).

6. Because the patient has an intraocular foreign body, patching the affected eye is appropriate pending exam by ophthalmology. Avoid use of Morgan Lens for irrigation. Apply topical anesthetics and topical NSAIDs for pain management. Apply topical antibiotics for infection prophylaxis.

7. Fluorescein staining in conjunction with a blue light is used to check for foreign bodies in the eye.

8. The second patient, the 65-year-old female, has risk factors for acute angle-closure glaucoma and presents with an onset of pain that occurred when transitioning from a dark to a light environment. The first patient's symptoms are more consistent with a corneal abrasion or foreign body.

9. The ED physician will order another medication to reduce intraocular pressure, like IV acetazolamide or mannitol. The nurse should prepare to administer the ordered medication.

10. Acute iritis can take several weeks to resolve. The patient will require use of topical steroids to decrease inflammation and mydriatic ophthalmic drops to prevent the onset of secondary glaucoma. The mydriatic drops will alter the appearance of the pupil, making it larger. Follow-up with ophthalmology is essential to monitor for secondary complications that can lead to permanent vision loss.

11. Uveitis is treated with mydriatic ophthalmic drops and topical corticosteroids.

12. This patient appears to have risk factors of diabetes, hypertension, and possible A-fib or vascular disease. These conditions increase risks for development of thrombolytic and atheroembolisms, which can occlude the retinal arteries.

13. A dilated fundoscopic exam would show red fovea and optic disc pallor and edema.

14. High myopia, or nearsightedness, is a risk factor for retinal detachment. High myopia occurs when the shape of the eye is elongated from front to back, causing tension and stretching of the retinal structure. The stretching can cause a hole or break in the retinal tissue, allowing fluid to enter between the layers, ultimately causing the retina to detach.

15. This patient exhibits signs consistent with an open global rupture. The nurse should initiate NPO status and obtain intravenous access. Pain and nausea should be managed to avoid vagal stimulus. Eye shield may be placed to discourage eye manipulation or movements. Head of bed should be elevated to 30 degrees and bedrest status maintained.

16. Hyphema may cause an increase in intraocular pressure that must be monitored closely and treated if applicable. Bedrest, keeping HOB elevated ≥ 45 degrees, and avoiding use of anticoagulant medications and alcohol are standards of care.

17. Ulcerative keratitis presents with a crescent-shaped inflammation of the epithelial layer that may progress to a white or cloudy spot on the cornea.

18. This patient's symptoms and history are consistent with an infectious corneal ulcer related to contact use. Contact lenses can transfer bacteria to the surface of the eye and essentially trap it under the contact for a prolonged period of time. The patient already had a breach in surface integrity from the preexisting abrasion.

18 ENVIRONMENT EMERGENCIES

BCEN OUTLINE: ENVIRONMENT EMERGENCIES

- *Burns*
- Chemical exposure (e.g., organophosphates, cleaning agents)
- Electrical injuries
- Envenomation emergencies
- *Submersion injury*
- *Temperature-related emergencies*
- Animal bites (e.g., rabies, infection)

Burns

Pathophysiology

Burns are trauma to the skin or underlying tissue caused by heat, radiation, electricity, or chemical exposure. The heat causes protein denaturation of the cells that leads to coagulative necrosis, platelet aggregation, and vessel constriction. *The inflammatory response to the injury creates a fluid shift that can result in hypovolemia and reduced cardiac output ("burn shock").* Damage to large areas of skin also puts patients at risk of hypothermia.

Burns are classified by depth as first degree, second degree, and third degree.

- **Superficial** (first degree): Damage is limited to the epidermis and does not result in blisters (e.g., sunburn).

- **Partial-Thickness** (second degree): Damage includes the dermis and epidermis accompanied by severe pain.

- **Full-Thickness** (third degree): All layers of the skin are damaged and there is likely underlying tissue damage. The patient may not feel pain in areas of significant nerve damage.

Burns are described by the **total body surface area (TBSA)** involved. TBSA is calculated by assigning a numerical value to the areas that are burned; the rule of 9s is the most commonly used method.

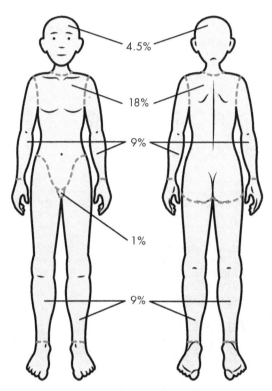

Figure 18.1. Rule of 9s for Calculating Total Body Surface Area (TBSA) of Burns

Physical Examination

- **Superficial** (first degree): Damage is limited to the epidermis and does not result in blisters (e.g., sunburn).

- **Partial-Thickness** (second degree): Damage includes the dermis and epidermis accompanied by severe pain.

- **Full-Thickness** (third degree): All layers of the skin are damaged and there is likely underlying tissue damage. The patient may not feel pain in areas of significant nerve damage.

Diagnostic Tests

- labs to monitor for hypovolemia, electrolyte imbalances, metabolic acidosis, and renal dysfunction
- ABGs and carboxyhemoglobin to monitor pulmonary function

Management

- priority: ABCs and IV access for fluids
  - look for signs of airway compromise (e.g., burns to the face, soot in the nose or mouth, singed nasal hair, or coughing due to smoke inhalation)
  - edema may develop quickly and obstruct the airway
- remove hot jewelry and clothing
- cool burns with cool water or saline-soaked gauze
- calculate TBSA (used to correct hypovolemia)
- *IV lactated Ringer's per Parkland formula*:
  - $4 \text{ ml} \times \text{TBSA (\%)} \times \text{body weight (kg)}$
  - Give 50% in first 8 hours; then 50% in next 16 hours.
  - Formula time starts at the time the burn happens.
  - Expected urine output is $0.5 - 1.0 \text{ ml/kg/hr}$ in adults and $1.0 - 1.5 \text{ ml/kg/hr}$ in children < 30 kg.
- analgesics
- clean wounds and apply sterile dressing
- topical antibiotic (e.g., silver sulfadiazine)
- escharotomy to remove constricting areas of eschar as needed
- full-thickness burns require hospitalization for excision and grafting

QUICK REVIEW QUESTIONS

1. What is the expected urine output for adults who are receiving IV fluids per the Parkland formula?

   _____

2. A patient presents to the ED with second-degree burns on their legs. The nurse establishes that the patient is breathing and has a pulse. What should the nurse prepare to do next?

   _____

→

CONTINUE

Chemical Exposure

Pathophysiology

Chemical burns result from contact with acids (e.g., hydrofluoric acid), alkalis (e.g., ammonia, cement), or organic compounds (e.g., phenol, gasoline). The injury will depend on the how the patient was exposed, what chemical they were exposed to, and the length of time of the exposure. Chemicals will continue to cause tissue damage as long as they have been removed, so early decontamination is critical.

Chemical burns may take several days for to slough, making them difficult to assess their severity. They should be assumed to be partial- or full-thickness during acute care.

The **safety data sheets (SDS)** (formally known as material safety data sheets [MSDS]) for a chemical agent will include information on toxicology, first aid, and exposure control.

Management

- consult poison control and/or SDS
- *__decontaminate the affected areas__*
    - remove patient's clothing
    - brush off dry chemicals
    - irrigate burn with water
- fluid resuscitation and wound care (as described in "Burns" above)
- hydrofluoric acid
    - administration of calcium gluconate (topically, subcutaneously, or intravenously)
    - monitor for dysrhythmias and electrolyte imbalances
- phenol: swab affected area with polyethylene glycol (PEG) and irrigate with water

> **QUICK REVIEW QUESTION**
>
> 3. A construction worker presents to the ED with intense pain and erythema on the lower legs. He states that he spent the previous day mixing concrete and did not wear lower-leg protection. What priority intervention should the nurse anticipate?

Electrical Injuries

Pathophysiology

Generated electrical energy causes external and internal injury from the electrical current running through the body. Injuries will vary depending on the intensity of the current, voltage, resistance, the length of time exposed, entry and exit locations, and the tissue and organs affected by the electrical current. Generated electrical injury can result in skin burns, damage to internal organs or tissue, respiratory arrest, or cardiac arrhythmias/arrest.

Physical Examination

- burns at the entry and exit points with a clean line of demarcation
- involuntary muscular contractions
- dyspnea
- seizures, confusion, or loss of consciousness
- paralysis
- dysrhythmias
- signs and symptoms of rhabdomyolysis or compartment syndrome in severe cases

Management

- priority: ABCs
- follows ALS protocols for respiratory/cardiac arrest
- IV fluids
  - *__standard burn fluid-resuscitation protocols are not used as there is usually more damage than is seen on surface burns__*
  - IV fluid treatment goal is to maintain urine output of 75 – 100 ml/hr
- analgesics
- monitor cardiac and kidney function
- head-to-toe assessment for injuries secondary to falls

QUICK REVIEW QUESTIONS

4. A conscious patient comes into the ED and states that he touched a live electrical wire. He has a small injury on his left hand and a small exit injury on the bottom of his left foot, but reports he feels no other symptoms. Why would the nurse proceed with a full electrical injury workup?

_____

5. A patient is brought into the ED with severe burns to the bilateral upper extremities and torso. Per order, a Foley catheter is placed and the nurse notes 30 mL of dark, tea-colored urine. What order would be expected?

_____

HELPFUL HINT:

Common complications of lightning strikes include keraunoparalysis, cardiac arrest, and neurological symptoms. Lightning strikes do not usually cause burns, rhabdomyolysis, or internal organ or tissue damage.

HELPFUL HINT:

In patients with electrical injuries, subcutaneous or deeper tissue damage is often greater than the areas indicated by the line of demarcation.

Envenomation Emergencies

Pathophysiology

Most animal bites or stings do not require emergency care and can be managed with OTC analgesics. However, emergent care may be required for exposure to lethal venom or for anaphylaxis.

HELPFUL HINT:

Coral snake venom contains a neuro-toxin that can cause weakness, paralysis, and respiratory arrest. All patients with coral snake bites should be monitored for at least 12 hours.

HELPFUL HINT:

Compression of most bites is contraindicated because it may keep the poison in the area, increasing localized damage.

TABLE 18.1. Diagnosis and Management of Envenomation Emergencies

Animal	Physical Examination	Treatment and Management
Snake	varies depending on snake species general s/s: nausea and vomiting, tachycardia, diaphoresis coagulation abnormalities weakness and lethargy confusion	ABCs antivenom supportive treatment for s/s
Spider	brown spider bites: delayed pain; ecchymosis and erythema; central blood-filled lesion that ruptures, leaving an ulcer widow spider bites: immediate pain; muscle cramping and weakness; diaphoresis; hypertension; tachycardia	wound care analgesics excision of brown spider bite opioids and benzodiazepines for symptomatic widow bites antivenom for widow bites only in patients at high risk for severe systemic response
Scorpion	immediate pain possible numbness or stinging muscular spasms or weakness restlessness or anxiety tachycardia hypertension increased respiration	supportive treatment for s/s antivenom only for patients with severe symptoms
Bee, Wasp, Hornet, or Fire Ant	immediate pain, burning, and itching erythema and edema	remove stinger if still in place ice, antihistamines, or NSAIDs for pain

6. What symptoms should the nurse expect to see at the site of a brown recluse spider bite?

_____

7. What interventions should the nurse anticipate for a patient with a coral snake bite?

_____

Submersion Injury

Pathophysiology

A **submersion injury** is a respiratory injury or impairment that occurs as a result of being submerged in a substance (usually water, but it can be other liquids or solids like grain). The respiratory impairment resulting from submersion leads to hypoxemia, which in turn can lead to organ failure. Common complications include dysrhythmias, ARDS, and cerebral edema.

Physical Examination

- change in LOC
- cool, clammy, pale skin
- wheezing or crackles
- signs and symptoms of respiratory failure

Diagnostic Tests

- ABG shows metabolic acidosis

Management

- follow ALS protocols for respiratory/cardiac arrest
- priority: treatment of hypoxemia
  - _**start patient on 100% oxygen**_; titrate down based on serial ABG results
  - intubation and mechanical ventilation may be needed
- nebulized bronchodilators to relieve bronchospasms or wheezing
- manage hypothermia (See "Temperature-Related Emergencies" next)

HELPFUL HINT:

Physical examination of submersion injury is not necessarily immediate; some respiratory damage may take up to 6 hours to produce symptoms.

8. A patient who was found floating in a body of water is admitted to the ED. The patient is currently on 100% O_2 and the current PaO_2 is 45%. What procedure should the nurse prepare for?

_____

9. What is the primary concern with submersion injuries?

_____

Temperature-Related Emergencies

HYPOTHERMIA

Pathophysiology

Hypothermia occurs when core body temperature drops below 35°C (95°F), causing a reduction in metabolic rate and in respiratory, cardiac, and neurological functions. When body temperature drops below 30°C (86°F), thermoregulation ceases.

During hypothermia, diuresis and systemic fluid leakage into the interstitial space can lead to hypovolemia. Vasoconstriction due to the cold can mask this hypovolemia. When the patient is rewarmed and the vessels dilate, the patient will go into shock or cardiac arrest if the fluid volume is not replaced.

Physical Examination

- mild hypothermia: 32 – 35°C (90 – 95°F)
- moderate hypothermia: 28 – 32°C (82 – 90°F)
- severe hypothermia: < 28°C (82°F)
- intense shivering that lasts until core body temperature drops below 31°C (87.8°F)
- lethargy, clumsiness, confusion, agitation, or hallucinations
- hypotension

Diagnostic Tests

- decreased cardiac function
  - initial bradycardia and slow A-fib, then V-fib or asystole

☐ ECG: will read as injury due to myocardial infarction, but will show a *J wave or Osborn wave*

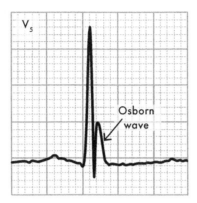

Figure 18.2. Osborn or J Wave

Management

- first line: prevent further heat loss by removing wet/cold clothing and insulating patient
- mild hypothermia: passively rewarm patients at a rate of 1°C per hour with an insulated blanket and warmed fluids.
- **severe hypothermia: active core warming**
  ☐ inhalation: oxygen at 40°C – 45°C (104°F – 113°F) delivered via oxygen mask or ET tube
  ☐ infusion: IV fluids or blood products at 40°C – 42°C (104°F – 107.6°F)
  ☐ lavage: closed thoracic lavage through 2 thoracic tubes at 40°C – 45°C (104°F – 113°F)
  ☐ extracorporeal core rewarming (ECR): not often performed as it requires a specialist and prearranged protocol
- fluid resuscitation: 1 – 2 L (for adults) or 20 ml/kg (for pediatrics) of 0.9% saline solution heated to 40°C – 42°C (104°F – 107.6°F) via IV
- CPR for V-fib or asystole: defibrillation once body temperature > 30°C (86°F)

QUICK REVIEW QUESTIONS

10. A 22-year-old patient who fell asleep in the snow has been brought into the ED. The patient is lethargic, shivering, and has slurred speech. The patient's temperature is 91°F (32.7°C). What warming technique should the nurse perform first?

11. A patient is admitted to the ED. The patient fell through ice and was submerged in the water for 20 minutes. The patient is unresponsive and has been intubated. How would the nurse prepare oxygen for administration?

HELPFUL HINT:

It is better to apply the heat to the core of the body. Heat applied to extremities may increase metabolic demand, which can strain the depressed cardiovascular system.

HELPFUL HINT:

Afterdrop is a decrease in body temperature caused by the return of cooled blood from the extremities; it may be accompanied by a drop in blood pressure (rewarming shock). It can be minimized by rewarming the core before the extremities.

LOCAL COLD-RELATED EMERGENCIES

- **Frostbite** is injury to the dermis and underlying tissue due to cold. The exposure to cold leads to cellular damage, impairment of the vascular system, and an inflammatory response.
    - Symptoms (early stage): cold and white skin; numbness, tingling, or throbbing in affected area
    - Symptoms (mild stage): skin hard or frozen to the touch; skin red and blistered when warmed and thawed
    - Symptoms (severe stage): blue, blotchy, or white skin; black necrotic areas; blood-filled blisters as skin warms; damage to underlying tissue

- **Immersion foot** is an injury that results from prolonged exposure to a cold and wet environment of a limb that had little or no mobility. The limb will be numb, cold, pale, clammy, and swollen. Severe cases may present with ulcers, eschar, or muscle atrophy.

- Management of frostbite and immersion foot
    - ***rewarm affected area until it is red in color: warm water, heated to 104°F – 108°F (40°C – 42°C), in a basin or bath***
    - analgesics (pain during rewarming may be severe)
    - wound care as necessary, including debridement

- **Chilblains** is an inflammatory response that occurs in the skin and small blood vessels after repeated exposure to cold but not freezing temperatures. It is most common in women, underweight patients, and patients with Raynaud's disease.
    - Symptoms: red or purple bumps on the skin that can be painful or swollen; complaints of itchy feeling; blistering or ulceration (severe case)
    - Management: passive rewarming of affected area; topical corticosteroids; daily nifedipine for recurrent chilblains

QUICK REVIEW QUESTIONS

12. A patient presents to the ED complaining of both hands being numb. The nurse observes that the patient's hands are blue and establishes that the patient has been outside without gloves for several hours. What intervention should the nurse prepare for?

   _____

13. Why is rubbing or massage contraindicated to warm extremities with frostbite?

   _____

Heat-Related Injuries

- **Heat cramps** (exercise-associated muscle cramps) occur when exercise or physical exertion leads to a profuse loss of fluids and sodium through sweating. The resulting hyponatremia causes muscle cramps.
  - Diagnosis: sudden onset of severe spasmodic muscle cramps in extremities; may progress to carpopedal spasms, which can incapacitate the hands or the feet
  - Management: keep patient cool; oral fluids (solution of 1 L of water with 10 g of sodium or commercial sports drinks); IV fluids if patient cannot tolerate fluids by mouth (1 – 2 L of 0.9% saline solution); stretch the affected muscle (firm, passive stretching)

- **Heat exhaustion** occurs when the body is exposed to high temperatures, leading to dehydration. It is <u>not</u> a result of deficits in thermoregulation or the central nervous system.
  - Diagnosis: temperature elevated but < 104°F (40°C); diaphoresis; dizziness and weakness; tachycardia; hypertension; headache; nausea and vomiting; syncope
  - Management: cool with ice packs; oral fluids (solution of 1 L of water with 10 g of sodium or commercial sports drinks); IV fluids if patient cannot tolerate fluids by mouth (1 – 2 L of 0.9% saline solution)

- **Heat stroke** (classic or exertional) results when the compensatory measures for ridding the body of excess heat fail, leading to an increased core temperature. Complications can include rhabdomyolysis, DIC, and acute kidney injury.
  - Diagnosis: ***temperature > 104°F (40°C)***; tachycardia and tachypnea; confusion or delirium; seizures; labs show organ dysfunction
  - Management: ***cool rapidly with ice bath or ice packs*** to 102°F (38.9°C); aggressive fluid resuscitation; electrolytes as needed; management of complications (e.g., platelets, benzodiazepines)

HELPFUL HINT:

Antipyretics are not effective at reducing temperature during heat exhaustion/stroke and may worsen organ dysfunction.

QUICK REVIEW QUESTION

14. A 16-year-old male athlete collapsed during practice and was brought to the ED. His vital signs are as follows:

temperature	105.5°F
HR	120 bpm
RR	22 breaths per minute
BP	95/62 mm Hg

    What priority intervention should the nurse anticipate?

_____

Animal Bites

- The most common cause of **animal bites** are domesticated dogs and cats, but bites may also come from wild animals such as bats, raccoons, and skunks.
  - Animal bites can cause punctures, lacerations, fractures, and crush injuries.
  - Wounds caused by animal bites are also at high risk for infection.
- Management: wound care, antibiotics for high-risk bite wounds, immunizations as indicated
- High-risk bite wounds include: cat and human bites, bites to the hand or foot, puncture wounds, damage to deep structures, and wounds to immunocompromised patients
- **Rabies** is a virus that causes encephalitis. It is carried in the saliva of infected animals and is transmitted during animal bites.
  - Management of animal bite: clean wound with soap and water or BZK wipes; *__rabies vaccine and rabies immune globulin (RIG)__*; once rabies has advanced, there is no curative treatment
  - Diagnosis of rabies: fatigue; fever; headache; confusion; agitation; hallucinations; insomnia; excessive salivation; hydrophobia; ascending paralysis; positive fluorescence antibody test from biopsy of skin near the nape of neck

QUICK REVIEW QUESTION

15. What interventions should the nurse expect to provide for a patient with an open wound caused by a bat bite?

_____

ANSWER KEY

1. The expected urine output for adults who are receiving IV fluids per the Parkland formula is 0.5 – 1.0 mL/kg/hr.

2. The nurse should establish IV access and prepare for fluid resuscitation.

3. The patient likely has burns from cement, an alkali. The nurse should prepare to decontaminate the area by irrigating with water.

4. The total amount of internal damage cannot be judged based on external damage. Internal injury or organ dysfunction could still be present even when the patient has little to no external damage and is presenting asymptomatically.

5. The nurse should expect to administer an IV fluid bolus followed by a continuous rate.

6. Symptoms of a brown recluse spider bite include ecchymosis and erythema and a central blood-filled lesion that ruptures, leaving an ulcer.

7. Interventions for a coral snake bite include management of ABCs, close respiratory and neurological monitoring, and possible administration of antivenom.

8. The nurse should prepare the patient to be intubated.

9. The primary concern for patients with submersion injuries is the prevention of tissue damage due to hypoxemia.

10. The nurse should remove the patient's wet clothes and wrap the patient in an insulated blanket.

11. The oxygen needs to be heated to 40°C – 45°C (104°F – 113°F) before being administered to this patient.

12. The nurse should gather materials to immerse the patient's hands in warm water.

13. Rubbing or massaging extremities with frostbite may cause further damage to tissue.

14. The patient is hyperthermic and does not require immediate respiratory intervention. The priority intervention will be rapid cooling with an ice bath or ice packs.

15. The nurse should clean the wound with soap and water or BZK wipes and then administer rabies vaccine and rabies immune globulin.

19 TOXICOLOGY

Acids and Alkalis

Pathophysiology

Acids are compounds that release hydrogen ions and taste sour; **alkalis** are compounds that accept hydrogen ions and are slippery or soapy. On the pH scale (1 to 14), acids have a value lower than 7, alkalis have a value greater than 7, and 7 is neutral. Ingestion of acids and alkalis is most common in young children. Ingestion in adults is usually linked to severe mental illness or suicidal behaviors.

- Common household acids: swimming pool and toilet cleaners, battery acid, anti-rust cleaners
- Common household alkalis: common bleach, drain cleaner

  Ingestion of acids usually causes injuries to the upper respiratory tract as the pain and sour taste prompt gagging or spitting, which may lead to aspiration. The acid may also cause coagulative necrosis in the stomach. *Alkali ingestion will cause liquefactive necrosis in the esophagus and will continue to cause damage until it has been neutralized.*

Physical Examination

- drooling
- dysphagia

- excessive thirst
- visible oral burns
- GI pain
- emesis (can appear brown)
- bleeding in mouth, throat, or stomach
- signs and symptoms of esophageal perforation
- stridor or dyspnea

Diagnostic Tests

- upper GI endoscopy to evaluate damage

HELPFUL HINT:

An endoscopy is usually performed on asymptomatic patients if they have ingested acids or alkalis to assess for damage in the GI tract.

Management

- manage airway; intubation for patients with severe oropharyngeal edema or necrosis
- supportive care for symptoms: analgesics, IV fluids
- contraindicated treatments include
  - gastric emptying by emesis
  - activated charcoal
  - neutralizing agents
  - gastric lavage
  - nasogastric tube
- immediate surgery for perforation or necrosis

QUICK REVIEW QUESTION

1. A 15-year-old patient is brought to the ED by her mother, who states that the patient mistook a bottle of ammonia for lemonade and drank it. The mother is very upset that the emergency room staff is not trying to make the patient throw it back up to get it out of her system. How do you explain this action to the patient's mother?

★ # Carbon Monoxide

Pathophysiology

Carbon monoxide (CO) displaces oxygen from hemoglobin, which prevents the transport and utilization of oxygen throughout the body. Mild **CO poisoning** can be resolved in the ED; severe CO poisoning can lead to myocardial ischemia, dysrhythmias, pulmonary edema, and coma. Sources of CO include smoke from fires, malfunctioning heaters and generators, and motor vehicle exhaust. CO poisoning and cyanide poisoning often occur together.

Physical Examination

- headache
- altered LOC or confusion
- dizziness
- visual disturbances
- dyspnea on exertion
- nausea and vomiting
- muscle weakness and cramps
- syncope, seizure, or coma

Diagnostic Tests

- _CO-oximetery: normal range is <3% (<12% for smokers)_

Management

- _100% oxygen through non-rebreather_
- hyperbaric oxygen may be used to treat patients with
  - □ carboxyhemoglobin level greater than 25%
  - □ cardiopulmonary complications
  - □ loss of consciousness
  - □ severe metabolic acidosis

HELPFUL HINT:

Pulse oximeters do not differentiate between oxyhemoglobin and carboxyhemoglobin, so patients with CO poisoning will often have normal pulse oximetry readings.

QUICK REVIEW QUESTION

2. For patients with CO poisoning, what carboxyhemoglobin level indicates a need for hyperbaric oxygen?

Cyanide

Pathophysiology

Cyanide interferes with the production of ATP in mitochondria. **Cyanide poisoning** is rare but usually fatal without medical intervention. Sources of cyanide include smoke from fires, medications (e.g., sodium nitroprusside), and pits/seeds from the family Rosaceae (which includes bitter almonds, apricots, peaches, and apples).

Physical Examination

- bitter almond smell on breath
- anxiety or agitation
- headache
- confusion
- bloody emesis
- diarrhea
- flushed, red skin
- tachycardia and tachypnea
- hypertension

Management

- decontaminate patient
- 100% oxygen through a non-rebreather; intubation usually required
- IV fluids
- activated charcoal if airway is not compromised
- *cyanide antidotes include: **hydroxocobalamin, amyl nitrite, sodium nitrite, and sodium thiosulfate***

QUICK REVIEW QUESTION

3. A patient presents to the ED with nonspecific symptoms, including confusion, headache, and vomiting. What situations in a patient's history should alert the ED nurse to the possibility of cyanide poisoning?

ANSWER KEY

1. Inducing vomiting is contraindicated when a patient ingests a caustic agent. Causing regurgitation will re-expose the upper GI tract to the caustic agent.

2. A carboxyhemoglobin level greater than 25% indicates a need for hyperbaric oxygen.

3. Nurses should consider cyanide toxicity when patients present to the ED after being around a fire: inhaled fumes from burning polymer products such as vinyl and polyurethane will produce cyanide poisoning. Cyanide toxicity can also be caused by a nitroprusside IV infusion.

20 COMMUNICABLE DISEASES

Isolation Precautions

Isolation precautions are used to prevent the spread of infection. The precautions are guidelines set by organizations like the World Health Organization (WHO) and the Centers for Disease Control (CDC) to prevent the transmission of microorganisms that are responsible for causing infection. There are two tiers of isolation precautions: the first tier is standard precautions, and the second tier consists of three transmission precautions (airborne, droplet, and contact).

Standard Precautions

- Assume that all patients are carrying an infectious microorganism.
- Practice hand hygiene.
  - Use soap and water when hands are visibly soiled.
  - Use antimicrobial foam or gel if hands are not visibly soiled.

HELPFUL HINT:

Antimicrobial foams and gels are not effective against some infectious agents, such as *C. difficile*.

- Wear gloves.
  - Gloves must be discarded between each patient visit.
  - Gloves may need to be discarded when soiled and a new pair donned.
  - Practice hand hygiene after removing gloves.
- Prevent needle sticks.
  - Immediately place used needles in puncture-resistant containers.
  - Recap using mechanical device or one-handed technique.
- Avoid splash and spray: wear appropriate PPE if there is a possibility of body fluids splashing or spraying.

Airborne Precautions

- Patient should be placed in a private room with a negative-pressure air system and the door kept closed.
- Wear N-95 respirator mask: put it on before entering the room, and keep it on until after leaving the room.
- Place N-95 or surgical mask on patient during transport.
- Examples of diseases requiring airborne precautions include chicken pox, measles, and tuberculosis. The precautions are also used for COVID-19 patients undergoing aerosol-generating procedures (e.g., intubation).

Droplet Precautions

- Place patient in a private room; the door may remain open.
- Wear appropriate PPE within 3 feet of patient.
- Wash hands with antimicrobial soap after removing gloves and mask, before leaving the patient's room.
- Place surgical mask on patient during transport.
- Examples of diseases requiring droplet precautions include influenza, pertussis, and COVID-19.

Contact Precautions

- Place the patient in a private room; the door may remain open.
- Wear gloves.
  - Change gloves after touching infected materials.
  - Remove gloves before leaving patient's room.

- Wear gown; remove before leaving patient's room.

- Use patient-dedicated equipment if possible; community equipment is to be used clean and disinfected between patients.

- During transport, keep precautions in place and notify different areas as needed.

- Examples of diseases requiring contact precautions include C. *difficile*, MRSA, and noroviruses.

QUICK REVIEW QUESTION

1. The nurse is assigned to a patient who has a positive diagnosis of measles. What PPE should the nurse wear?

C. Difficile

Pathophysiology

Clostridium difficile (commonly called **C. diff**) is an acute bacterial infection in the intestine most commonly seen after antibiotic use. The antibiotics disrupt the normal intestinal flora, allowing the antibiotic-resistant C. *diff* spores to proliferate in the intestines. The bacterium releases a toxin that causes the intestine to produce yellow-white plaques on the intestinal lining. The C. *diff* infection can produce inflammation in the intestines, resulting in toxic colitis (toxic megacolon) or pseudomembranous colitis, and may also lead to perforation and sepsis.

HELPFUL HINT:

Proton inhibitors and H2 blockers have both been shown to be risk factors for C. *diff* infection.

Transmission and Precautions

- fecal to oral transmission

- use contact precautions

- do not use foams and gels (they will not kill the spores)

- environmental cleanse of a 1:10 bleach-to-water solution

Physical Examination

- foul-smelling diarrhea 5 – 10 days after start of antibiotic

- signs and symptoms of toxic colitis: tenesmus, rectal bleeding, abdominal distension and tenderness

Diagnostic Tests

- enzyme immunoassay (EIA): most commonly run diagnostic test
- PCR test on the stool specimen: most sensitive and specific diagnostic test

Management

- antibiotic-induced *C. diff*: stop current use of antibiotics if possible
- oral antibiotics; IV if oral antibiotics cannot be tolerated
  - □ vancomycin (Vancocin)
  - □ fidaxomicin (Dificid)
  - □ metronidazole (Flagyl)

QUICK REVIEW QUESTION

2. A patient is admitted to the ED with a suspected *C. difficile* infection. What PPE should the nurse use?

Vaccine-Preventable Diseases

CHICKEN POX

Pathophysiology

Chicken pox (varicella zoster virus) is a viral infection that infects the conjunctiva or the mucous membranes of the upper respiratory tract. The infection then spreads, causing the hallmark rash of small, itchy, fluid-filled blisters all over the body.

Transmissions and Precautions

- person to person through direct contact or airborne droplets
- airborne, droplet, and contact precautions

Physical Examination

- itchy rash that forms small fluid-filled blisters that eventually scab
- mild headache
- moderate fever
- fatigue

Diagnostic Tests

- varicella titer test on a blood sample
- Tzanck test performed on a swab sample of the lesion area

Management

- supportive care for symptoms (systemic antihistamines, colloidal oatmeal baths)
- antivirals in severe cases

QUICK REVIEW QUESTION

3. The nurse is preparing to discharge a 2-year-old patient diagnosed with chicken pox. What information about OTC medications should the nurse include in his teaching?

HELPFUL HINT:

Children with viral infections should not be given aspirin: it increases these children's risk of developing Reye's syndrome, a life-threatening encephalopathy linked to viral infections and aspirin use.

DIPHTHERIA

Pathophysiology

Diphtheria is an infection caused by the bacterium *Corynebacterium diphtheriae*. The bacterium enters through the pharynx or the skin and releases a toxin that causes inflammation and necrosis.

Transmissions and Precautions

- person to person through respiratory droplets (pharyngeal infection)
- person to person skin contact (skin infection)
- droplet, contact precautions

Physical Examination

- white or gray glossy exudate in the back of the throat
- mild sore throat and hoarseness
- serosanguinous or purulent discharge
- difficulty swallowing or getting food stuck in throat
- visibly swollen neck (bull neck)
- stridor

- low-grade fever
- skin infection: non-specific symptoms

Diagnostic Tests

- positive culture from swab

Management

- diphtheria antitoxin (IM or IV)
- antibiotics (penicillin, erythromycin)
- clean skin infection with soap and water
- diphtheria vaccination after recovery

QUICK REVIEW QUESTION

4. The nurse is discharging a 4-year-old patient diagnosed with diphtheria. What instructions should she provide to the parents about vaccinations?

MEASLES
Pathophysiology

Measles is an acute, highly contagious infection caused by a paramyxovirus. The virus enters through the upper respiratory tract or conjunctiva and spreads systemically through the lymph nodes, triggering a systemic inflammatory response. Infants, elderly patients, and immunocompromised patients are more likely to experience serious complications such as pneumonia and encephalitis.

Transmissions and Precautions

- person to person through respiratory droplets that can live in the air or on hard surfaces for up to 2 hours
- airborne, droplet, and contact precautions

Physical Examination

- fever
- cough
- runny nose and conjunctivitis
- sore throat

- Koplik spots
- red, blotchy rash (usually starts on the face and spreads cephalocaudally)

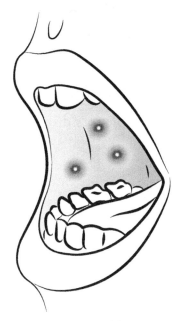

Figure 20.1. Koplik Spots

Diagnostic Tests

- positive PCR or serum measles IgM antibody

Management

- vitamin A
- antivirals (ribavirin) for high-risk patients
- supportive care for symptoms
- prophylaxis for high-risk contacts (MMR vaccine or immune globulin)

QUICK REVIEW QUESTION

5. A 3-year-old patient presents to the ED with a fever and cough. What other physical findings should lead the nurse to suspect measles?

Mumps
Pathophysiology

Mumps is an acute infection caused by a paramyxovirus. The virus causes an inflammatory response that results in swelling of the salivary glands (usually the parotid glands). Possible complications include epididymo-orchitis, meningitis, encephalitis, and hearing loss.

Transmissions and Precautions

- person to person through respiratory droplets in close proximity
- droplet precautions

Physical Examination

- fever
- salivary gland edema
- parotitis
- pain when chewing or swallowing
- swelling in submandibular glands or tongue

Diagnostic Tests

- positive serum IgM or PCR

Management

- supportive care for symptoms (acetaminophen, warm/cold packs for swelling)

QUICK REVIEW QUESTION

6. A nurse is assessing a patient and notes a temperature of 102°F (38.9°C) and swelling in the patient's neck under the jawline. The patient also reports that their throat burned this morning when they drank their orange juice. Which diagnostic test should the nurse anticipate will be ordered?

Pertussis
Pathophysiology

Pertussis (whooping cough) is an infection caused by the bacterium *Bordetella pertussis* that causes a mucopurulent sanguineous exudate that can compromise the respiratory tract.

Transmissions and Precautions

- person to person through respiratory droplets in close proximity
- droplet precautions

Physical Examination

- paroxysmal or spasmodic cough ("whoop") that ends in a prolonged, high-pitched inspiration

Diagnostic Tests

- PCR on nasal or throat swab

Management

- antibiotics (erythromycin, azithromycin)
- supportive care for symptoms, including suctioning

QUICK REVIEW QUESTION

7. A mother brings her 2-year-old into the ED with complaints of a persistent cough and hoarseness. What tests should the nurse anticipate to determine if the child has pertussis?

Influenza

Pathophysiology

Influenza (flu) is a group of contagious viruses that cause respiratory symptoms and fever. Four types of human influenza viruses have been identified (A, B, C, and D); only types A and B cause severe illness in people. Flu is a common seasonal illness that tends to be more widespread during the fall and winter. However, infection may occur at any time of the year.

Symptoms of flu typically appear suddenly and can range from mild to life-threatening. For most people, flu is a self-limiting infection that does not require emergent care. High-risk patients may develop severe complications, including pneumonia, sepsis, myositis, seizure, and encephalopathy. Risk factors for severe flu complications include:

- age of < 2 years or > 65 years
- being immunocompromised
- pregnancy
- asthma or chronic lung disease

- diabetes
- obesity
- heart, liver, kidney, or metabolic disorders

Transmissions and Precautions

- transmission through mucous membrane contact and respiratory droplets
- contact and droplet precautions

Physical Examination

- fever
- headache
- myalgia
- nonproductive cough
- sore throat
- nausea and vomiting

Diagnostic Tests

- rapid influenza diagnostic test or molecular assay (more reliable)

Management

- pharmacological management of symptoms
  - □ antipyretics
  - □ cough suppressant
  - □ antiemetics
- antiviral drugs administered to high-risk patients and patients with symptom onset of < 48 hours previous

TABLE 20.1. Antiviral Treatments for Flu

Drug	Notes
Oseltamivir	recommended for ages 2 years and older may cause nausea and vomiting
Zanamivir	for ages 7 and older risk of bronchospasm
Peramivir	approved for ages 2 and older may cause diarrhea
Baloxavir	for ages 12 and older

- monitor for and manage complications
- isolate until symptoms resolve or at least 24 hours after fever has gone

QUICK REVIEW QUESTION

8. A 54-year-old woman with COPD arrives at the ED with a fever, dyspnea, a productive cough, and a general feeling of malaise. A rapid influenza test is positive. What antiviral drug would be contraindicated for this patient?

Multi-Drug Resistant Organisms

- **Methicillin-resistant *Staphylococcus aureus* (MRSA)** is a bacterial infection caused by a strain of *Staphylococcus* ("staph") that is resistant to many of the antibiotics normally used to treat staph infections, including the beta-lactam agents ampicillin, amoxicillin, methicillin, penicillin, and cephalosporin.
  - ☐ Diagnosis: red area on the skin; swelling; pain; warm to the touch; pus or drainage from bumps on skin; fever; positive culture of MRSA bacterium
  - ☐ Management: antibiotics (trimethoprim, sulfamethoxazole, clindamycin linezolid)

- **Vancomycin-resistant enterococci (VRE)** is a bacterial infection caused by strains of enterococci bacteria that are resistant to vancomycin.
  - ☐ Diagnosis: s/s of wound infection, pneumonia, UTI, meningitis, or sepsis; culture and sensitivity
  - ☐ Management (general): antibiotics (amoxicillin, ampicillin, gentamicin, penicillin, piperacillin, streptomycin)
  - ☐ Management (skin infections): daptomycin, linezolid, tedizolid, tigecycline
  - ☐ Management (intra-abdominal infections): piperacillin-tazobactam, imipenem, meropenem

HELPFUL HINT:

Alcohol-based wipes are not sufficient to kill the bacteria that cause VRE on equipment and hard surfaces. Germicidal wipes should be used instead.

QUICK REVIEW QUESTION

9. Which antibiotics should NOT be used to treat patients with methicillin-resistant *Staphylococcus aureus* (MRSA)?

Tuberculosis

Pathophysiology

Tuberculosis (TB) is a chronic, progressive bacterial infection of the lungs. There is an initial asymptomatic infection followed by a period of latency that may develop into active disease. Active TB produces granulomatous necrosis, more commonly known as lesions. The rupturing of the lesions in the pleural space can cause empyema, bronchopleural fistulas, or a pneumothorax.

Transmission and Precautions

- person to person through respiratory droplets
- airborne precautions

Physical Examination

- prolonged productive cough
- fever and fatigue
- night sweats
- hemoptysis
- dyspnea

Diagnostic Tests

HELPFUL HINT:

TB skin tests do not distinguish latent TB infection from active TB disease.

- TB skin test (Mantoux skin test)
- CXR showing multinodular infiltrate near the clavicle

Management

- supportive treatment for symptoms
- 2 months of treatment with: isoniazid (INH), rifampin (RIF), pyrazinamide (PZA), ethambutol (EMB)
- after 2 months of treatment, PZA and EMB discontinued after 2 months; INH and RIF continue for another 4 – 7 months

QUICK REVIEW QUESTION

10. A patient in the ED complains of a cough that has lasted for several weeks and also states that they have been waking up at night covered in sweat. Which diagnostic test should the nurse prepare for?

Hemorrhagic Fevers

Pathophysiology

Viral hemorrhagic fevers (VHFs) are caused by several distinct groups of RNA viruses with the potential to cause severe, emergent disease. Hemorrhagic fevers are rare in the US and are usually diagnosed in travelers returning from areas where the viruses are endemic. Symptoms will develop within 1 to 3 weeks of exposure.

TABLE 20.2. Geographic Range of Hemorrhagic Fevers	
Virus	**Endemic in**
Crimean-Congo Hemorrhagic Fever (CCHF)	sub-Saharan Africa, the Middle East, Eastern Europe, Central Asia, and the Balkans
Dengue Fever	Central and South America, India, and Southeast Asia
Ebola	sub-Saharan Africa
Lassa	West Africa
Marburg	sub-Saharan Africa
Yellow Fever	tropical areas of Africa and South America

Transmission and Precautions

- person-to-person transmission through contact with bodily fluids or mucous membranes
- patients with suspected VHF infection should be isolated
- PPE: gown, mask, face shield, and gloves required

Physical Examination

- most common presentation
  - high fever
  - myalgia
  - abdominal pain
  - vomiting or diarrhea
  - bleeding or hemorrhage
- hantavirus pulmonary syndrome (HPS): abrupt-onset VHF symptoms followed by respiratory distress
- hemorrhagic fever with renal syndrome (HFRS)

- early symptoms include facial flushing, eye irritation and redness and petechiae rash
- late symptoms are hypovolemic shock and acute kidney failure that causes extreme fluid overload

Management

- treatment for VHFs is supportive (e.g., antipyretics, fluid replacement)
- no antiviral treatment is available for most VHFs

QUICK REVIEW QUESTION

11. A patient with a known exposure to hantavirus is being monitored. The patient states that their eyes feel grainy. What complication should the nurse be concerned about?

ANSWER KEY

1. The nurse should use gloves and an N-95 respirator.

2. *C. difficile* requires contact protections, so the nurse should use gloves and an isolation gown.

3. The nurse should tell the parents not to give aspirin to a child with chicken pox. Aspirin increases these children's risk of developing Reye's syndrome, a life-threatening encephalopathy linked to viral infections and aspirin use.

4. The patient will need to be given the diphtheria vaccine once he has recovered. The parents should make sure that anyone who comes in close contact with the child also has an up-to-date diphtheria vaccine.

5. Conjunctivitis, Koplik spots, and a red, blotchy rash on the face are all signs of measles.

6. The nurse should anticipate drawing a blood sample for lab testing to confirm mumps.

7. The diagnostic tests for pertussis include nasopharyngeal culture and PCR testing. The PCR test is preferred because it is the most sensitive.

8. Zanamivir is not recommended for patients with respiratory issues, due to the side effect of bronchospasm.

9. MRSA is resistant to beta-lactam agents, including ampicillin, amoxicillin, methicillin, penicillin, and cephalosporin.

10. The nurse should prepare the patient for a chest X-ray to confirm tuberculosis.

11. Hemorrhagic fever with renal syndrome is a serious, emergent complication that can develop early and present as red, irritated eyes; flushing of the face; and development of rash from petechiae and purpura.

21 PROFESSIONAL ISSUES

BCEN OUTLINE: PROFESSIONAL ISSUES

- Nurse
- Patient
- System

Nurse

IMPAIRED NURSE AND DRUG DIVERSION

Drug diversion is the abuse or unlawful distribution of prescription medication. Addiction is the most common reason nurses divert drugs, but medications may also be diverted for sale or use by others. Common categories of diverted drugs include opioids, benzodiazepines, antipsychotics, and amphetamines. Drug diversion usually occurs via one of the following methods:

- taking unused medications (particularly by ordering excessive PRN drugs)
- not administering drugs to patients or administering a substitute

Drug diversion presents a threat to patient safety. Using drugs at work may impair the nurse's job performance, and patient comfort and health are at risk if drugs are not administered properly.

Nurses should follow facility policy for reporting suspected drug diversion and impaired nurses. Management is obligated by law to report drug and alcohol abuse to the state board of nursing; in most states, they are also obligated to report to local law enforcement. Most states offer protection and rehabilitation for nurses that self-report drug and alcohol abuse.

HELPFUL HINT:

Always follow the chain of command to report a nurse who appears to be impaired.

QUICK REVIEW QUESTION

1. A nurse notes that her coworker has slurred speech, smells of alcohol, and keeps falling asleep. She asks him if he is feeling ill. He responds that he is just tired and offers to pass medications to both of their patients so that he can "get up and move around." What should the nurse do in this situation?

Workplace Violence

According to OSHA, **workplace violence** includes both threats and acts of physical or mental abuse during working hours or within the health care facility. Workplace violence may include harassment, intimidation, and threatening disruptive behavior.

Violence includes behaviors like verbal assault and physical striking. Even if no injury results from such behaviors, they are still considered violent.

Workplace violence is not limited to onsite workers. Patients, visitors, vendors, or any other individual or group that is connected with the facility can be the perpetrators or victims of workplace violence.

Workplace violence can sometimes be prevented before it starts. Some guidelines for **prevention** include:

- Read and understand the facility's workplace violence policies and procedures.
- Participate in training and education on violence awareness.
- Immediately report any suspected or known workplace violence.
- Do not accept workplace violence as a normal occurrence in the health care environment: develop zero-tolerance policies.
- Be aware of exits, emergency phone numbers, and unit safe rooms.
- Use screening tools to identify violent behaviors early on.

Sometimes workplace violence cannot be avoided. Still, **de-escalation** methods to decrease the likelihood of severe violence may be used in some situations.

- A potentially violent individual typically exhibits five types of behaviors:
    1. anxiety
    2. defensiveness
    3. verbal threats
    4. physical threats
    5. assault

- Early intervention may be possible for an individual exhibiting anxiety and/or defensiveness.
- De-escalation tactics for individuals demonstrating anxiety and defensiveness include:
  - using nonjudgmental and empathetic language
  - keeping a safe distance from the patient
  - discussing feelings
  - setting limits and expectations for appropriate behavior
  - allowing the patient time for quiet reflection and to make decisions

If the nurse feels unsafe or threatened, or if a person's behavior has escalated to verbal threats, the nurse should call for help per facility policies (e.g., code gray, behavioral alert). This indicates a violent or dangerous situation and alerts security and coworkers.

Any experienced or witnessed incident of violence or threat of violence must be **reported** to management.

- Report violent incidents to local authorities per state laws.
- Offer support to coworkers to create a culture that encourages voluntary reporting.

QUICK REVIEW QUESTION

2. A patient's family member has been insulting and berating a new nurse. The nurse reports this incident to his manager. What steps should the nurse manager take?

_____

STRESS MANAGEMENT

ED nurses work in a high-stress environment and are exposed to many difficult and emotionally disturbing situations.

- **Compassion fatigue** occurs with repeated exposure to situations involving traumatized, vulnerable, or distressed individuals. The caregiver may feel pain, distress, and suffering similar to what the patient is exhibiting.
- **Moral distress** is when the nurse's personal beliefs, morals, and perceived obligations clash with the ethical duties they encounter while caring for others.
- Both compassion fatigue and moral distress can lead to depression, fatigue, burnout, and post-traumatic stress disorder.
- Potential triggers of compassion fatigue and moral distress include:
  - end-of-life care
  - futile care

- inappropriate uses of staffing and supply resources
- inadequate pain relief
- false hope
- communications that give false hope

- Working in the fast-paced environment of the ED exacerbates compassion fatigue and moral distress due to many factors:
  - inadequate staffing
  - working overtime
  - high-stress situations
  - influxes of patients

Nurses often express concern that patients do not receive appropriate or adequate care. Furthermore, not knowing the patient's outcome once they are admitted to the facility or discharged can lead to unresolved questions and stress.

- **Symptoms** of stress include:
  - sleep disturbances
  - emotional unbalance
  - difficulty making decisions
  - self-isolation
  - emotional and physical fatigue, lethargy
  - lack of interest in previous hobbies and enjoyable activities
  - impulsive behaviors
  - alcohol and drug abuse
  - blaming self and others

The nurse can take personal steps to manage stress. Similarly, the health care facility may implement systemic changes for **stress management**.

- Personal methods of stress management include:
  - discuss feelings with others
  - seek assistance, if needed (psychiatric, psychological, counseling)
  - participate in regular exercise
  - manage stress with healthy behaviors

- Systemic methods of stress management include:
  - implement healthy work environment initiatives
  - consult the ethics committee for guidance and advice when encountering moral distress situations
  - Management may consider increasing staff during busy times, rotating staff to ensure breaks are taken, and staff debriefings after code situations.

Just Culture

Just Culture refers to an environment of shared responsibility. Its purpose is to:

- determine the systematic reasons for undesirable events
- adjust systems to promote safety

Rather than blaming an individual for a systems error, the organization seeks to improve the system to prevent the error from reoccurring and to improve quality and patient safety.

- Employees can report safety concerns in a nonpunitive way and even anonymously.
- All employees, management, and administration can access a computer reporting system.
    - Reports, often called **variances**, may be logged under the employee's name or ID, or completed anonymously.
- Staff are encouraged to report:
    - errors
    - complications
    - sentinel events
    - safety concerns
- When completing a variance, employees must answer questions about the event, including:
    - time
    - place
    - staff involved
    - whether a patient was affected
    - a description of what occurred
- Variances are then automatically sent to the involved managers for review. The review process generally involves departments beyond the home unit.

Patient

DISCHARGE PLANNING

- In the ED, **discharge planning** generally involves arranging for follow-up care either with primary care services or specialty care consultations.
    - Patients discharged from the ED are considered stable and should not require extensive discharge planning services.
- **Care coordination** is the organization of patient care activities between two medical entities (ED and primary care, community care, etc.).
    - Effective care coordination can help prevent overreliance on ED and urgent care settings.
- Depending on the patient's diagnosis, discharge planning is effective in the early stages if patients are being admitted to the facility.
- The ED nurse should report to the unit nurse any social or economic concerns that may impact a patient's care:
    - lack of insurance
    - homelessness
    - living alone
- Patients with new diagnoses (like MI, CHF, COPD) should receive educational pamphlets that describe the disease, treatment, and prognosis to the patient and family.

    When concerns of patient care beyond the facility are expected, consultations to rehabilitation, dietary, social services, and other specialty services are better facilitated early on.

- The ED nurse should consider potential consultation needs and query providers for orders as soon as possible.

HELPFUL HINT:

Emergency nurses can offer community resources to patients who are experiencing homelessness or who otherwise require assistance, but these needs should not prevent an otherwise healthy patient from being discharged.

PALLIATIVE CARE

Palliative care is for patients whose serious illness limits their daily lives. Palliative care focuses on improving patients' quality of life and alleviating their pain and symptoms. It can be administered at any age and phase of a disease and may last the duration of the patient's life.

- The conditions with the highest rates of palliative care include:
    - cardiovascular disease
    - cancer
    - chronic respiratory diseases
    - AIDS
    - diabetes
- Unlike hospice care, active treatment may continue in palliative care.
- Palliative care may be initiated for people at any age and at any stage of a chronic, severe disease or illness.

The palliative care team is multidisciplinary and applies a holistic approach to manage the physical, mental, emotional, social, and spiritual needs of the patient.

- Palliative care may include any intervention that promotes an improved quality of life based on patient presentation. It is aimed at alleviating or improving:
    - pain
    - depression and anxiety
    - dyspnea
    - nausea/vomiting
    - nutritional intake
    - ROM and mobility
    - social support (e.g., group therapy)

QUICK REVIEW QUESTION

6. A 32-year-old patient receiving dialysis has unmanageable pain that is affecting her ability to perform ADLs and to fully participate in her child's life. The nurse asks if the patient has considered palliative care. The patient replies, "I am too young and not ready to die yet." What should the nurse explain to the patient?

_____

PATIENT SAFETY

The ED is a high-risk environment. Special considerations and skills are needed to ensure that patients and staff remain safe and to treat and prevent emergent conditions. Following safety protocols and national guidelines prevents some of the most common patient safety concerns.

Potential **patient safety** issues in the ED include patient falls, medication errors, and the safety of moderately ill patients in waiting rooms.

- **Preventing falls** in the ED is a difficult endeavor due to the chaotic and fast-paced nature of the environment. Communication with the patient, provision of call lights, nonslip footwear, and hourly rounding are good ways to mitigate the risk of patient falls. Bed and chair alarms should be used when appropriate.

- **Medication errors** in emergency situations or resuscitation efforts are more likely to occur in the ED. Drills and practice in these situations allow the nurse to be confident and efficient in administering emergency drugs. Use facility safety checks and barcode medication administration per protocol.

- ED **overcrowding** can lead to poor patient outcomes in the waiting room before a patient can be seen. Hourly rounding and reassessment of patients can prevent deterioration or waiting room deaths.

- Follow **SBAR** recommendations to ensure that adequate and appropriate handoffs are given during shift change and when the patient is admitted to the facility.

- Develop protocols to enhance patient safety by:
  - enforcing standing orders for time-sensitive conditions that require urgent treatment (e.g., stat ECG for chest pain)
  - decreasing time to treat
  - initiating testing and treatment early on
  - creating a safety checklist
  - using translation services when language barriers are identified
  - ensuring staffing matrix is sufficient for patient load
  - starting sepsis protocol while the patient is in the ED

QUICK REVIEW QUESTION

7. A family member approaches the ED nurse to ask when their husband will be seen. The patient came to the department for dizziness and nausea; now he is complaining of chest pain. What safety initiative would be most appropriate for this patient?

TRANSITION OF CARE

Transition of care is the process of moving patients from one care setting to another. Key considerations for transition of care include:

- accessibility of services
- information sharing and communication

- community partnerships
- care coordination
- health care utilization and costs
- safety

SBAR (**S**ituation, **B**ackground, **A**ssessment, and **R**ecommendation) handoff is a reporting tool used during shift change, when a patient is being admitted, or when an acute change in the patient's condition needs to be communicated to the care team.

- **S**ituation: nurse's name, patient's name and location, any current problems
- **B**ackground: diagnosis, history, and current care plan
- **A**ssessment: relevant vital signs and diagnostic testing
- **R**ecommendation: recommendations for further testing, changes to care plan, or transfers

QUICK REVIEW QUESTION

8. EMS is en route with a patient who has dyspnea and a cardiac history of A-fib. ETA is 15 minutes. Vital signs include BP 102/65, HR 165, and a temperature of 102.6°F. Initially, the patient was emergently treated for SVT and administered adenosine, with no effect. The family stated the patient has had a productive cough for the past week and a headache. What other important information should be shared before arrival at the ED?

ABUSE AND NEGLECT

Abuse is the intentional infliction of injury on another person. **Neglect** occurs when a person fails to meet the needs of a someone in their care; this may be a child, an elderly person, or a person with disabilities.

Child abuse and neglect, intimate partner violence, and **elder neglect** may lead victims to seek acute care. Nurses must be able to recognize the signs of abuse and neglect during assessment. These include:

- bruises, lacerations, burns, or fractures
- injuries inconsistent with the provided history
- patient anxiety around caregivers or partners
- patients expressing concerns about confidentiality
- caregivers or partners who stay very close to the patient or interfere with care

There are laws to protect vulnerable populations unable to protect themselves or adequately meet their own essential needs. Covered entities

HELPFUL HINT:

The **Child Abuse Prevention and Treatment Act** mandates the reporting of cases of child abuse. Failure to report suspected cases of child abuse could result in a misdemeanor.

are required to report known or suspected cases of child (under 18) or elder (over 60) abuse or neglect to social services or another agency designated to handle this issue.

Most states also have laws protecting individuals aged 18 – 59 with known disabilities that prevent them from caring for or protecting themselves. The offenses that must be reported include physical, emotional, psychological, financial, and sexual abuse or exploitation; neglect; and abandonment.

The requirements for reporting intimate partner violence vary from state to state. While it is mandatory for health care providers to report suspected cases to the police, the specifications of who is a mandatory reporter and what must be reported vary.

When signs of abuse or neglect are seen, the ED nurse should follow the facility's reporting policy.

QUICK REVIEW QUESTION

9. A parent brings a 3-year-old child with a broken arm to the ED. While assessing the patient, the nurse notices bruising in various stages of healing on the child's upper body. The parent says the child is clumsy and fell off a swing. What action should the nurse take next?

HUMAN TRAFFICKING

Human trafficking is the illegal exploitation of human beings for monetary or sexual gain. According to the US Department of Homeland Security, trafficking in persons means using "force, fraud, or coercion to obtain some type of labor or commercial sex act." The main types of human trafficking are forced labor, domestic servitude, and commercial sex acts. Human trafficking is against the law.

Sex trafficking includes inducing people to perform commercial sexual acts. If the victim is under 18, no force or coercion need be used for the act to be considered trafficking. Forced labor includes the recruitment, harboring, transportation, provision, or obtaining of a person for labor or services. Traffickers use force, fraud, or coercion to subject people to involuntary servitude, peonage, debt bondage, or slavery.

- Certain conditions may make an individual more vulnerable to becoming a trafficking victim:
  - □ poverty
  - □ lack of education
  - □ living in a rural location
  - □ being a migratory worker
  - □ belonging to an indigenous tribe

- belonging to the LGBTQ community
- lack of social support system, especially among girls aged 12 – 16
- disability
- history of abuse

- Nurses should be alert to **signs** of human trafficking, including:
  - bruising, cuts, burns, and other evidence of unexplained injuries
  - depression and anxiety
  - suicidal thoughts and self-harm behavior
  - flat affect
  - PTSD
  - alcohol and drug abuse
  - answers to health questions that do not make sense or seem scripted
  - fearful behavior with lack of eye contact

  Any signs or suspicions of abuse of elders, minors, or incompetent individuals should be reported per state law and hospital policy.

- If patients are in immediate or emergent danger, contact law enforcement per facility policy.

- If a patient discloses that they are being trafficked:
  - The nurse should inform their supervisor.
  - The patient should be encouraged to contact the National Human Trafficking Resource Center (NHTRC) hotline at 1-888-373-7888 and be given privacy to do so.

- Document all information in cases of suspected trafficking.

QUICK REVIEW QUESTION

10. A 63-year-old woman is brought to the ED for a laceration and large bruise on her left leg. The patient is accompanied by her employer. The patient does not speak English well. Both the employer and the patient state that the patient fell on the stairs while cleaning. The nurse requests privacy to assess the patient. The patient discloses that the employer keeps her as a maid without pay. What should the nurse do?

System
DELEGATION OF TASKS TO ASSISTIVE PERSONNEL

Delegation means empowering another person with responsibility to take an action. Certain tasks in the ED may be delegated to assistive personnel, depending on their scope of practice.

Local organizational policies, state nurse practice acts, and professional association practice guidelines all govern delegation of tasks in the health care setting.

Registered nurses in the ED may delegate tasks to the following licensed personnel:

- paramedics and EMTs working in the ED
- LPNs/LVNs
- medical assistants
- nursing assistants
- technicians

Tasks must be delegated under the following conditions:

- The nurse ultimately remains responsible for the completion of the task and its outcome.
- Delegation should account for the scope of practice and, to the extent possible, the skills and abilities of the individual to whom the task is delegated.

QUICK REVIEW QUESTION

11. When is it NOT appropriate for a nurse to delegate a task to licensed personnel?

DISASTER MANAGEMENT AND MASS CASUALTY

Disaster management in the context of emergency nursing includes considerations for mass casualty incidents, natural disasters, pandemic/epidemic illness, and decontamination of patients. **Disaster preparedness** is usually managed in the form of large-scale drills or tabletop exercises to determine how to mitigate weaknesses and identify needs in disaster management plans.

Many organizations use the **incident command system (ICS)** promoted by FEMA to manage disaster situations. Each role in the ICS is preassigned and drilled in preparation for disaster events. Organizations may customize the hierarchy below the general staff to fit the needs of their own system.

The following are four steps to disaster management and preparedness.

- Mitigation: Identify vulnerabilities to threats or weaknesses in current plans.
- Preparedness: Develop mutual aid agreements, create disaster management plans, determine supply thresholds and needs, consider stockpiles, and establish a command-and-control structure.

- Response: Warn (notify), isolate (during the disaster), and rescue (following the disaster).

- Recovery: Inventory supplies and resources, relieve staff members present during the isolation phase, incorporate records into the EMR, implement CISM program if needed, and activate employee assistance programs if needed.

Mass casualty incidents (MCIs) are characterized by a rapid influx of patients that overwhelms the resources available in the ED, resulting in the activation of a contingency plan to bring more resources (staff, supplies, etc.) where they are needed. Examples of MCIs include mass shootings, sudden onset of contagious disease (e.g., COVID-19 pandemic), MVCs involving buses or a large number of vehicles, train and airplane accidents, and biological/chemical accidents or attacks.

Decontamination must be performed by trained or certified individuals with a strong working knowledge of contaminants. Decontamination areas must be set up a good distance from any entrance into a hospital to avoid cross contamination of the area and building.

- The **hot zone** of care is the point of entry to the decontamination process following an incident.
  - □ Patients triaged as immediate, delayed, or non-ambulatory will be decontaminated first.
  - □ Patients are triaged in the hot zone and have their clothes removed as they approach the warm zone.

- The **warm zone** is where active decontamination occurs. Decontamination usually includes the use of water, but this will depend on the chemical, biological, or radioactive agent the patient is exposed to.

- The **cold zone** is the point of exit from the decontamination area. The patient enters the cold zone and may be treated onsite or transported to an appropriate level of care.

QUICK REVIEW QUESTION

12. A nurse is preparing to receive patients who have been exposed to a chemical from a work-related accident. What should occur after the patients are triaged and as they are moved to the warm zone for decontamination?

_____

ANSWER KEY

1. The nurse should decline the offer of help and report to management that she suspects her coworker may be impaired.

2. The nurse manager should tell the family member that their behavior is a form of workplace violence and explain that it will not be tolerated. If the family member continues the behavior, security should be notified to escort them out of the building.

3. The nurse could ask the ethics committee for assistance with this patient's care plan and to debrief after caring for the patient.

4. The UAP should fill out a variance using the safety reporting system so that maintenance can investigate the cause of the fall and prevent it from reoccurring.

5. The nurse should offer the patient community resources, like information about shelters that provide short-term living assistance for people experiencing homelessness. A health care facility is not obligated to admit a patient who is medically cleared for discharge because they do not have a home.

6. The nurse should educate the patient on the difference between hospice and palliative care. Palliative care can start at any age and phase of a disease; it is intended to relieve the symptoms that affect quality of life.

7. Chest pain is a medical emergency. The patient should be seen immediately and given an ECG. Creating and implementing protocols for emergent conditions that require immediate action are a national guideline for patient care.

8. Although the patient has a cardiac history, the symptoms (dyspnea, tachycardia, and fever) may indicate a respiratory infection. EMS should indicate whether the patient has had any known exposure to COVID-19 so that the ED can initiate precautions for the patient.

9. The nurse should look for other signs of suspected abuse and report immediately to the charge nurse or nurse manager and the attending physician. It is the nurse's responsibility to ensure that suspected child abuse is reported to the appropriate state authorities under the Child Abuse Prevention and Treatment Act.

10. The nurse should inform their supervisor and provide the patient with the contact information for the National Human Trafficking Resource Center. Accommodations should be made for the patient to call in privacy while in the ED.

11. Tasks outside the scope of practice or skills and abilities of other licensed personnel should never be delegated.

12. After a patient is triaged and moved from the hot zone to the warm zone, the nurse must ensure that the patient's clothes are removed.

22 Practice Test

READ THE QUESTION, AND THEN CHOOSE THE MOST CORRECT ANSWER.

1. The ED nurse is caring for a patient with a subdural hematoma sustained in an automobile accident. The patient currently has an ICP of 22 mmHg. Which of the following would NOT be an appropriate intervention?

   A. BMP and CBC

   B. lumbar puncture

   C. mechanical ventilation

   D. Foley catheter placement

2. Which of the following substances is contraindicated for an 80-year-old patient with acute heart failure?

   A. dopamine

   B. adrenaline

   C. digoxin

   D. dobutamine

3. Which observation in a patient with abdominal aortic aneurysm indicates the need for immediate treatment?

   A. complaints of yellow-tinted vision

   B. hemoptysis

   C. urinary output of 75 mL/hr per urinary catheter

   D. complaints of sudden and severe back pain and dyspnea

4. The nurse is evaluating patients for risk of heparin-induced thrombocytopenia (HIT). Which patient is at greatest risk for HIT, based on the nurse's assessment?

    A. a male patient who just completed a 1-week course of heparin

    B. a male patient taking enoxaparin for management of unstable angina

    C. a female patient receiving heparin for postsurgical thromboprophylaxis

    D. a female patient taking enoxaparin to prevent clots following a mild myocardial infarction

5. During cardiac assessment of a patient with pericarditis, the nurse should expect to hear

    A. mitral regurgitation.

    B. S3 gallop.

    C. S4 gallop.

    D. pericardial friction rub.

6. Complications resulting from an untreated/undertreated high-velocity injection injury may be minimized by

    A. educating the patient to return if signs of infection appear.

    B. administering prophylactic antibiotics.

    C. obtaining a surgical consultation and exploration.

    D. immobilizing the extremity involved.

7. A patient arrives in the ED with midsternal chest pain radiating down the left arm and left jaw. He slumps to the floor and is unresponsive, pulseless, and apneic. High-quality compressions are started, and the patient's ECG shows the following rhythm. What is the priority nursing intervention?

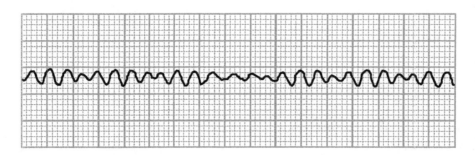

    A. administer a fluid bolus of 1 L normal saline

    B. defibrillate with 200 J

    C. administer 1 mg epinephrine IV

    D. insert an advanced airway

8. A patient comes to the ED complaining of intermittent nausea and vomiting for the past month. She states that she has pain in the abdomen that is relieved by eating. She began having diarrhea the day before. Medical history shows that the patient takes naproxen daily for arthritis. The nurse should assess for

    A. obesity.

    B. appendicitis.

    C. hypertension.

    D. gastritis.

9. An infant's parents bring him to the ED because of bloody, mucous stools. The child cries constantly and pulls his knees up to his chest. Which of the following findings would be the most critical?

    A. vomiting

    B. diarrhea

    C. abdominal swelling

    D. a lump in the abdomen

10. A patient with abdominal pain and possible appendicitis wants to leave the ED. What should the nurse do next?

    A. Inform the patient he will be involuntarily committed to the hospital if he tries to leave.

    B. Inform the physician of the patient's wish to leave.

    C. Warn the patient he will die if he leaves the department.

    D. Give the patient directions to the exit.

11. The current American Heart Association (AHA) guidelines for CPR on an adult patient with 2 rescuers is

    A. 30 compressions : 2 ventilations.

    B. 15 compressions : 2 ventilations.

    C. 30 compressions : 1 ventilation.

    D. 15 compressions : 1 ventilation.

12. A patient in the ED is diagnosed with a right ventricular infarction with hypotension. The nurse should prepare to administer which of the following to treat the hypotension?

    A. normal saline fluid boluses 1 to 2 L

    B. dopamine (Intropine) at 10 mcg/kg/min

    C. D5W fluid boluses titrate 3 L

    D. furosemide drip at 20 mg/hr

13. Which lab results confirm a diagnosis of carbon monoxide toxicity in a nonsmoking adult?

   A. COHb 0.8%

   B. COHb 8%

   C. $PaCO_2$ 38

   D. $PaCO_2$ 41

14. A 43-year-old female patient comes to the ED with complaints of vaginal discharge with itching and burning. The nurse notes a non-odorous white discharge that resembles cottage cheese. The nurse should prepare to treat the patient for which of the following?

   A. bacterial vaginosis

   B. trichomoniasis vaginitis

   C. *Candida vulvovaginitis*

   D. *Neisseria gonorrhoeae*

15. An 82-year-old patient presents to triage with a complaint of diarrhea for the past 3 days. She tells the triage nurse that she is on her third day of antibiotics. Which precautions should the nurse implement?

   A. airborne precautions

   B. contact precautions

   C. droplet precautions

   D. contact and droplet precautions

16. A 20-year-old female patient comes to the ED complaining of a green-gray frothy malodorous vaginal discharge and vaginal itching. The wet prep shows only WBCs. The nurse should prepare to assess for

   A. trichomoniasis.

   B. bacterial vaginosis.

   C. herpes simplex virus.

   D. chlamydia.

17. The nurse is performing an abdominal assessment on a patient with suspected heart failure. The patient asks the nurse the reason for assessing the abdomen. Which of the following would be the best response from the nurse?

   A. "Sometimes the medications used in heart failure will cause stomach upset."

   B. "Hepatomegaly, or an enlarged liver, is common in heart failure."

   C. "I am checking to see if you are constipated."

   D. "Heart failure can lead to appendicitis."

18. When trying to find a piece of glass in the soft tissue of the lateral thigh, which assessment technique should the nurse avoid?

    A. deep tissue palpation

    B. visual inspection

    C. palpation of distal pulses

    D. CSM of extremity

19. A patient's cardiac monitor shows the rhythm below. He is awake and alert but is pale and confused. His blood pressure reads 64/40 mm Hg. What is the priority nursing intervention for this patient?

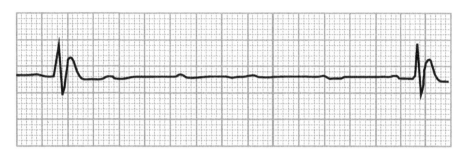

    A. defibrillate at 200 J

    B. prepare for transcutaneous pacing

    C. administer epinephrine 1 mg

    D. begin CPR

20. A patient who is 28 weeks pregnant presents to the ED with a malodorous vaginal discharge, a temperature of 102.3°F (39°C), and no complaints of uterine contractions. These signs and symptoms are most indicative of which of the following?

    A. septic spontaneous abortion

    B. ectopic pregnancy

    C. missed abortion

    D. abdominal trauma

21. Which of the following lab values should the nurse expect to order for a patient receiving IV heparin therapy for a pulmonary embolism?

    A. hematocrit

    B. HDL and LDL

    C. PT and PTT

    D. troponin level

22. A patient is being treated for rapidly evolving disseminated intravascular coagulation (DIC) in the ED. Which of the following lab values would the nurse expect?

    A. increased hemoglobin

    B. decreased D-dimer

    C. increased platelets

    D. decreased fibrinogen

23. The nurse is caring for a patient with Guillain–Barré syndrome who is at risk for autonomic dysfunction. The nurse should monitor the patient for

    A. trigeminy.

    B. heart block.

    C. atrial flutter.

    D. tachycardia.

24. Which of the following procedures can be performed under procedural sedation in the ED?

    A. perimortem cesarean section

    B. synchronized cardioversion

    C. dilatation and curettage

    D. open fracture reduction

25. A nurse notes crackles while assessing lung sounds in a child with pneumonia. How would the nurse classify this respiratory disorder?

    A. upper airway disorder

    B. lower airway disorder

    C. lung tissue disorder

    D. disordered control of breathing

26. The ECG in the exhibit supports the diagnosis of

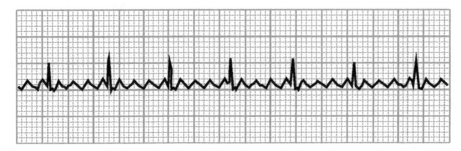

    A. atrial flutter.

    B. atrial fibrillation.

    C. torsades de pointes.

    D. ventricular fibrillation.

27. A patient who was playing basketball outside all day has been drinking only water to stay hydrated. He suddenly became confused, complained of a headache, and collapsed. The nurse should suspect

    A. hyperkalemia.

    B. hyponatremia.

    C. hypernatremia.

    D. hypokalemia.

28. Which of the following medications should a nurse anticipate administering to an 18-month-old patient with a barking cough first?

    A. epinephrine 0.01 mg/kg IV stat

    B. nebulized epinephrine breathing treatment

    C. albuterol breathing treatment

    D. dexamethasone PO or IV

29. Classic signs of Bell's palsy include

    A. facial droop, dysphagia, dysarthria.

    B. facial droop, confusion, ataxia.

    C. hemiparalysis, photophobia, headache.

    D. tinnitus, nausea, vertigo.

30. Which of the following is most likely to be found in a patient with left-sided heart failure?

    A. jugular vein distention

    B. crackles

    C. hepatomegaly

    D. ascites

31. Localized pain and edema associated with systemic fever and left shift differential may be indicative of

    A. foreign body infection of surgical hardware.

    B. superficial foreign body.

    C. buckle fracture.

    D. Achilles tendon rupture.

32. The most common site of injection injuries is

    A. the second digit of the nondominant hand.

    B. the first digit of the nondominant hand.

    C. the second digit of the dominant hand.

    D. the first digit of the dominant hand.

33. A 12-year-old patient is brought to the ED after falling 15 feet out of a tree. She is complaining of severe pain in the right side of the chest and severe dyspnea. Upon auscultation, the nurse notes absent breath sounds on the right and should suspect

    A. pneumothorax.

    B. foreign body lodged in the right side of the chest.

    C. hematoma.

    D. pleural effusion.

34. A patient with a subarachnoid hemorrhage from a fall at home arrives at the ED. When reviewing the medical orders, which medication order should prompt the nurse to notify the health care provider?

    A. warfarin

    B. morphine

    C. nimodipine

    D. a stool softener

35. Which symptom, identified by the patient, is the most common and consistent with a myocardial infarction?

    A. palpitations

    B. lower extremity edema

    C. feeling of pressure in the chest

    D. nausea

36. A patient arrives to the ED with a grossly deformed shoulder injury obtained while surfing. Suspecting a dislocation, which nursing intervention should the nurse initiate immediately?

    A. elevate the extremity

    B. put patient on NPO status

    C. apply ice

    D. provide ice chips

37. Which of the following statements should be included in the discharge instructions for a patient who has been prescribed carbamazepine to control seizures?

    A. Avoid exposure to sunlight.

    B. Limit foods high in vitamin K.

    C. Do not take on an empty stomach.

    D. Use caution when driving or operating machinery.

38. The nurse is caring for a patient with a traumatic brain injury who has a Glasgow Coma Scale (GCS) of 7. The nurse should anticipate the need to

A. bolus with NS via IV.

B. assist patient to chair.

C. assist with intubation.

D. apply 2L O_2 via nasal cannula.

39. The nurse is caring for a patient who just had a lumbar puncture to rule out meningitis. Which assessment finding would prompt the nurse to notify the health care provider?

A. The patient is drinking fluids.

B. The patient is lying flat in the bed.

C. The patient's pain scale is 3 out of 10.

D. The patient complains of severe headache.

40. A patient presents with signs and symptoms characteristic of myocardial infarction (MI). Which of the following diagnostic tools should the nurse anticipate will be used to determine the location of the myocardial damage?

A. electrocardiogram

B. echocardiogram

C. cardiac enzymes

D. cardiac catheterization

41. The ED nurse is waiting for a bed for a 72-year-old patient with Alzheimer's disease who has episodes of confusion. Which of the following will be included in the plan of care for this patient?

A. prescribe haloperidol to prevent agitation

B. provide toileting every 2 hours

C. use restraints at night to prevent wandering

D. allow choices when possible to promote feelings of respect

42. A 16-year-old patient arrives to the ED after ingesting an entire bottle of acetaminophen 4 hours before. The most appropriate intervention is

A. administration of N-acetylcysteine.

B. endotracheal intubation.

C. administration of naloxone.

D. gastric lavage.

43. A patient with emphysema comes to the ED complaining of dyspnea. The nurse should assist the patient into which of the following positions?

    A. lying flat on the back

    B. in a prone position

    C. sitting up and leaning forward

    D. lying on the side with feet elevated

44. A patient with severe dementia is brought to the ED for urinary retention. The patient repeatedly asks for her mother, who passed away many years ago. Which technique should the nurse use when the patient asks for her mother?

    A. confrontation

    B. reality orientation

    C. validation therapy

    D. seeking clarification

45. The nurse sees a bedbug on the personal linens of a child transported from the home setting to the ED via ambulance. What is the most appropriate action?

    A. Place the patient on airborne precautions.

    B. File a report with the local child welfare agency.

    C. Wash the patient thoroughly and replace all linens and clothing items with hospital-provided materials.

    D. Ask the parents to provide new clothing and linen from the home.

46. The nurse is caring for a patient with suspected diverticulitis. The nurse should anticipate all of the following findings EXCEPT

    A. fever.

    B. anorexia.

    C. lower abdominal pain.

    D. low WBC count.

47. A patient presents to the ED with abdominal pain and is found to have an incarcerated hernia. The patient is prepared for surgery. Which assessment finding by the nurse should be reported immediately to the health care provider?

    A. a burning sensation at the site of the hernia

    B. sudden nausea and vomiting with increased pain since arrival

    C. a palpable mass in the abdomen

    D. pain that occurs when bending over or coughing

48. EMS arrives to the ED with a stable adult patient who has a clear developmental delay. Emergent intervention is not needed upon arrival. What should the ED nurse do before treating the patient?

A. Call the legal guardian of the patient to obtain consent for care.

B. Continue to care for the patient.

C. Obtain consent for care from the patient.

D. Obtain permission from the hospital legal department to care for the patient.

49. A patient arrives at the ED complaining of severe pain to the right lower abdominal quadrant. The patient states that the pain is worse with coughing. The nursing assessment reveals that pain is relieved by bending the right hip. The patient has not had a bowel movement in three days. The nurse should anticipate all of the following interventions EXCEPT

A. IV fluids.

B. morphine 2mg IV.

C. STAT MRI of abdomen.

D. maintain NPO status.

50. A patient is admitted to the ED with an acute myocardial infarction (MI). The nurse is preparing the patient for transport to the cardiac catheterization laboratory. An alarm sounds on the cardiac monitor, and the patient becomes unresponsive. V-fib is noted. The nurse should anticipate doing which of the following first?

A. beginning high-quality CPR

B. defibrillation at 200 J

C. administering epinephrine 1 mg

D. placing an IV

51. A nursing home patient with an enterocutaneous fistula caused by an acute exacerbation of Crohn's disease arrives at the ED. The nursing priority is to

A. administer antibiotics.

B. preserve and protect the skin.

C. apply a wound VAC to the area.

D. provide quiet times for relaxation.

52. A patient with cardiogenic shock is expected to have

A. hypertension; dyspnea.

B. decreased urine output; warm, pink skin.

C. increased urine output; cool, clammy skin.

D. hypotension; weak pulse; cool, clammy skin.

53. A patient in the ED with chronic pain is requesting more intravenous pain medication for reported 10/10 pain. The physician will not give any more medication. How should the nurse approach this patient?

   A. Inform the patient that it is the physician's decision.

   B. Discuss chronic pain relief and realistic expectations with the patient.

   C. Ignore the patient's pain complaint.

   D. Discuss drug-seeking concerns with the patient.

54. Which appearance is most consistent with an avulsion?

   A. open wound with presence of sloughing and eschar tissue

   B. skin tear with approximated edges

   C. shearing of the top epidermal layers

   D. separation of skin from the underlying structures that cannot be approximated

55. The ED nurse receives a patient with blunt-force abdominal injury due to a knife wound. On inspection, a common kitchen knife is found in the patient's abdomen in the upper right quadrant. The patient is rapidly placed on a non-rebreather mask, two large-bore IVs are started, and labs are drawn. No evisceration is noted. Which should the nurse do next?

   A. Notify next of kin.

   B. Estimate blood loss.

   C. Stabilize the knife with bulky dressings.

   D. Attempt to gently pull the knife straight out.

56. In a hypothermic patient, hypovolemia occurs as the result of

   A. diuresis and third spacing.

   B. shivering and vasoconstriction.

   C. diaphoresis and dehydration.

   D. tachycardia and tachypnea.

57. A 14-year-old male patient is brought to the ED, stating he woke up in the middle of the night with sudden, severe groin pain and nausea. The pain persists despite elevation of the testes. These findings most likely indicate

   A. testicular torsion.

   B. epididymitis.

   C. UTI.

   D. orchitis.

58. A 16-year-old patient is brought to the ED complaining of abdominal pain, nausea, and sharp constant pain on both sides of the pelvis. She has a history of pelvic inflammatory disease and is not sexually active. The nurse notes a purulent vaginal discharge. These signs and symptoms are most indicative of which condition?

    A. ectopic pregnancy

    B. tubo-ovarian abscess

    C. diverticulitis

    D. ruptured appendix

59. A patient who is 9 weeks pregnant comes to the ED with complaints of abdominal cramping. During the physical assessment the nurse notes slight vaginal bleeding and a large, solid tissue clot. These findings most likely indicate

    A. septic spontaneous abortion.

    B. incomplete spontaneous abortion.

    C. threatened abortion.

    D. complete spontaneous abortion.

60. A 4-month-old infant is brought to the ED with croup. Which of the following medications will the nurse administer in order to decrease inflammation?

    A. ipratropium

    B. albuterol

    C. corticosteroids

    D. antibiotics

61. A 21-year-old male patient reports to the ED with complaints of burning on urination and urethral itching. During the assessment, the nurse notes a mucopurulent discharge and no lesions. These signs and symptoms are most indicative of which of the following?

    A. chlamydia

    B. syphilis

    C. HPV

    D. herpes simplex virus

62. The mother of a 3-year-old patient diagnosed with varicella asks for the best at-home treatment. Which of the following treatments is NOT appropriate for the nurse to suggest?

    A. oral antihistamines

    B. colloidal oatmeal baths

    C. acetaminophen

    D. aspirin

63. A full-term neonate is delivered in the ED. After stimulation and suctioning, the infant is apneic with strong palpable pulses at 126/minute. The nursing priority is to

   A. rescue breaths at 12 – 20 breaths per minute.

   B. rescue breaths at 40 – 60 breaths per minute.

   C. insert endotracheal intubation.

   D. insert an LMA.

64. A pediatric patient in cardiopulmonary arrest has had a 40-minute resuscitation attempt in the ED. The ED nurse feels that the resuscitation is reaching the point of concern for medical futility. What is the nurse's responsibility at this time?

   A. Tell the parents to order the resuscitation attempt to be stopped.

   B. Suggest that the team leader consider ending the resuscitation.

   C. Order the team to stop the resuscitation.

   D. Continue with the resuscitation and allow the team leader to decide when to stop.

65. After an emergent delivery, a full-term infant is apneic with a pulse rate of 48 bpm. The infant has not responded to chest compressions. The nurse should prepare to administer

   A. atropine 0.5 mg/kg.

   B. epinephrine 0.01 – 0.03 mg/kg.

   C. sodium bicarbonate 1 to 2 mEq/mL.

   D. dobutamine drip.

66. Which treatment is appropriate for a minor blunt injury resulting in intact skin, ecchymosis, edema, and localized pain and tenderness?

   A. fasciotomy and opioid pain medications

   B. rest, ice, compression, elevation, and opioid pain medications

   C. rest, ice, compression, elevation, and use of NSAIDs

   D. immobilization and use of NSAIDs

67. A patient with depression and Alzheimer's disease presents to the ED complaining of abdominal pain. In reviewing the patient's health care orders, which medication should prompt the nurse to notify the health care provider?

   A. sertraline

   B. paroxetine

   C. memantine

   D. amitriptyline

68. A 14-year-old patient arrives to the ED with delirium, respiratory distress, and headache. Upon examination of the airway, the nurse notes a burn to the roof of the patient's mouth. What does the nurse suspect?

  A. ingestion of a hot beverage

  B. inhalation of chemicals from a compressed gas can

  C. ingestion of dry ice

  D. marijuana use

69. The nurse is caring for a patient who was brought to the ED with seizures. The patient begins having a seizure. The nursing priority is

  A. padding the bed rails.

  B. inserting a tongue blade.

  C. administering IV diazepam.

  D. turning the patient to his side.

70. A patient who is 32 weeks pregnant is having profuse bright red painless vaginal bleeding after being in a motor vehicle crash (MVC). The nurse should prepare to treat her for

  A. abruptio placentae.

  B. placenta previa.

  C. ectopic pregnancy.

  D. complete abortion.

71. A 30-week pregnant patient comes to the ED after falling down a flight of steps. She complains of uterine tenderness, and a small amount of dark bloody vaginal drainage is noted. The nurse should suspect

  A. abruptio placenta.

  B. placenta previa.

  C. incomplete spontaneous abortion.

  D. complete spontaneous abortion.

72. The ED nurse is caring for a patient with schizophrenia. The patient appears to be looking at someone and asks the nurse, "Aren't you going to speak to Martha?" No one else is in the room. Which response by the nurse is appropriate?

  A. "There's nobody there."

  B. "I will find a blanket for Martha."

  C. "Is Martha going to stay a while?"

  D. "Does Martha ever tell you to hurt yourself or others?"

73. A patient in the ED is having difficulty breathing and is diagnosed with a large pleural effusion. The nurse prepares her for which of the following procedures?

    A. pericardiocentesis

    B. chest tube insertion

    C. thoracentesis

    D. pericardial window

74. When caring for a patient with esophageal varices, the nurse should first prepare to administer

    A. phenytoin

    B. octreotide

    C. levofloxacin

    D. pantoprazole

75. The ED nurse is caring for a patient who is deeply depressed following the death of her mother. She tells the nurse, "I just lost my world when Mom died. She was my anchor, and now I have no one." Which response by the nurse is the most appropriate?

    A. "You will feel better in time."

    B. "You should join a grief support group."

    C. "I felt the same way when my mother died."

    D. "You're feeling lost since your mother died."

76. A patient is admitted to the ED with chest pain. A 12-lead ECG is performed with ST elevations noted in leads II, III and aVF. The nurse should prepare to administer

    A. nitrates.

    B. diuretics.

    C. morphine.

    D. IV fluids.

77. A 20-year-old male college student arrives to the ED during spring break complaining of a headache, fever, nausea, and vomiting. He shows the ED nurse a petechial rash on his trunk and chest. Which of the following should the nurse suspect?

    A. influenza

    B. pertussis

    C. meningitis

    D. scabies

78. A patient comes to the ED with complaints of nausea and vomiting for 3 days. His ECG reading is shown in the exhibit. The nurse should suspect

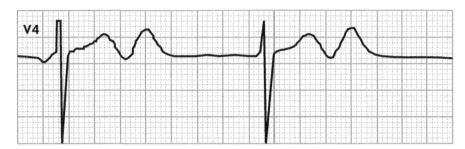

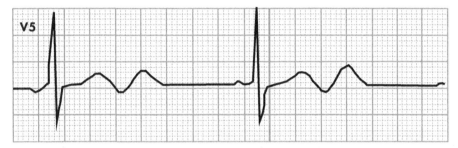

    A. hyperkalemia.

    B. hypokalemia.

    C. hypercalcemia.

    D. hypocalcemia.

79. An ED nurse is caring for a patient who was injured during a violent crime. Which of the following is a priority in evidence collection and care?

    A. chain of custody

    B. chain of evidence

    C. photographing of evidence

    D. documenting of evidence

80. A patient is brought to the ED following a motor vehicle crash. He was driving without a seat belt and was hit with the steering wheel on the left side of his chest. He complains of severe chest pain and dyspnea. During assessment, the nurse is unable to hear breath sounds on the left. The nurse should prepare to assist with immediate

    A. endotracheal intubation.

    B. chest compressions.

    C. chest tube insertion.

    D. thoracotomy.

81. Epistaxis occurring from Kiesselbach's plexus is controlled by all methods EXCEPT

 A. cauterization of a visualized vessel.

 B. high Fowler's position leaning forward and applying continuous pressure to the midline septum.

 C. nasal packing with hemostatic material.

 D. endoscopic litigation.

82. Which of the following interventions is NOT appropriate for a patient with adrenal hypofunction?

 A. peripheral blood draws

 B. low-sodium diet

 C. blood glucose monitoring

 D. hydrocortisone therapy

83. A patient is brought to the ED with dyspnea, headache, light-headedness, and diaphoresis. A diagnosis of hyperventilation syndrome is made. The nurse is aware that hyperventilation syndrome can present with signs and symptoms similar to which of the following?

 A. pneumonia

 B. bronchitis

 C. pulmonary embolism

 D. pneumothorax

84. Which test should a nurse expect before a health care provider prescribes risperidone to manage psychotic symptoms?

 A. a cardiac workup

 B. comprehensive metabolic panel (CMP)

 C. creatinine clearance

 D. complete blood count (CBC)

85. The nurse is caring for a patient who says he wants to commit suicide. He has a detailed, concrete plan. The nurse places the patient on suicide precautions, which include a 24-hour sitter. The patient becomes angry and refuses the sitter. Which action is the most appropriate?

 A. place the patient in soft wrist restraints

 B. have security sit outside the patient's door

 C. assign a sitter despite the patient's refusal

 D. allow the patient to leave against medical advice (AMA)

86. Which laboratory finding indicates that a 62-year-old male patient is at risk for ventricular dysrhythmia?

   A. magnesium 0.8 mEq/L

   B. potassium 4.2 mmol/L

   C. creatinine 1.3 mg/dL

   D. total calcium 2.8 mmol/L

87. A patient presents to the ED with chest pain, dyspnea, and diaphoresis. The nurse finds a narrow complex tachycardia with a HR of 210 bpm, BP of 70/42 mm Hg, and a RR of 18. The nurse should anticipate which priority intervention?

   A. administer adenosine 6 mg IV

   B. defibrillate at 200 J

   C. administer amiodarone 300 mg IV

   D. prepare for synchronized cardioversion

88. A patient is brought to the ED in supraventricular tachycardia (SVT) with a rate of 220. EMS has administered 6 mg of adenosine, but the patient remains in SVT. What is the next intervention the nurse should anticipate?

   A. administer 12 mg adenosine IV

   B. administer 1 mg epinephrine IV

   C. administer 300 mg amiodarone IV

   D. administer 0.5 atropine IV

89. A 6-year-old child is admitted to the ED with an acute asthma attack. A pulse oximetry is attached with a reading of 91%. The nursing priority is to

   A. administer dexamethasone.

   B. provide supplemental oxygen.

   C. prepare for immediate endotracheal intubation.

   D. administer a nebulized albuterol treatment.

90. A patient is admitted to the ED with a sickle cell crisis. The nurse should prepare to administer which of the following blood products?

   A. warm packed RBCs

   B. whole blood

   C. fresh frozen plasma (FFP)

   D. cryoprecipitate

91. Which complication of compartment syndrome would the nurse suspect if urinalysis reveals myoglobinuria?

    A. disseminated intravascular coagulation (DIC)

    B. rhabdomyolysis

    C. Volkmann's contracture

    D. sepsis

92. A patient presents to the ED with complaints of substernal sharp, tearing knifelike chest pain radiating to the neck, jaw, and face. Morphine sulfate is given with no relief of the pain. These signs and symptoms are most indicative of which of the following?

    A. myocardial infarction (MI)

    B. pericarditis

    C. pneumonia

    D. acute aortic dissection

93. A patient is admitted to the ED with a potassium level of 6.9. Which of the following medications could have caused her electrolyte imbalance?

    A. bumetanide

    B. captopril

    C. furosemide

    D. digoxin

94. A patient presents to the ED with a bleeding laceration to the arm and a history of idiopathic thrombocytopenic purpura (ITP). The nurse should anticipate which treatment to be ordered?

    A. cryoprecipitate

    B. fresh frozen plasma (FFP)

    C. platelets

    D. protamine sulfate

95. Which of the following is usually associated with variant (Prinzmetal's) angina?

    A. cyanide poisoning

    B. gastroesophageal reflux

    C. Raynaud's phenomena

    D. beta-blocker toxicity

96. Hyperglycemic hyperosmolar state (HHS) is most often caused by

    A. inadequate glucose monitoring.

    B. dehydration.

    C. noncompliance with insulin therapy.

    D. a breakdown of ketones.

97. Fluoxetine for moderate depression is contraindicated in patients with

   A. arthritis.

   B. migraines.

   C. glaucoma.

   D. appendicitis.

98. A patient presents to the ED with severe throbbing fingers after coming home from the gym. Upon observing thin, shiny skin, pallor, and thick fingernails, the nurse should suspect

   A. acute arterial injury.

   B. acute arterial occlusion.

   C. peripheral venous thrombosis.

   D. peripheral vascular disease.

99. Which of the following IV solutions should be administered to a patient with diabetic ketoacidosis (DKA) who is placed on an insulin drip?

   A. lactated Ringer's

   B. normal saline

   C. normal saline with potassium

   D. normal saline with dextrose

100. EMS brings in a patient with a history of alcohol abuse, homelessness, and poor adherence to antiseizure medications. The patient has experienced 3 seizures in 30 minutes. These findings support the diagnosis of

   A. atonic seizure.

   B. tonic–clonic seizure.

   C. status epilepticus.

   D. simple partial seizure.

101. When taking the history of a patient with suspected pancreatitis, the nurse should expect to find

   A. the patient feels better when lying supine.

   B. the patient has a history of alcohol abuse and peptic ulcer disease.

   C. the pain is described as a sharp, burning sensation.

   D. the pain began gradually and radiated to the right lower abdomen.

102. A pediatric patient is being resuscitated in a trauma bay, and his father wants to be in the room. What should the nurse do?

   A. Tell the father he may not be in the trauma room during resuscitation.

   B. Allow the father in the trauma room with a knowledgeable staff member for support.

   C. Ask the father to stand just outside the trauma room.

   D. Call the legal department for advice.

103. A patient arrives to the ED after an attempted suicide by a self-inflicted gunshot wound. He is determined to be brain dead, but his life can be sustained for organ procurement. The patient is identified as an organ donor. Which of the following is the next step for the ED nurse?

    A. notify local organ procurement organization

    B. remove all life-supporting interventions

    C. perform postmortem care on the patient

    D. complete the death certificate

104. When caring for a patient with thyroid storm, the nurse should first prepare to administer which medication?

    A. propylthiouracil (PTU)

    B. epinephrine

    C. levothyroxine

    D. atropine

105. A patient arrives to the ED with a sheriff escort after being found in a street acting erratically and shouting. She is unkempt and not appropriately dressed for the weather. She states that she wants to commit suicide. What can the ED nurse expect to happen to the patient?

    A. She will be given benzodiazepines for anxiety and discharged.

    B. She will be medically cleared and brought to jail.

    C. She will be involuntarily committed.

    D. She will be voluntarily admitted to the hospital.

106. A patient with a blood glucose reading of 475 mg/dL presents to the ED with Kussmaul respirations, nausea, and vomiting, and a pH of 7.3. The nurse should expect to treat which condition?

    A. myxedema coma

    B. hyperosmolar hyperglycemic state (HHS)

    C. pheochromocytoma

    D. diabetic ketoacidosis (DKA)

107. The nurse is using the Glasgow Coma Scale (GCS) to assess a patient who fell in a parking lot. The patient opens his eyes to sound, localizes pain, and makes incoherent sounds when spoken to. Which GCS score will the nurse document?

    A. 9

    B. 10

    C. 11

    D. 12

108. A patient arrives to the ED with a complaint of sore throat and fever. Which of the following findings is the most immediate concern?

   A. visualized white abscess on the soft palate

   B. patchy tonsillar exudate

   C. petechiae on the hard palate

   D. lymphedema

109. A patient in the ED is diagnosed with ulcerative colitis (UC). Which dietary changes can the nurse recommend to help manage symptoms?

   A. Eat a high-fiber diet.

   B. Limit coffee to two cups daily.

   C. Avoid lactose-containing foods.

   D. Consume dried fruit several times a week.

110. A 32-year-old female patient comes to the ED with complaints of abdominal pain. She describes the pain as sharp and states it began suddenly during intercourse. The pain is worse with movement, and there is no vaginal discharge noted. These findings support the diagnosis of

   A. ectopic pregnancy.

   B. ruptured appendix.

   C. ruptured ovarian cyst.

   D. STD.

111. Which of the following signs or symptoms should lead a nurse to suspect septic shock?

   A. WBC of 2,500

   B. serum lactate level of 2.6

   C. decrease in neutrophils

   D. increase in RBCs

112. A patient is admitted to the ED with nausea, vomiting, and diarrhea for 3 days and signs of severe dehydration. The nurse starts an IV and prepares to administer which fluid replacement?

   A. hypertonic solution

   B. isotonic crystalloid

   C. hypotonic solution

   D. colloid solution

113. The nurse is reviewing the history of a patient with heart failure. Which of the following coexisting health problems will cause an increase in the patient's afterload?

   A. diabetes

   B. endocrine disorders

   C. hypertension

   D. Marfan syndrome

114. The nurse is caring for a patient who presented to the ED with a subarachnoid hemorrhage. While taking the patient's history, what symptoms would the nurse expect to see with this patient?

   A. sudden food cravings

   B. rash on the lower trunk

   C. Battle's sign

   D. a severe, sudden headache

115. The nurse is discharging a patient who has been prescribed medications to control progressive MS. Which statement by the patient indicates a need for further teaching by the nurse?

   A. "I will wear an eye patch on alternating eyes if I have double vision."

   B. "I will clear rugs and extra furniture from my walking paths at home."

   C. "I hope I feel like going to Disney World this summer with my grandchildren."

   D. "I will call my doctor if I have any signs or symptoms of infection, such as fever."

116. Lower abdominal pain that is worsened with movement, a non-malodorous vaginal discharge, a fever, and tachycardia are usually associated with

   A. appendicitis.

   B. pelvic inflammatory disease.

   C. ectopic pregnancy.

   D. STI.

117. Which prescription would the nurse anticipate administering to a patient with no known medication allergies who presents with orofacial edema, halitosis, and a complaint of tasting pus in the mouth?

   A. nystatin

   B. sodium fluoride drops

   C. penicillin V potassium

   D. saliva substitute

118. A patient with a myocardial infarction (MI). The patient has received nitroglycerin sublingual and is still experiencing chest pain. The nurse should prepare to administer

    A. hydromorphone.

    B. meperidine.

    C. morphine sulfate.

    D. acetaminophen.

119. A patient presents to the ED with complaints of dizziness and fatigue and a past medical history of HIV. She states she is noncompliant with her antiviral medications. Her temperature is 101.2°F (38.4°C), BP 100/72 mm Hg, HR 130 bpm, RR 22, and O_2 96%.

    Which of the following orders would be the priority intervention?

    A. administering an antibiotic

    B. administering acetaminophen

    C. administering prescribed antivirals

    D. administering 2 units of packed RBCs

120. The nurse is caring for a patient who suffered a head injury following a fall off a ladder. The nurse assesses the patient for signs of increased intracranial pressure (ICP). Which finding by the nurse is a LATE sign of increased ICP?

    A. headache

    B. restlessness

    C. dilated pupils

    D. decreasing LOC

121. An 11-month-old infant is brought to the ED with a barking cough, a respiratory rate of 66, substernal retractions, and copious nasal secretions. Which of the following positions will best facilitate the child's breathing?

    A. sitting upright in a parent's lap

    B. on a stretcher in a prone position

    C. reverse Trendelenburg

    D. semi-Fowler's

122. Which of the following statements would be included in the discharge teaching for a patient with ulcerative colitis (UC)?

    A. "Hemorrhage is a potential complication."

    B. "Patients may have 5 – 6 loose stools per day."

    C. "Patients with UC are more likely to have fistulas."

    D. "Many times, surgery is needed to treat symptoms."

123. Which pain characteristics are associated with inflammation of the fifth cranial nerve?

   A. progressive onset, bilateral, throbbing

   B. abrupt onset, unilateral, hemifacial spasm

   C. intermittent, circumoral, shooting

   D. paroxysmal, bilateral, paresthesia

124. Two weeks post–left-sided myocardial infarction (MI) a patient presents to the ED with dyspnea and cough with hemoptysis. The nurse should suspect the patient has developed

   A. pneumonia.

   B. over-coagulation.

   C. pulmonary edema.

   D. ruptured ventricle.

125. A patient arrives to the ED with altered mental status, blood pressure of 70/40, and declining vital signs. Her husband states that she does not wish to be resuscitated. What should the ED nurse do?

   A. Tell the patient that the physician will decide her advance directive status.

   B. Ask the spouse for the advanced directive paperwork.

   C. Document the patient's advanced directive wishes and honor the request in case resuscitation is needed.

   D. Inform the patient that advanced directives are not used in EDs.

126. A family in the ED must decide whether to withdraw care for a family member with no advance directive. Which person would NOT be consulted as a part of a multidisciplinary team to make this decision?

   A. chair of ethics committee

   B. legal department

   C. critical care physician

   D. pharmacist

127. A 2-year-old child presents to the ED with septal deviation and a visualized foreign body in the right naris. Which nursing intervention is most appropriate?

   A. instructing the parent to perform nasal positive pressure

   B. instructing the child to blow his nose

   C. instructing the parent to perform oral positive pressure

   D. restraining the child for forceps retraction

128. Which treatment is contraindicated for a corneal abrasion?

    A. application of ophthalmic lubricating solution

    B. application of topical anesthetics

    C. patching the affected eye

    D. wearing glasses instead of contact lenses

129. The ED nurse is caring for a patient with delirium who tells the nurse, "There are snakes crawling up on my bed." How should the nurse respond?

    A. "That's just the wrinkles in your blanket."

    B. "I will see if I can move you to another room."

    C. "I will call maintenance to come and remove them."

    D. "I know you're scared, but I don't see any snakes on your bed."

130. The nurse is caring for a patient who has been prescribed rasagiline mesylate for Parkinson's disease. Which medication on the patient's current record should prompt the nurse to notify the health care provider?

    A. baclofen

    B. amantadine

    C. benztropine

    D. isocarboxazid

131. Which medication would the nurse anticipate administering to a patient with a periorbital vesicular rash along the trigeminal nerve?

    A. acyclovir

    B. erythromycin

    C. ketorolac

    D. ciprofloxacin

132. The nurse is caring for a patient who presents to the ED with the following arterial blood gas (ABG) results:

> pH 7.32
> $PaCO_2$ 47 mm Hg
> HCO_3 24 mEq/L
> PaO_2 91 mm Hg

The nurse should expect the patient to present with

    A. chest pain.

    B. nausea and vomiting.

    C. deep, rapid respirations.

    D. hypoventilation with hypoxia.

133. Management of acute iritis includes

    A. topical mydriatic ophthalmic drops and topical corticosteroids.

    B. copious irrigation.

    C. IV mannitol and acetazolamide.

    D. topical anesthetics and topical antibiotics.

134. Discharge teaching for a patient diagnosed with ulcerative keratitis is effective if she states which of the following?

    A. "There is no need to follow up with an ophthalmologist."

    B. "I will stop the antibiotic drops tomorrow if the pain is better."

    C. "I will wear glasses and not contacts for at least two weeks."

    D. "I need to stay home from work until the infection clears because I am highly contagious."

135. The nurse is caring for a patient with a history of cirrhosis who arrived at the ED with a new onset of confusion. The patient's skin is jaundiced. Labs are as follows:

Ammonia 130 mcg/dL
ALT 98 U/L
Blood glucose 128

The nurse should prepare to administer

    A. lactulose.

    B. bisacodyl.

    C. mesalamine.

    D. insulin 2 units.

136. Which of the following is a clinical feature of an open globe rupture?

    A. cherry red macula

    B. rust ring

    C. pale optic disc

    D. afferent pupillary defect

137. Dopamine (Intropin) is ordered for a patient with heart failure because the drug

    A. lowers the heart rate.

    B. opens blocked arteries.

    C. prevents plaque from building up.

    D. increases the amount of oxygen delivered to the heart.

138. Which statement regarding tourniquet use to control hemorrhagic bleeding for a partial limb amputation is correct?

   A.   A commercially available tourniquet that is at least 2 inches wide with a windlass, a ratcheting device to occlude arterial flow, is recommended.

   B.   Tourniquet application is never recommended even when direct pressure does not control blood loss from an extremity.

   C.   Tourniquets properly applied in the prehospital setting should always be removed upon arrival to the ED, regardless if there is adequate team support to manage bleeding.

   D.   Time of tourniquet application should be noted clearly on the device and should not exceed 4-hour intervals before reassessment of bleeding.

139. Which of the following will confirm the diagnosis of a pulmonary embolism?

   A.   chest X-ray

   B.   D-dimer

   C.   fibrin split products

   D.   CT angiography

140. The nurse is caring for a patient with a history of schizophrenia, alcohol abuse, bipolar disorder, and noncompliance with treatment and medications. The patient has also been arrested in the past for violent behavior. Which action by the nurse is the most important when caring for a potentially violent patient?

   A.   treat the patient with courtesy and respect

   B.   always maintain an open pathway to the door

   C.   be sure the patient swallows his pills and does not "cheek" them

   D.   ask permission from the patient before drawing blood or performing other invasive procedures

141. A 13-year-old female arrives to the ED complaining of chest pain. A physical exam reveals tenderness along the fourth, fifth, and sixth ribs. Which diagnosis does the nurse suspect?

   A.   myocardial infarction

   B.   Ludwig's angina

   C.   pleurisy

   D.   costochondritis

142. Which of the following describes the characteristics of a flail chest?

   A.   The chest sinks in with inspiration and out with expiration.

   B.   Only the right side of the chest has movement.

   C.   Movement is noted on the left side of the chest only.

   D.   There is no movement noted on either side of the chest.

143. The ED nurse is providing discharge teaching to a patient newly diagnosed with migraines who has been given a prescription for sumatriptan. Which of the following statements indicates the patient understands the discharge teaching?

    A.   "This medication is safe to take while pregnant."

    B.   "I will report chest pain immediately to my physician."

    C.   "I will take my blood pressure medicine before I take sumatriptan."

    D.   "I will take this medication 15 minutes after I feel a migraine starting."

144. A 4-year-old child was in a bicycle accident and presents with oral lacerations and complete dental avulsions to the 2 top front teeth. The best initial management by the health care provider is

    A.   immediate replantation of the avulsed teeth.

    B.   laceration repair.

    C.   replantation of the avulsed tooth after soaking for 30 minutes in Hank's solution.

    D.   dental consult.

145. Diagnostic findings common with gouty arthritis include

    A.   hyperammonemia.

    B.   hyperbilirubinemia.

    C.   hyperuricemia.

    D.   hyperhomocysteinemia.

146. Which dressing would be most appropriate for a patient with a partial thickness wound to the epidermis?

    A.   transparent dressing

    B.   occlusive dressing

    C.   nonstick adherent dressing

    D.   bulky dressing

147. A patient arrives to the ED from a house fire. The nurse notes soot at the opening of her mouth and both nares. What is the primary concern for this patient?

    A.   total body surface areas covered in burns

    B.   airway edema related to inhalation injury

    C.   foreign body ingestion during the fire

    D.   trauma as a result of rescue from the fire

148. Which intervention is contraindicated for a patient with acute angle glaucoma?

    A. administration of ophthalmic beta blocker

    B. maintaining patient in a supine position

    C. dimming lights in the room or providing a blindfold for comfort

    D. administration of IV mannitol

149. Which of the following chest X-ray readings is consistent with acute respiratory distress syndrome (ARDS)?

    A. bilateral, diffuse white infiltrates without cardiomegaly

    B. bilateral, diffuse infiltrates with cardiomegaly

    C. tapering vascular shadows with hyperlucency and right ventricular enlargement

    D. prominent hilar vascular shadows with left ventricular enlargement

150. Which positive toxicology result would the nurse suspect in a patient with a MRSA-positive infectious abscess of the right antecubital space?

    A. alcohol

    B. opioid

    C. benzodiazepine

    D. tetrahydrocannabinol (THC)

151. A patient arrives to the ED after taking a sedative and subsequently becoming confused and disoriented. His temperature is 96.2°F (35.6°C), pulse is 47 bpm with distant heart tones, and BP is 82/65 mm Hg. He states that he is currently receiving thyroid replacement therapy. The nurse should suspect

    A. allergic reaction to the sedative.

    B. thyroid storm.

    C. myxedema coma.

    D. acute stroke.

152. The health care provider orders xylocaine with epinephrine to be prepared for a patient with a

    A. 2 cm laceration to the penile shaft.

    B. 2 cm laceration above the right eyebrow.

    C. 3 cm laceration to the left index finger.

    D. 7 cm laceration to the left forearm.

153. Which is the most appropriate post-exposure rabies prophylaxis treatment for an animal bite in a patient not previously vaccinated?

   A. rabies vaccine on days 0, 3, 7, and 14

   B. human rabies immune globulin injected into the wound bed

   C. human rabies immune globulin injected into the wound bed and rabies vaccine on days 0, 3, 7, and 14

   D. tetanus 0.5 mL via intramuscular injection

154. A child is admitted to the ED with wheezing on exhalation, use of accessory muscles, using 1-word sentences, and tripod positioning. The nurse should suspect

   A. pneumonia.

   B. pneumonitis.

   C. foreign body aspiration.

   D. asthma.

155. Which of the following IV medications should a nurse anticipate administering to a patient experiencing a severe anaphylactic reaction to a bee sting?

   A. epinephrine 1:1000 0.3 – 0.5 mL

   B. diphenhydramine 25 – 50 mg

   C. Solu-Medrol 125 mg

   D. theophylline 6mg/kg

156. The best medical management for carbon monoxide toxicity is

   A. hydroxocobalamin

   B. hyperbaric oxygen

   C. N-acetylcysteine

   D. sodium bicarbonate

157. A patient presents to the ED with complaints of severe headache, irritability, confusion, and lethargy. During triage he mentions that he has spent the last several days in his shop with a wood-burning stove. The ED nurse should be concerned for which of the following?

   A. migraine headache

   B. stroke

   C. carbon monoxide poisoning

   D. allergic reaction

158. The nurse is reviewing the laboratory results of a patient with renal failure and notes a serum potassium level of 7.2. The nurse should prepare to administer which of the following medications to protect cardiac status?

    A. aspirin

    B. insulin

    C. calcium gluconate

    D. digoxin

159. A college student arrived at the ED with suspected meningitis, and a positive diagnosis was confirmed via lumbar puncture. Which of the following findings suggests that she may have developed hydrocephalus?

    A. sluggish pupillary response

    B. inability to wrinkle the forehead

    C. inability to move the eyes laterally

    D. inability to move the eyes downward

160. Appropriate discharge teaching for a patient with diverticular disease includes instructions to

    A. avoid foods high in sodium.

    B. consume clear liquids until pain subsides.

    C. limit alcohol to one glass per day.

    D. include strawberries to get enough vitamin C.

161. Which neurological assessment finding commonly occurs in a patient struck by lightning?

    A. tic douloureux

    B. ascending paralysis

    C. Bell's palsy

    D. keraunoparalysis

162. A patient presents to the ED with confusion, anxiety, irritability, and a slight tremor. During assessment, she states she drinks two or more bottles of wine per day. Which of the following questions is important to ask?

    A. Do you drink any other alcoholic drinks on a regular basis?

    B. When was your last drink?

    C. When was your first drink?

    D. Have you ever experienced alcohol withdrawal?

163. A 34-year-old patient attempted suicide by consuming his grandmother's oral antidiabetic agent. Administration of glucose has been unsuccessful in reversing the effect of the medication. Which antidote should the nurse expect to administer next?

    A. flumazenil

    B. acetylcysteine

    C. octreotide

    D. methylene blue

164. A patient presents to triage with a complaint of cough lasting three weeks without improvement. The patient confirms recent travel to a developing country, and states she has had fevers and chills for the last three days. The nurse should suspect

    A. herpes zoster.

    B. tuberculosis.

    C. influenza.

    D. hepatitis C.

165. A woman arrives to the ED with her 5-year-old child, whom she discovered eating her nifedipine. She does not know how many pills the child consumed. The nursing priority is to

    A. place a referral to child protective services.

    B. obtain a 12-lead ECG.

    C. place the child on oxygen.

    D. ask the child how many she took.

166. A 10-year-old child presents to triage with conjunctivitis, cough, and a rash in the back of his mouth. During the assessment, the patient's father indicates that the child is not vaccinated. These findings most likely indicate

    A. varicella.

    B. mumps.

    C. measles.

    D. pertussis.

167. Which of the following medications should the nurse expect to administer to a patient who chronically abuses alcohol?

    A. naloxone

    B. thiamine

    C. flumazenil

    D. vitamin K

168. A 35-year-old patient in the ED has been diagnosed with herpes zoster. Which of the following statements should the nurse include in her discharge teaching?

- **A.** Herpes zoster occurs any time after an initial varicella infection and may recur several times.
- **B.** The varicella vaccine is known to cause latent herpes zoster when administered to children.
- **C.** Herpes zoster outbreaks are caused by a latent virus, so it is not contagious.
- **D.** The zoster vaccine should not be given to patients who have had a herpes zoster outbreak.

169. A 7-year-old unvaccinated child arrives to the ED. The nurse suspects diphtheria, based on which of the following symptoms?

- **A.** thick gray membrane covering the tonsils and pharynx
- **B.** temperature of 104°F (40°C) or greater
- **C.** macular rash on the thorax and back, along the dermatomes
- **D.** cluster headache with nausea and symptoms of an aura

170. Which of the following statements from a nurse demonstrates that his participation in a Critical Incident Stress Debriefing (CISD) session was effective?

- **A.** He agrees to meet with the manager regarding the incident.
- **B.** He agrees to attend future debriefing sessions as needed.
- **C.** He agrees to schedule an appointment for further counseling.
- **D.** He provides the incident details before departing the debrief.

171. The ED nurse's responsibility to practice quality nursing care is achieved through which of the following?

- **A.** reading research articles
- **B.** participating in Evidence-Based Practice (EBP) projects
- **C.** participating in research studies
- **D.** participating in grand rounds

172. Nurses managing patient transitions of care in the ED should consider all of the following characteristics EXCEPT

- **A.** accessibility of services.
- **B.** safety.
- **C.** community partnerships.
- **D.** patient income.

173. What is the appropriate ratio of compressions to ventilations for a full-term neonate who is apneic with a pulse rate of 50 bpm?

    A. 30:2

    B. 15:1

    C. 15:2

    D. 3:1

174. Which of the following interventions is NOT necessary for a patient who has died in the ED and is not in a vegetative state?

    A. maintaining the head of the bed at 20 degrees

    B. instilling artificial tears in eyes to preserve tissue

    C. taping eyes closed with paper tape

    D. inserting Foley catheter to decompress the bladder

175. A 24-year-old male patient arrives at the ED with a complaint of a 1-month history of a rash that is annular, with raised margins and centralized clearing. Which of the following dermal infections does the nurse expect?

    A. scabies

    B. ringworm

    C. impetigo

    D. cellulitis

ANSWER KEY

1. **B**

   Rationale: Lumbar punctures are contraindicated for patients with increased ICP because of the risk of brain shift caused by the sudden release of CSF pressure. Severe brain shift can result in permanent damage. BMP and CBC labs are routinely monitored in patients with increased ICP. Mechanical ventilation and Foley catheter placement are commonly ordered for patients with increased ICP.

   Objective: Neurological Emergencies

   Subobjective: Increased Intracranial Pressure (ICP)

2. **C**

   Rationale: Adrenaline, dopamine, digoxin, and dobutamine are all positive inotropes and can be helpful in the management of heart failure. However, digoxin is not recommended in the treatment of acute heart failure in an 80-year-old patient as elderly patients are more susceptible to digoxin toxicity.

   Objective: Cardiovascular Emergencies

   Subobjective: Heart Failure

3. **D**

   Rationale: Sudden back pain and dyspnea indicate rupture of the aneurysm, which is an emergency. The nurse should notify the health care provider, monitor neurological and vital signs, and remain with the patient. Yellow-tinted vision is a finding of digitalis toxicity. Hemoptysis a sign of pulmonary edema. Urinary output of 75 mL/hr is normal.

   Objective: Cardiovascular Emergencies

   Subobjective: Aneurysm/Dissection

4. **C**

   Rationale: Increased risk factors for heparin-induced thrombocytopenia (HIT) include being female and heparin use for postsurgical thromboprophylaxis. HIT is more common in patients who have been on unfractionated heparin or who have used heparin for longer than 1 week. Enoxaparin is a low-molecular-weight heparin, which carries a lower risk of

causing HIT. It is often prescribed for patients with unstable angina to help increase blood flow through the heart.

   Objective: Cardiovascular Emergencies

   Subobjective: Thromboembolic Disease

5. **D**

   Rationale: A pericardial friction rub is heard in pericarditis due to the inflammation of the pericardial layers rubbing together. Mitral regurgitation does not occur in pericarditis. An S3 gallop is heard in heart failure. S4 gallop is heard in cardiomyopathies and congenital heart disease.

   Objective: Cardiovascular Emergencies

   Subobjective: Pericarditis

6. **C**

   Rationale: High-velocity injection injuries damage underlying tissue and often result in necrosis and compartment syndrome and may require amputation. Obtaining a surgical consultation and exploration minimizes the risk of long-term complications. While administering prophylactic antibiotics, providing patient education, and immobilizing the affected extremity are correct nursing interventions, they alone will not minimize the risk for complications.

   Objective: Wound

   Subobjective: Injection Injuries

7. **B**

   Rationale: The patient is in V-fib and is pulseless. After CPR is started, the next priority intervention is defibrillation. Epinephrine should not be administered until after defibrillation. Inserting an advanced airway may be indicated but is not the priority. A fluid bolus is not a priority for a patient in V-fib.

   Objective: Cardiovascular Emergencies

   Subobjective: Cardiopulmonary Arrest

8. **D**

   Rationale: The patient has signs and symptoms of gastritis. Pain relievers such as naproxen can inflame the lining of the stomach and lead to gastritis. Tobacco use, radiation, and viral or bacterial infection are also risk factors. Obesity, appendicitis, and hypertension are not associated with naproxen.

Objective: Gastrointestinal Emergencies

Subobjective: Gastritis

9. **C**

Rationale: The infant has signs of intussusception, in which part of the intestine telescopes into another area of the intestine. Abdominal swelling in a child with intussusception is a sign of peritonitis, which can be life-threatening. Vomiting, diarrhea, and a lump in the abdomen are expected findings in a child with intussusception.

Objective: Gastrointestinal Emergencies

Subobjective: Intussusception

10. **B**

Rationale: The physician will counsel the patient on the risks associated with leaving against medical advice (AMA). Whenever possible, the patient should be counseled by the physician, sign AMA paperwork, and then leave the department. A patient with appendicitis will not be involuntarily committed. It is not appropriate to tell a patient he will die if he leaves, although he should be informed of possible negative consequences. The patient should speak with the physician before he tries to leave.

Objective: Professional Issues

Subobjective: Patient (Discharge Planning)

11. **A**

Rationale: Current 2015 guidelines for CPR from the AHA is 30 compressions to 2 ventilations for adult patients with 2 rescuers.

Objective: Cardiovascular Emergencies

Subobjective: Cardiopulmonary Arrest

12. **A**

Rationale: Fluid boluses of 1 to 2 L normal saline should be used to treat hypotension. The patient is dehydrated at the cellular level and needs fluid resuscitation. Furosemide is used

as a diuretic and would further dehydrate the patient, exacerbating the issue. Inotropes such as dopamine are used to promote cardiac contractility and will not hydrate the patient. D5W is not indicated because it is not an isotonic solution that will add to the systemic fluid volume.

Objective: Cardiac Emergencies

Subobjective: Acute Coronary Syndromes

13. **B**

Rationale: An elevated carboxyhemoglobin (COHb) level of 2% or higher for nonsmokers and 10% or higher for smokers strongly supports a diagnosis of carbon monoxide poisoning. COHb may be measured with a fingertip pulse CO-oximeter or by serum lab values. $PaCO_2$ measurements remain normal (38 – 42).

Objective: Environmental

Subobjective: Chemical Exposure

14. **C**

Rationale: A non-odorous white "cottage cheese"–appearing vaginal discharge describes *Candida vulvovaginitis*. Bacterial vaginosis presents with thin white, gray, or green discharge and a fishy odor. *Trichomoniasis* vaginitis typically presents with thin discharge and itching or burning of the genital area. *Neisseria gonorrhoeae* usually does not cause any symptoms but may have dysuria and thin discharge.

Objective: Gynecological

Subobjective: Infection

15. **B**

Rationale: The nurse should place the patient on contact precautions with concern for *C. difficile*. The other levels of precautions are not appropriate based on the information presented.

Objective: Communicable Diseases

Subobjective: C. Difficile

16. **A**

Rationale: A greenish-gray frothy malodorous vaginal discharge and itching are signs and symptoms of *trichomoniasis*.

Bacterial vaginosis would present with a thin discharge and presence of clue cells on the wet prep. Herpes would most likely present with lesions upon inspection. Chlamydia would not cause frothy discharge.

Objective: Gynecological

Subobjective: Infection

17. B

Rationale: Hepatomegaly is seen in patients with right-sided heart failure due to vascular engorgement. Heart failure does not lead to appendicitis. Constipation is not directly a result of heart failure and therefore is not a priority assessment consideration. Stomach upset is a common side effect of many medications but is not a cause for focused or priority assessment.

Objective: Cardiac Emergencies

Subobjective: Heart Failure

18. A

Rationale: Deep tissue palpation should be avoided to minimize the risk of injury to the nurse and to prevent advancement of the foreign body deeper into the tissue structure.

Objective: Wound

Subobjective: Foreign Bodies

19. B

Rationale: The patient is unstable in a third-degree or complete heart block, so transcutaneous pacing is indicated.

Objective: Cardiovascular Emergencies

Subobjective: Dysrhythmias

20. A

Rationale: The patient's symptoms are signs of a septic abortion. An ectopic pregnancy typically presents with vaginal bleeding and pain without fever. A missed abortion may have no other symptoms except a brown discharge. The symptoms are not indicative of abdominal trauma.

Objective: Obstetrical

Subobjective: Threatened/Spontaneous Abortion

21. C

Rationale: PT (prothrombin time) and PTT (partial thromboplastin time) are blood tests that monitor effectiveness of anticoagulant therapy. Hematocrit measures packed RBCs and is not a specific study of anticoagulant effectiveness. HDL and LDL are components of cholesterol measurement. Troponin levels measure myocardial muscle injury.

Objective: Respiratory Emergencies

Subobjective: Pulmonary Embolism

22. D

Rationale: The patient who is diagnosed with disseminated intravascular coagulation (DIC) has both a clotting and bleeding problem. Increased PT/PTT, elevated D-dimer levels, decreased platelets, decreased hemoglobin, and a decreased fibrinogen level are all expected lab values for this patient.

Objective: Medical Emergencies

Subobjective: Blood Dyscrasias

23. B

Rationale: Symptoms of autonomic dysfunction include heart block, bradycardia, hypertension, hypotension, and orthostatic hypotension. Deficits in CN X (vagus nerve) contribute to the development of autonomic dysfunction. Trigeminy, atrial flutter, and tachycardia are not symptoms of autonomic dysfunction.

Objective: Neurological Emergencies

Subobjective: Guillain–Barré Syndrome

24. B

Rationale: Procedural sedation is appropriate for synchronized cardioversion. A perimortem cesarean section typically is done emergently. Open fracture reductions should occur in the operating room, as should dilatation and curettage.

Objective: Professional Issues

Subobjective: Patient (Pain Management and Procedural Sedation)

25. C

Rationale: Lung tissue disorders include pneumonia and pulmonary edema. Examples of lower airway disorders are bronchiolitis and asthma. An upper airway disorder would be croup, anaphylaxis, or foreign body obstruction. Disordered control of breathing means an irregular, slow breathing pattern with a neurological component, such as a seizure.

Objective: Respiratory Emergencies

*Subobjective:*Infections

26. **A**

Rationale: In atrial flutter, there are no discernible P waves, and a distinct sawtooth wave pattern is present. The atrial rate is regular, and the PR interval is not measurable. In atrial fibrillation, the rhythm would be very irregular with coarse, asynchronous waves. Torasades de pointes, or "twisting of the points," is characterized by QRS complexes that twist around the baseline and is a form of polymorphic ventricular tachycardia. It may resolve spontaneously or progress to ventricular fibrillation, which is emergent, as the ventricles are unable to pump any blood due to disorganized electrical activity. Untreated, it quickly leads to cardiac arrest.

Objective: Cardiovascular Emergencies

Subobjective: Dysrhythmias

27. **B**

Rationale: The patient has been playing sports, sweating and replacing lost fluid with only water, which can cause hyponatremia. A loss of sodium will cause neurological effects such as confusion, seizures, and coma. The symptoms are not indicative of a potassium imbalance. Hyperkalemia would cause thirst and nausea/vomiting.

Objective: Medical Emergencies

Subobjective: Electrolyte/Fluid Imbalance

28. **B**

Rationale: A barking cough is a symptom of croup, and nebulized epinephrine is the treatment of choice. IV epinephrine is not indicated in croup; it is more often used in anaphylaxis and resuscitation efforts. Albuterol has a primary effect on lower lung structures and will not improve symptoms of croup. Dexamethasone is indicated for croup but is not the priority intervention.

Objective: Respiratory Emergencies

Subobjective: Infections

29. **A**

Rationale: Bell's palsy is caused by an inflammation of the seventh cranial nerve and presents with facial paralysis and weakness.

Objective: Maxillofacial

Subobjective: Facial Nerve Disorders

30. **B**

Rationale: Left-sided heart failure manifestations include pulmonary symptoms such as crackles and dyspnea. Right-sided heart failure causes systemic congestion, leading to hepatomegaly, dependent edema, jugular vein distention, and ascites.

Objective: Cardiovascular Emergencies

Subobjective: Heart Failure

31. **A**

Rationale: Foreign body infections and cellulitis of surgical hardware sites present with local pain and systemic infectious indicators such as fever, edema, warmth, and elevated WBCs with left shift in neutrophils.

Objective: Orthopedic

Subobjective: Foreign Bodies

32. **A**

Rationale: The second digit of the nondominant hand is the most common site, as these types of injuries are usually self-inflicted.

Objective: Wound

Subobjective: Injection Injuries

33. **A**

Rationale: Absent or decreased breath sounds are present in a pneumothorax. A nurse would be able to visualize a foreign body on the right side of chest while doing the initial assessment. Hematoma and pleural effusion are both associated with decreased breath sounds, not with absent sounds.

Objective: Respiratory Emergencies

Subobjective: Pneumothorax

34. A

Rationale: Warfarin is an anticoagulant commonly prescribed for patients with A-fib. Any anticoagulant must be given cautiously to patients with subarachnoid hemorrhage due to the increased risk of bleeding. Morphine is commonly prescribed for pain, and nimodipine is given to treat or prevent cerebral vasospasm. Stool softeners are given to reduce the need to strain during a bowel movement.

Objective: Neurological Emergencies

Subobjective: Trauma

35. C

Rationale: An uncomfortable feeling of pressure, squeezing, fullness, or pain in the center of the chest is the predominant symptom of a myocardial infarction (MI), particularly in women. Palpitations indicate a dysrhythmia. Edema in the lower extremities is a later sign of cardiac failure. A feeling of nausea is not common with MI.

Objective: Cardiovascular Emergencies

Subobjective: Acute Coronary Syndrome

36. B

Rationale: NPO status is essential for all suspected surgical cases. Elevation is limited with regard to injury. Ice, while therapeutic, would not be a priority intervention.

Objective: Orthopedic

Subobjective: Fractures/Dislocations

37. D

Rationale: Carbamazepine may cause dizziness or drowsiness. The patient should use caution while driving or operating machinery until he understands how the medication will affect him. There is no contraindication to sunlight exposure with this medication. Dietary concerns with carbamazepine are limited to consulting the health care provider before taking with grapefruit juice.

Objective: Neurological Emergencies

Subobjective: Seizure Disorders

38. C

Rationale: A Glasgow Coma Scale (GCS) of 7 indicates that the patient is experiencing deficits in eye opening, motor response, and verbal response. As the GCS drops, the patient is less alert and able to follow commands. Patients with a GCS of 7 will require intubation to maintain oxygenation. The lower the GCS, the less likely the patient is to fully recover without permanent deficits. An IV bolus will not negate the need for assisted breathing. This patient will be unable to get up to a chair. As the GCS drops, a nasal cannula becomes ineffective at providing oxygenation.

Objective: Neurological Emergencies

Subobjective: Trauma

39. D

Rationale: A severe headache indicates increased intracranial pressure (ICP), a complication of lumbar puncture. The health care provider should be notified immediately. Other indications of increased ICP are nausea, vomiting, photophobia, and changes in LOC. The patient should be encouraged to increase fluid intake unless contraindicated. The patient will remain flat and on bed rest following the procedure, per agency and health care provider guidelines. Minor pain controlled with analgesics is not a concern but should be monitored for changes.

Objective: Neurological Emergencies

Subobjective: Meningitis

40. A

Rationale: The electrocardiogram (ECG) is most commonly used to initially determine the location of myocardial damage. An echocardiogram is used to view myocardial wall function after a myocardial infarction (MI) has been diagnosed. Cardiac enzymes will aid in diagnosing an MI but will not determine the location. While not performed initially, cardiac catheterization determines coronary artery disease and would suggest the location of myocardial damage.

Objective: Cardiovascular Emergencies

Subobjective: Acute Coronary Syndrome

41. B

Rationale: As Alzheimer's disease progresses, confusion increases. Providing regular toileting can prevent possible falls that result when to hurrying to the bathroom to maintain continence. Haloperidol should be used with extreme caution in geriatric patients with Alzheimer's. Restraints can increase confusion in these patients and should be used only per facility guidelines. Offering too many choices can overwhelm the patient and lead to increased confusion and frustration.

Objective: Neurological Emergencies

Subobjective: Alzheimer's Disease/Dementia

42. **A**

Rationale: N-acetylcysteine is the antidote for acetaminophen toxicity and is administered to patients with hepatotoxic levels of serum acetaminophen levels. Intubation is not indicated, and naloxone is not the correct antidote. Gastric lavage is not indicated in this circumstance.

Objective: Communicable Diseases

Subobjective: Overdose and Ingestion

43. **C**

Rationale: The patient with emphysema can gain optimal lung expansion by sitting up and leaning forward. Lying in a prone position, flat on the back, or on the side with feet elevated will further potentiate any airway obstruction and effort, exacerbating the problem.

Objective: Respiratory Emergencies

Subobjective: Chronic Obstructive Pulmonary Disease

44. **C**

Rationale: Validation therapy is used with patients with severe dementia when reality orientation is not appropriate. The nurse may ask the patient what her mother looks like or what she is wearing but does not argue about whether her mother is living. This allows the nurse to acknowledge the patient's concerns while avoiding confrontation or encouraging further belief that her mother is alive. Confrontation may cause the patient with dementia to react inappropriately and is used only when the nurse has established patient trust. Reality orientation works best with patients in the early stages of dementia. Seeking clarification will only cause more confusion because the nurse is asking the

patient to explain something, which can lead to patient frustration.

Objective: Neurological Emergencies

Subobjective: Alzheimer's Disease/Dementia

45. **C**

Rationale: The patient should be thoroughly washed, and all linens and clothing items should be replaced with hospital-provided materials to prevent spread of bedbugs. All home-provided clothing and linens must be double-bagged and either disposed of or placed in a dryer on hot setting for 30 minutes. The presence of bedbugs is not necessarily a sign of abuse or neglect and therefore does not warrant a call to child welfare services. Contact precautions would be most appropriate.

Objective: Environmental

Subobjective: Parasite and Fungal Infestations

46. **D**

Rationale: A patient with diverticulitis would be expected to have lower abdominal pain with anorexia and fever in addition to an elevated WBC count.

Objective: Gastrointestinal Emergencies

Subobjective: Diverticulitis

47. **B**

Rationale: An increase in pain with nausea and vomiting are signs that an incarcerated hernia may be causing a bowel obstruction and should be reported immediately. The other findings are expected in a patient with a hernia and do not need to be immediately reported to the health care provider.

Objective: Gastrointestinal Emergencies

Subobjective: Hernia

48. **A**

Rationale: If the patient has diminished decisional capacity due to a developmental delay, the legal guardian must consent to any intervention for the patient unless there is an emergent issue.

Objective: Professional Issues

Subobjective: System (Patient Consent for Treatment)

49. C

Rationale: This patient is experiencing appendicitis. Pain that is relieved by bending the right hip suggests perforation and peritonitis. The patient would not need an abdominal MRI based on her symptoms. The patient will need surgery, so maintaining NPO status and administering IV fluids are a priority. Morphine will be given for pain.

Objective: Gastrointestinal Emergencies

Subobjective: Acute Abdomen

50. A

Rationale: The first priority for an unresponsive patient in V-fib is performing high-quality CPR. The patient should then be prepared to be defibrillated. Epinephrine should be administered after the patient has been defibrillated at least twice. IV access is not the initial priority.

Objective: Cardiovascular Emergencies

Subobjective: Dysrhythmias

51. B

Rationale: The nursing priority for patients with fistulas is preserving and protecting the skin. The nurse should inspect the skin frequently and assess for any redness, irritation, or broken areas. The skin should remain dry and intact. Antibiotics may be given but are not the first priority. Wound VACs should not be used simply to manage drainage or in patients with increased bleeding risk. Providing a quiet environment is important, but skin integrity is the first priority with this patient.

Objective: Gastrointestinal Emergencies

Subobjective: Inflammatory Bowel Disease

52. D

Rationale: Classic signs of cardiogenic shock include a rapid pulse that weakens; cool, clammy skin; and decreased urine output. Hypotension is another classic sign.

Objective: Cardiovascular Emergencies

Subobjective: Shock

53. B

Rationale: Having a frank, professional conversation regarding chronic pain relief is the nurse's priority. The nurse should not immediately assume the patient is drug-seeking, nor should the nurse ignore the patient's pain complaint.

Objective: Professional Issues

Subobjective:

Patient (Pain Management and Procedural Sedation)

54. D

Rationale: An avulsion is characterized by the separation of skin from the underlying structures that cannot be approximated.

Objective: Wound

Subobjective: Avulsions

55. C

Rationale: The priority for this patient is to prepare for surgical removal of the knife, so it should be stabilized with bulky dressings to avoid shifting as the patient is transported. The nurse should never attempt to remove an embedded object in a patient, as this is beyond the scope of practice for nursing. Blood loss may be estimated based on how many dressings or towels are saturated. Next of kin should be notified only after the patient is stabilized.

Objective: Gastrointestinal Emergencies

Subobjective: Abdominal Trauma

56. A

Rationale: Dysfunction of the renal cells and decreased levels of ADH hormone/vasopressin lead to diuresis, and fluid leakage into the interstitial spaces further contributes to hypovolemia. Shivering and vasoconstriction mask the symptoms of hypovolemia rather than contribute to it. Diaphoresis, dehydration, tachycardia, and tachypnea are all common symptoms of hyperthermia.

Objective: Environmental

Subobjective: Temperature-Related Emergencies

57. **A**

Rationale: A sudden, severe onset of testicular pain indicates the possibility of testicular torsion and a stat ultrasound should be ordered to confirm. Epididymitis typically presents gradually with unilateral pain and discharge, and pain is relieved with elevation of the testes. Sudden, severe pain is not an indication of UTI or orchitis.

Objective: Genitourinary

Subobjective: Testicular Torsion

58. **B**

Rationale: A purulent vaginal discharge with bilateral pelvic pain and nausea are symptoms of a tubo-ovarian abscess. An ectopic pregnancy would most commonly present with vaginal bleeding, not purulent discharge. A ruptured appendix would typically present as RLQ pain. Diverticulitis may cause abdominal pain and nausea but not purulent vaginal discharge.

Objective: Gynecological

Subobjective: Infection

59. **D**

Rationale: Abdominal cramping with vaginal bleeding and expulsion of tissue are signs of a complete spontaneous abortion. An incomplete spontaneous abortion would have retained tissue. Septic abortions are typically febrile. A threatened abortion may progress to a spontaneous abortion but would not result in passing a large solid tissue clot.

Objective: Obstetrical

Subobjective: Threatened/Spontaneous Abortion

60. **C**

Rationale: Corticosteroids will be administered to decrease inflammation of the airways. Albuterol and ipratropium are bronchodilators and do not address the swelling and inflammation caused by croup. Antibiotics are not indicated for croup.

Objective: Respiratory Emergencies

Subobjective: Infections

61. **A**

Rationale: Mucopurulent discharge, burning, and itching are symptoms of chlamydia. A herpes infection would have lesions. Syphilis typically presents with a small, painless sore. HPV typically presents asymptomatically but may also have warts.

Objective: Gynecological

Subobjective: Infection

62. **D**

Rationale: Aspirin is contraindicated for children with varicella because it can lead to Reye syndrome, a rare form of encephalopathy. Antihistamines, colloidal oatmeal baths, and non-aspirin antipyretics such as acetaminophen are all recommended in-home therapies to relieve symptoms.

Objective: Communicable Diseases

Subobjective: Childhood Diseases

63. **B**

Rationale: Current NRP guidelines (2015) recommend 40 – 60 breaths per minute for rescue breathing in the newborn. Rescue breaths at a rate of 12 – 20 are not adequate to provide enough ventilation for the neonate. Inserting an LMA or intubation may be indicated but is not the immediate nursing priority.

Objective: Obstetrical

Subobjective: Neonatal Resuscitation

64. **B**

Rationale: As a member of the team the nurse can suggest to the team leader to consider the futility of the resuscitation at that point. The nurse does not have the authority to end the resuscitation and should not advise the patient's parents to make that decision. Ethically, the nurse should speak up if he or she feels that the efforts are futile.

Objective: Professional Issues

Subobjective: Patient (End-of-Life Issues)

65. **B**

Rationale: The current (2015) guidelines for neonatal resuscitation recommend epinephrine to be administered at 0.01 – 0.03mg/kg. The other medication dosages are not appropriate as a first-line medication to be administered to a neonate with bradycardia.

Objective: Obstetrical

Subobjective: Neonatal Resuscitation

66. **C**

Rationale: Contusions accompanied by the symptoms mentioned should be treated with rest, ice, compression, and elevation. NSAIDs will provide appropriate pain relief; opioid therapy is not indicated for minor contusions.

Objective: Orthopedic

Subobjective: Trauma

67. **D**

Rationale: Amitriptyline is a tricyclic antidepressant. This class of drugs has anticholinergic effects, which frequently cause serious side effects. In older, confused patients such as those with Alzheimer's disease, amitriptyline can cause increased confusion, constipation, and urinary retention. Paroxetine and sertraline are SSRIs and may be given to patients with Alzheimer's. Memantine is an NMDA receptor antagonist prescribed to slow the progression of Alzheimer's.

Objective: Neurological Emergencies

Subobjective: Alzheimer's Disease/Dementia

68. **B**

Rationale: Adolescent patients presenting with frostbite burns to the roof of the mouth are most likely abusing inhalants, typically in the form of aerosols, glues, paints, and solvents. A hot beverage would not cause the other symptoms, nor would marijuana use. Dry ice would cause tissue injury to the entire mouth.

Objective: Communicable Diseases

Subobjective: Substance Abuse

69. **D**

Rationale: The patient should be turned on his side because he may lose consciousness and aspirate. The side-lying position facilitates the drainage of any oral secretions. Padded side rails may be used as part of seizure protocols, but turning the patient on his side is the priority. Tongue blades should never

be left at the bedside, as their use can chip teeth, which can be aspirated. Administering IV diazepam should be done only after the patient is turned to his side to avoid aspiration.

Objective: Neurological Emergencies

Subobjective: Seizure Disorders

70. **B**

Rationale: The patient has suffered trauma in the motor vehicle crash (MVC). The bright red painless vaginal bleeding is a sign of placenta previa. Abruptio placentae results in painful bleeding that is typically dark red. An ectopic pregnancy and complete abortion would not occur due to an MVC.

Objective: Obstetrical

Subobjective: Placenta Previa

71. **A**

Rationale: Abdominal tenderness and dark red vaginal bleeding are signs of abruptio placenta. Placenta previa would present with bright red painless bleeding. Spontaneous abortions typically do not occur after 20 weeks.

Objective: Obstetrical

Subjective: Abruptio Placenta

72. **D**

Rationale: Safety is the priority for patients with altered mental status. The nurse should ask if the patient is hearing voices telling him to harm himself or others. Simply saying that no one is there dismisses the patient's feelings. Offering to find a blanket validates the delusion that someone is there. Asking if Martha is staying also prevents reality orientation and may worsen the patient's confusion.

Objective: Psychosocial Emergencies

Subobjective: Psychosis

73. **C**

Rationale: A thoracentesis is performed to remove the fluid. A chest tube is used to decompress a hemothorax or pneumothorax and is not indicated in the presence of pleural effusion. A pericardial window is used to drain excess fluid from the pericardium, not the pleural space.

Objective: Respiratory Emergencies

Subobjective: Pleural Effusion

74. **B**

Rationale: Esophageal varices can lead to death via hemorrhage. Octreotide is a vasoconstrictor used to control bleeding before performing endoscopy. Phenytoin is an anticonvulsant, levofloxacin is an antibiotic, and pantoprazole is a proton pump inhibitor; none of these are indicated at this time.

Objective: Gastrointestinal Emergencies

Subobjective: Esophageal Varices

75. **D**

Rationale: "You're feeling lost since your mother died," uses the therapeutic technique of restating. The nurse repeats the patient's words back to her. This therapeutic communication technique allows the patient to verify that the nurse understood the patient and allows for clarification if needed. It also encourages the patient to continue. Telling the patient that she will feel better in time minimizes the patient's feelings and sounds uncaring. Telling the patient to join a grief support group forces the nurse's decision onto the patient. Stating shared feelings takes the focus from the patient to the nurse.

Objective: Psychosocial Emergencies

Subobjective: Depression

76. **D**

Rationale: The symptoms indicate right-sided myocardial infarction (MI), so IV fluids are the priority treatment for this patient. When treating patients with right ventricular infarction, nitrates, diuretics, and morphine are to be avoided due to their pre-load-reducing effects.

Objective: Cardiac Emergencies

Subobjective: Acute Coronary Syndromes

77. **C**

Rationale: The symptoms are characteristic of meningococcal meningitis, which is commonly contracted in crowded living

spaces such as college dorms. Influenza is characterized by upper-respiratory symptoms; scabies is a dermal infection; and pertussis is a respiratory illness.

Objective: Communicable Diseases

Subobjective: Childhood Diseases

78. **B**

Rationale: The patient has had nausea and vomiting, which can cause hypokalemia. A U wave can be noted on an ECG or cardiac monitor. Hyperkalemia would show peaked T waves. Hypercalcemia may produce a shortened QT interval, and hypocalcemia may show QT prolongation.

Objective: Medical Emergencies

Subobjective: Electrolyte/Fluid Imbalance

79. **A**

Rationale: Chain of custody is the concept of limiting the number of people handling and collecting evidence after a crime is committed. Nurses caring for patients and handling evidence should use local official documents to demonstrate the chain of custody for evidence and to document when it is given to authorities.

Objective: Professional Issues

Subobjective: Patient (Forensic Evidence Collection)

80. **C**

Rationale: The patient has a pneumothorax and will need a chest tube. Chest compressions are indicated only for cardiac arrest. Thoracotomy is done when there is severe trauma and impending or present cardiac arrest and is the final effort made to sustain life; it is associated with a low rate of successful outcomes. Endotracheal intubation is not indicated if the patient is able to protect his own airway, as is evidenced by his ability to communicate verbally.

Objective: Respiratory Emergencies

Subobjective: Pneumothorax

81. **D**

Rationale: Endoscopic litigation is indicated for *posterior* epistaxis stemming from the ethmoid or sphenopalatine arteries. Kiesselbach's plexus is the most common site of *anterior* epistaxis that responds to conventional treatments.

Objective: Maxillofacial

Subobjective: Epistaxis

82. **B**

Rationale: The patient with adrenal hypofunction should not be on a sodium-restrictive diet, as it may lead to an adrenal crisis. Peripheral blood draws, glucose monitoring, and hydrocortisone therapy are all appropriate for adrenal insufficiency.

Objective: Medical Emergencies

Subobjective: Endocrine Conditions

83. **C**

Rationale: Patients with hyperventilation syndrome will present with similar signs and symptoms as pulmonary emboli. Patients with a pneumothorax will present with absent breath sounds on the side of the injury, anxiety, and pain on inspiration. Pneumonia is characterized by fever, malaise, and crackles at the base of the lungs.

Objective: Respiratory Emergencies

Subobjective: Pulmonary Embolus

84. **A**

Rationale: Antipsychotics are used to treat psychotic symptoms such as hallucinations, paranoia, and delusions. They carry an increased risk of mortality, primarily from cardiovascular complications. A cardiac workup identifies any risk factors that would be a contraindication to antipsychotics. A comprehensive metabolic panel (CMP), creatinine clearance, and a CBC do not address the underlying risk of cardiovascular complications.

Objective: Psychosocial Emergencies

Subobjective: Psychosis

85. **C**

Rationale: The nurse should assign a sitter because the patient's safety is more important than his right to refuse care. Placing the patient in restraints does not guarantee his

safety and may escalate the situation. If the patient manages to get out of the restraints, he might hang himself with them. Having security sit outside the door does not provide direct observation of the patient and uses up a limited resource of the facility. Allowing the patient to leave against medical advice (AMA) leaves the nurse and the facility vulnerable to legal action if he commits suicide after leaving.

Objective: Psychosocial Emergencies

Subobjective: Suicidal Ideation

86. **A**

Rationale: Abnormalities in magnesium levels may put the patient at risk for ventricular dysrhythmia. A hypomagnesemia level of 0.8 mEq/L would be of concern (normal range is 1.5 – 2.5 mEq/L). The other values are within normal ranges.

Objective: Cardiovascular Emergencies

Subobjective: Dysrhythmias

87. **D**

Rationale: The patient is experiencing an unstable supraventricular tachycardia (SVT) with BP of 70/42 mm Hg and requires immediate synchronized cardioversion. Defibrillation is not indicated because the patient is awake and has an organized heart rhythm. Adenosine can be used in patients with stable SVT; however, this patient is not stable. Amiodarone is not indicated for unstable patients in SVT.

Objective: Cardiovascular Emergencies

Subobjective: Dysrhythmias

88. **A**

Rationale: The drug of choice for supraventricular tachycardia (SVT) is adenosine. The first dose of 6 mg has already been given, so the next appropriate dose would be 12 mg. The other options are not the next appropriate intervention for a patient in SVT.

Objective: Cardiovascular Emergencies

Subobjective: Dysrhythmias

89. B

Rationale: The goal for pulse oximetry readings is 94% – 99%. The nurse should apply supplemental oxygen for an SpO_2 below 94%. Albuterol and dexamethasone are appropriate for asthma but are not the priority intervention. Endotracheal intubation is needed only if a patient is unable to maintain their airway.

Objective: Respiratory Emergencies

Subobjective: Asthma

90. A

Rationale: The patient experiencing a sickle cell crisis needs fluid resuscitation with crystalloid solutions and the administration of warmed RBCs. Whole blood contains additional components such as plasma or platelets, which are not needed. Fresh frozen plasma and cryoprecipitate are not indicated for sickle cell crisis.

Objective: Medical Emergencies

Subobjective: Blood Dyscrasias

91. B

Rationale: Rhabdomyolysis is characterized by the breakdown of skeletal muscle with the release of myoglobin and other intercellular proteins and electrolytes into the circulation. The presence of myoglobin produces heme-positive results in the urinalysis.

Objective: Orthopedic

Subobjective: Trauma

92. D

Rationale: The sharp, tearing knifelike substernal chest pain with no relief from morphine is a hallmark sign of an aortic dissection. Pneumonia presents with pain related to coughing. Pain from a myocardial infarction (MI) or pericarditis would likely be relieved with doses of morphine sulfate.

Objective: Cardiovascular Emergencies

Subobjective: Aneurysm/Dissection

93. B

Rationale: Captopril is an ACE inhibitor, which can cause hyperkalemia. Bumetanide and furosemide are diuretics, which

would cause hypokalemia. Digoxin is an antidysrhythmic and can also cause hypokalemia.

Objective: Medical Emergencies

Subobjective: Electrolyte/Fluid Imbalance

94. C

Rationale: Patients with idiopathic thrombocytopenic purpura (ITP) have decreased platelet production, so platelets are the expected treatment. The other options are not indicated for this condition.

Objective: Medical Emergencies

Subobjective: Blood Dyscrasias

95. C

Rationale: Vasospastic disorders such as Raynaud's phenomena and migraine headaches are associated with variant (Prinzmetal's) angina.

Objective: Cardiac Emergencies

Subobjective: Chronic Stable Angina Pectoris

96. B

Rationale: Hyperosmolar hyperglycemic state (HHS) is often caused by dehydration, especially in patients over 65. Inadequate glucose monitoring and medication noncompliance are not the most common causes of HHS. A breakdown of ketones causing ketoacidosis would be found in diabetic ketoacidosis (DKA).

Objective: Medical Emergencies

Subobjective: Endocrine Conditions

97. C

Rationale: Fluoxetine is given cautiously to patients with glaucoma, due to the anticholinergic side effects. There are no current indications that this medication causes side effects with arthritis, migraines, or appendicitis.

Objective: Psychosocial Emergencies

Subobjective: Depression

98. D

Rationale: Throbbing fingers or toes after exercise accompanied with thin, shiny skin and thick fingernails are symptoms of peripheral vascular disease. Acute occlusion would present with pain and cyanosis distal to the occlusion. Venous thrombosis occurs more often in the lower extremities, and there is no information suggesting arterial injury.

Objective: Cardiovascular Emergencies

Subobjective: Peripheral Vascular Disease

99. C

Rationale: Insulin administration shifts potassium into the cells causing hypokalemia, so fluids with potassium are indicated for this patient. The other fluids are not indicated for this patient.

Objective: Medical Emergencies

Subobjective: Endocrine Conditions

100. C

Rationale: Status epilepticus occurs when a person experiences a seizure that lasts more than 5 minutes or has repeated episodes over 30 minutes. This is a medical emergency, as death can result if seizures last more than 10 minutes. Causes of status epilepticus include alcohol or drug withdrawal, suddenly stopping antiseizure medications, head trauma, and infection. Atonic seizures occur when the patient has a sudden loss of muscle tone for a few seconds, followed by postictal confusion. Tonic–clonic (grand mal) seizures last for only a few minutes. With a simple partial seizure, the patient remains conscious during the episode, which may be preceded by auras. Autonomic changes may occur, such as heart rate changes and epigastric discomfort.

Objective: Neurological Emergencies

Subobjective: Seizure Disorders

101. B

Rationale: Risk factors for pancreatitis include alcohol abuse, peptic ulcer disease, renal failure, vascular disorders, hyperlipidemia, and hyperparathyroidism. Patients often find relief in the fetal position, while the supine position worsens pain. The pain is severe and sudden and feels intense and boring, as if it is going through the body. Pain occurs in the mid-epigastric area or left

upper quadrant. Pain can radiate to the left flank, the left shoulder, or the back.

Objective: Gastrointestinal Emergencies

Subobjective: Pancreatitis

102. B

Rationale: Family member at the bedside for resuscitation has been demonstrated in the evidence as a preference for patients and families and should be offered when possible and appropriate. Family members should be present only if they are not disruptive to patient care.

103. A

Rationale: When an organ donor patient dies in the ED the nurse should first contact the organ procurement organization because of time sensitivity. Life-supporting interventions such as ventilators and medications should be continued until the organ procurement agency arrives. Postmortem care and completing the death certificate can be performed after organ procurement has taken place.

Objective: Professional Issues

Subobjective: Patient (End-of-Life Issues)

104. A

Rationale: Propylthiouracil (PTU) is the drug of choice in treating thyroid storm, as it inhibits the synthesis of thyroxine. Epinephrine and atropine are contraindicated for thyroid storm, as these patients already have a dangerously high heart rate. Levothyroxine would be indicated for myxedema coma.

Objective: Medical Emergencies

Subobjective: Endocrine Conditions

105. C

Rationale: The patient will be involuntarily committed because she is a threat to her own safety. She has not committed a crime. She will not be admitted voluntarily because she did not come to the hospital of her own volition.

Objective: Professional Issues

Subobjective: Patient (Transitions of Care)

106. D

Rationale: The patient is in acidosis and has Kussmaul respirations, which are indicative of diabetic ketoacidosis (DKA). Myxedema coma and pheochromocytoma would not cause these symptoms. Hyperosmolar hyperglycemic state (HHS) normally causes higher blood sugar levels and does not present in acidosis.

Objective: Medical Emergencies

Subobjective: Endocrine Conditions

107. B

Rationale: The Glasgow Coma Scale (GCS) is calculated as follows: opening eyes to sound (3), localizing pain (5), and making incoherent sounds (2) gives a GCS score of 10.

Objective: Neurological Emergencies

Subobjective: Trauma

108. A

Rationale: The patient is showing signs of peritonsillar abscess. Peritonsillar abscess is an emergent condition that occurs from the accumulation of purulent exudate between the tonsillar capsule and the pharyngeal constrictor muscle. Patchy tonsillar exudate, petechiae, and lymphedema are common findings with viral and bacterial strep throat infections.

Objective: Maxillofacial

Subobjective: Peritonsillar Abscess

109. C

Rationale: Foods high in lactose may be poorly tolerated by patients with ulcerative colitis (UC) and should be limited or avoided. High-fiber foods can aggravate GI symptoms in some patients and should be avoided. Caffeine is a stimulant that can increase cramping and diarrhea. Dried fruit stimulates the GI tract and can exacerbate symptoms.

Objective: Gastrointestinal Emergencies

Subobjective: Inflammatory Bowel Disease

110. C

Rationale: A sudden sharp pain in the pelvic region associated with sexual intercourse and no vaginal discharge is common with an ovarian cyst rupture. An ectopic pregnancy does not typically present with sudden pain, and there is usually vaginal bleeding. A ruptured appendix will cause constant pain to the RLQ and commonly causes a fever. The symptoms are not indicative of an STD.

Objective: Gynecological

Subobjective: Ovarian Cyst

111. B

Rationale: An elevation in serum lactate level will conclude the diagnosis of sepsis. The WBC count and neutrophil count would be increased. RBCs do not give adequate information to suspect sepsis.

Objective: Medical Emergencies

Subobjective: Sepsis and Septic Shock

112. B

Rationale: Dehydration requires an isotonic crystalloid solution, such as normal saline or lactated Ringer's, which will evenly distribute between the intravascular space and cells. Hypertonic solutions pull water from cells into the intravascular space, and hypotonic solutions move fluid from the intravascular space into the cells. Colloid solutions, such as albumin, draw fluid into intravascular compartments and would not be appropriate for this patient.

Objective: Medical Emergencies

Subobjective: Electrolyte/Fluid Imbalance

113. C

Rationale: A history of hypertension will cause an increase in afterload. Diabetes will cause complications with microvascular disease, leading to poor cardiac function. Endocrine disorders will cause an increase in cardiac workload. Marfan syndrome causes the cardiac muscle to stretch and weaken.

Objective: Cardiac Emergencies

Subobjective: Heart Failure

114. D

Rationale: Patients with subarachnoid hemorrhage commonly describe having the "worst headache of my life." Nausea and vomiting, not food cravings, may occur. There is no rash associated with subarachnoid hemorrhage. Battle's sign is a characteristic symptom of basilar skull fracture.

Objective: Neurological Emergencies

Subobjective: Trauma

115. C

Rationale: Several of the medications used to treat MS are immunosuppressants; therefore, the patient is more susceptible to infection while taking them. Patients should avoid crowds and anyone who appears to have an infection, such as the flu. Alternating an eye patch from one eye to the other every few hours can relieve diplopia. Patients with MS have alterations in mobility, and clearing walking paths in the home makes it safer to ambulate, especially with a walker or cane. If the patient suspects infection, he or she should notify the health care provider immediately.

Objective: Neurological Emergencies

Subobjective: Chronic Neurological Disorders

116. B

Rationale: The signs and symptoms of pelvic inflammatory disease are lower abdominal pain that worsens with movement, a temperature greater than 101.3°F (38.5°C), tachycardia, and non-malodorous vaginal discharge. Appendicitis does not cause vaginal discharge. Ectopic pregnancy typically causes vaginal bleeding. Most STIs present with malodorous discharge and do not cause fever and tachycardia.

Objective: Gynecological

Subobjective: Infection

117. C

Rationale: Penicillin V potassium for antibiotic therapy is indicated for the treatment of dental abscesses, a condition indicated by this patient's symptoms. Sodium fluoride drops are a supplement for children, nystatin is used to treat oral candida albicans infections, and saliva substitute is a rinse for dry mouth.

Objective: Maxillofacial

Subobjective: Dental Conditions

118. C

Rationale: Morphine sulfate is the analgesic of choice in acute coronary syndrome (ACS): it provides analgesic and sedation and also decreases preload and afterload. Morphine is administered to relieve pain as well as to decrease pain-related anxiety that can further exacerbate the symptoms of the myocardial infarction (MI). Meperidine is not indicated for use in MI. Hydromorphone is more appropriate for patients with no cardiac compromise, and acetaminophen is not indicated in MI.

Objective: Cardiovascular Emergencies

Subobjective: Acute Coronary Syndrome

119. A

Rationale: HIV patients with a fever are considered emergent, and a septic workup is expected. After drawing blood cultures, antibiotics should be the priority intervention. Acetaminophen may be administered but is not the priority. Taking the patient's antivirals after she has been noncompliant is not a priority. She does not need a blood transfusion.

Objective: Medical Emergencies

Subobjective: Immunocompromised

120. C

Rationale: Late signs of increased intracranial pressure (ICP) include dilated or pinpoint pupils that are sluggish or nonreactive to light. Headache, restlessness, and decreasing LOC are early signs of increased ICP.

Objective: Neurological Emergencies

Subobjective: Increased Intracranial Pressure (ICP)

121. A

Rationale: The child should remain with the parent in an upright position. Taking the child from the parent could cause anxiety and crying and worsen the respiratory distress.

Objective: Respiratory Emergencies

Subobjective: Infections

122. A

Rationale: Complications of ulcerative colitis (UC) include hemorrhage and nutritional deficiencies. Patients may have up to 10 – 20 bloody, liquid stools per day. Loose, non-bloody stools and fistulas are more common in patients with Crohn's disease. Surgery is rarely required for these symptoms.

Objective: Gastrointestinal Emergencies

Subobjective: Inflammatory Bowel Disease

123. B

Rationale: Trigeminal neuralgia pain has an abrupt onset, is unilateral along the branch of the fifth cranial nerve, and causes hemifacial spasms.

Objective: Maxillofacial

Subobjective: Facial Nerve Disorders

124. C

Rationale: The patient is experiencing symptoms of pulmonary edema, a complication of left-sided heart failure. Coagulation is not a secondary effect of myocardial infarction (MI). Pneumonia is not generally related to post–MI concerns. A ruptured ventricle would present symptoms closer to the time of injury.

Objective: Cardiovascular Emergencies

Subobjective: Heart Failure and Cardiogenic Pulmonary Edema

125. B

Rationale: Advance directives must be valid, up to date, and documented before they can be honored in the ED. The nurse can document the patient's wishes, but it is not official until the paperwork is present. The physician does not make that decision, and with the correct documentation, EDs will honor advance directives.

Objective: Professional Issues

Subobjective: Patient (End-of-Life Issues)

126. D

Rationale: A pharmacist would not be consulted in this situation. Other members of the team may include ED physicians, social workers, and hospital religious team members.

Objective: Professional Issues

Subobjective: Patient (End-of-Life Issues)

127. C

Rationale: Instruct the parent to perform oral positive pressure by sealing his or her mouth securely over the child's mouth and providing a short, sharp puff of air while simultaneously occluding the unaffected nostril.

Objective: Maxillofacial

Subobjective: Foreign Bodies

128. C

Rationale: Patching the affected eye decreases oxygen delivery to the cornea, delays wound healing, and creates an environment that increases the risk for infection.

Objective: Ocular

Subobjective: Abrasions

129. D

Rationale: When a patient is experiencing hallucinations, the nurse should acknowledge the patient's fear but reinforce reality. Telling the patient that it is the wrinkles in the blanket dismisses the patient's fear and does not reorient the patient. Offering to move the patient to another room accepts the snakes as real and does not help the patient with reality. Offering to call maintenance reinforces the patient's belief that the snakes are real.

Objective: Psychosocial Emergencies

Subobjective: Psychosis

130. D

Rationale: Isocarboxazid and other MAOI inhibitors should not be taken with rasagiline mesylate due to the risk of increased blood pressure and hypertensive crisis. The other medications are not contraindicated for this patient: baclofen relieves muscle spasms, benztropine is an older drug that treats severe motor symptoms such as rigidity and tremors, and amantadine is an antiviral drug often prescribed with carbidopa and levodopa to reduce dyskinesias.

Objective: Neurological Emergencies

Subobjective: Chronic Neurological Disorders

131. A

Rationale: Herpes zoster infection of the facial nerves commonly involves the eyelid and surrounding structures. Treatment is palliative, using antiviral medications such as acyclovir.

Objective: Ocular

Subobjective: Infections

132. D

Rationale: These ABGs indicate acute respiratory acidosis. Common signs of respiratory acidosis include hypoventilation with hypoxia, disorientation, and dizziness. Untreated respiratory acidosis can progress to ventricular fibrillation, hypotension, seizures, and coma. Deep, rapid respirations and nausea and vomiting are signs of metabolic acidosis. Chest pain is not a symptom of respiratory acidosis.

Objective: Respiratory Emergencies

Subobjective: Chronic Obstructive Pulmonary Disorder

133. A

Rationale: Iritis is treated with topical mydriatic ophthalmic drops to dilate the pupil, topical corticosteroids to reduce inflammation, and referral to ophthalmology within 24 hours.

Objective: Ocular

Subobjective: Infections

134. C

Rationale: Patients with ulcerative keratitis MUST NOT use contact lenses until the infection has resolved and been cleared by an ophthalmologist. The patient should complete the full course of prescribed antibiotics. Not all ulcers are contagious, so she could safely return to work after 24 hours of antibiotic use.

Objective: Ocular

Subobjective: Ulcerations/Keratitis

135. A

Rationale: The patient's ammonia level and ALT are elevated, which is expected with cirrhosis. Lactulose is given to lower ammonia levels in patients with cirrhosis. Bisacodyl is a laxative and is not indicated for this patient.

Mesalamine is an anti-inflammatory given for ulcerative colitis. The patient's blood glucose is not elevated enough to require 2 units of insulin.

Objective: Gastrointestinal Emergencies

Subobjective: Cirrhosis

136. D

Rationale: Clinical open globe rupture features include afferent pupillary defect, impaired visual acuity, gross deformity of the eye, and prolapsing uvea.

Objective: Ocular

Subobjective: Trauma

137. D

Rationale: Dopamine (Intropin) is a positive inotrope, which will increase cardiac contractility and cardiac output, decrease the myocardial workload, and improve myocardial oxygen delivery.

Objective: Cardiovascular Emergencies

Subobjective: Heart Failure

138. A

Rationale: A commercially available tourniquet at least 2 inches wide with a windlass or ratcheting device is recommended for both prehospital and in-hospital use. The nurse should never remove a tourniquet without team support to control hemorrhagic bleeding. Assessment occurs in 2-hour intervals.

Objective: Orthopedic

Subobjective: Amputation

139. D

Rationale: Only the CT angiography will confirm the diagnosis. D-dimer may be increased in the presence of pulmonary embolism (PE) but is not a stand-alone indicator for definitive diagnosis. A chest X-ray will rule out other disease processes but does not rule in a PE. Fibrin split products are measured in the presence of disseminated intravascular coagulation and are not relevant for the concern of PE.

Objective: Respiratory Emergencies

Subobjective: Pulmonary Embolism

140. B

Rationale: When caring for mentally unstable or possibly violent patients, staff safety is the primary concern. The nurse should avoid getting blocked into a corner between the patient and the door. If possible, the patient should be in a room near the nurses' station, and the nurse should notify someone before entering the room. Bringing another nurse or patient care technician can also maintain safety. All patients should be treated with courtesy and respect, especially someone who may be prone to paranoia. It may be necessary to observe the patient closely for "cheeking" pills instead of swallowing them. Some medications may be ordered in IV form to ensure that the patient receives the medication if he has surreptitiously avoided swallowing pills in the past. Always ask permission before touching or approaching the patient to avoid startling him. If the patient refuses medications or blood draws, do not argue. Chart the refusal in the medical record and notify the health care provider.

Objective: Psychosocial Emergencies

Subobjective: Aggressive/Violent Behavior

141. D

Rationale: Costochondritis occurs from localized inflammation of the joints attaching the ribs to the sternum and most commonly presents in females ages 12 to 14.

Objective: Orthopedic

Subobjective: Costochondritis

142. A

Rationale: In a flail chest there is asymmetrical movement of the chest wall. Ribs are completely broken and cause abnormal movement of the chest wall. As the patient breathes in, the flail segment will sink in; as the patient breathes out, the segment will bulge outward.

Objective: Respiratory Emergencies

Subobjective: Trauma

143. B

Rationale: Chest pain can occur with the first dose of sumatriptan and should be reported immediately. Sumatriptan may not be safe for pregnant women, so the patient should be coached on using an effective birth control method while taking it. Most triptans are contraindicated with hypertension and would not be prescribed if the patient is taking antihypertensives due to the risk of coronary vasospasm. The medication should be taken as soon as the first symptoms of migraine appear.

Objective: Neurological Emergencies

Subobjective: Headache

144. B

Rationale: Avulsed primary teeth are not replanted because of the potential for subsequent damage to the developing permanent tooth and the increased frequency of pulpal necrosis. Best initial management would be to repair the lacerations.

Objective: Maxillofacial

Subobjective: Dental Conditions

145. C

Rationale: Gouty arthritis characteristically occurs in patients with hyperuricemia, which causes high levels of uric acid in the blood from breakdown of purines. Hyperammonemia is the presence of an excess of ammonia in the blood. Hyperbilirubinemia is too much bilirubin in the blood. Hyperhomocysteinemia is a marker for the development of heart disease.

Objective: Orthopedic

Subobjective: Inflammatory Conditions

146. C

Rationale: Nonstick adherent dressing such as a Band-Aid or Telfa pad is the appropriate choice.

Objective: Wound

Subobjective: Abrasions

147. B

Rationale: There should be a high index of suspicion that the patient experienced an inhalation injury, and measures should be taken to protect her airway. Burns and trauma are secondary concerns to airway compromise. Soot at the mouth opening suggests smoke inhalation, not foreign body ingestion.

Objective: Respiratory Emergencies

Subobjective: Inhalation Injuries

148. C

Rationale: Dimming lights or providing a blindfold are contraindicated, as low lighting will increase pupillary size, creating an increase in intraocular pressure. Pupil size should remain constricted through use of bright lighting and miotic ophthalmic drops.

Objective: Ocular

Subobjective: Glaucoma

149. A

Rationale: The typical chest radiography for a patient with adult respiratory distress syndrome (ARDS) is bilateral, diffuse white infiltrates without cardiomegaly. Options C and D show results for abnormal heart tissue but not for lung tissue and do not give any information about infiltrates.

Objective: Respiratory Emergencies

Subobjective: Respiratory Distress Syndrome

150. B

Rationale: Many opioid substances are commonly injected, resulting in abscess formation from use of non-sterile equipment and aseptic technique. Cocaine, amphetamines, and other substances may also be injected. Alcohol, benzodiazepine, and tetrahydrocannabinol use may be co-occurring in the patient, but these substances are not commonly injected.

Objective: Wound

Subobjective: Infections

151. C

Rationale: The patient is hypotensive, hypothermic, and bradycardic. He has ingested thyroid replacement medications and sedatives, which can lead to a myxedema coma. The symptoms are not indicative of an allergic reaction or an acute stroke. A thyroid storm would show increased heart rate, temperature, and blood pressure.

Objective: Medical Emergencies

Subobjective: Endocrine Conditions

152. D

Rationale: Epinephrine is never used for lacerations of the fingers, toes, face, or penis.

Objective: Wound

Subobjective: Lacerations

153. C

Rationale: Post-exposure prophylaxis in a patient who has not been vaccinated must consist of both immunoglobin and vaccine therapy. While up-to-date tetanus immunization should be considered, it is a targeted vaccine against infection by *Clostridium tetani*.

Objective: Environmental

Subobjective: Vector-Borne Illnesses

154. D

Rationale: The child is presenting with signs of asthma exacerbation. Symptoms of foreign body aspiration are consistent with acute airway obstruction to include respiratory distress and drooling. Pneumonitis would present with chest pain and dyspnea but not these acute symptoms. Pneumonia is characterized with crackles in the lower lobes and decreased oxygen saturation.

Objective: Respiratory Emergencies

Subobjective: Asthma

155. A

Rationale: The patient will need epinephrine administered immediately. Most anaphylactic deaths occur due to a delay in epinephrine administration. Diphenhydramine and Solu-Medrol are indicated for minor allergic reactions. Theophylline is typically used to treat asthma and is not indicated for anaphylaxis.

Objective: Medical Emergencies

Subobjective: Allergic Reactions and Anaphylaxis

156. B

Rationale: Hyperbaric oxygen is used to treat severe carbon monoxide toxicity.

Hydroxocobalamin is a cyanide-binding agent. *N*-acetylcysteine restores depleted hepatic glutathione, reversing effects of acetaminophen toxicity. Sodium bicarbonate is standard treatment for salicylate toxicity.

Objective: Environmental

Subobjective: Chemical Exposure

157. C

Rationale: Patients presenting with vague neurological symptoms may be difficult to diagnose. The history and information leading up to presentation in the department is vital in determining differential diagnoses. This patient is not presenting with stroke-like symptoms. The symptoms are similar to those of a migraine; however, the history makes carbon monoxide poisoning more likely. The patient is not demonstrating stroke or allergic reaction symptoms.

Objective: Toxicology

Subobjective: Carbon Monoxide

158. C

Rationale: Calcium gluconate is administered to the patient with hyperkalemia for cardiac and neuromuscular protection. Aspirin is used for acute coronary syndrome but would not be a first-line drug for this condition. Insulin and dextrose may be given to lower potassium levels but do not function to protect cardiac status. Digoxin is an antidysrhythmic and is not indicated for hyperkalemia.

Objective: Medical Emergencies

Subobjective: Renal Failure

159. C

Rationale: Monitoring neurological status is the most important nursing intervention for patients with meningitis. Deficits of cranial nerve VI prevent lateral eye movement, which is an indicator of hydrocephalus. Other indicators of hydrocephalus include urinary incontinence and signs of increased intracranial pressure (ICP). Declining LOC is the first sign of increased ICP, and the nurse must be sensitive to even small changes in LOC. The other findings do not indicate increasing ICP.

Objective: Neurological Emergencies

Subobjective: Increased Intracranial Pressure (ICP)

160. B

Rationale: Patients with diverticular disease should remain on clear liquids until pain has subsided. For maintenance, they will need to eat 25 to 35 grams of fiber daily to provide bulk to the stool. Patients should avoid high-sodium foods and alcohol, which irritates the bowel. Strawberries contain seeds that may block a diverticulum and should be avoided, along with nuts, corn, popcorn, and tomatoes.

Objective: Gastrointestinal Emergencies

Subobjective: Diverticulitis

161. D

Rationale: Keraunoparalysis is a condition specific to lightning strikes, resulting from vasoconstriction in the tissues surrounding entry and exit points. Ascending paralysis is a common finding in Guillain–Barré syndrome. Bell's palsy and tic douloureux are both facial nerve disorders.

Objective: Environmental

Subobjective: Electrical Injuries

162. B

Rationale: The patient's last drink is important to determine the possibility of withdrawal or delirium tremens. The other questions are relevant but are not the priority based on the patient's presentation.

Objective: Communicable Diseases

Subobjective: Withdrawal Syndrome

163. C

Rationale: Octreotide is used for overdoses refractory to glucose administration. It stimulates the release of insulin from the beta islet cells of the pancreas. Flumazenil is the antidote for benzodiazepine overdose. Acetylcysteine is used for acetaminophen overdose, and methylene blue is used for nitrites and anesthetics overdose.

Objective: Communicable Diseases

Subobjective: Overdose and Ingestion

164. B

Rationale: Tuberculosis is characterized by a cough lasting 2 – 3 weeks or more, fever, chills, night sweats, and fatigue. The recent travel to a developing country is a concern for potential infectious disease. The other conditions have similar symptoms, but the travel and chronic cough indicate strong concern for pulmonary tuberculosis.

Objective: Communicable Diseases

Subobjective: Tuberculosis

165. B

Rationale: Calcium channel blockers can cause symptoms in children with doses as low as 1 tablet. Rapid deterioration may occur if the tablets are short acting. A 5-year-old may not accurately count or recollect the number of tablets consumed. A referral to child protective services should be made if there is a reasonable suspicion for the need but is not a priority intervention. Oxygen should be provided only if pulse oximetry is less than 92%.

Objective: Communicable Diseases

Subobjective: Overdose and Ingestion

166. C

Rationale: The rash, conjunctivitis, and cough are indicative of measles, and the patient's vaccination status makes this diagnosis even more likely. Varicella is characterized by vesicular rash on the trunk and face; mumps, by nonspecific respiratory symptoms and edema in the parotid gland; and pertussis is a respiratory disease with a specific "whoop"-sounding cough.

Objective: Communicable Diseases

Subobjective: Childhood Diseases

167. B

Rationale: People who chronically abuse alcohol are deficient in thiamine and are given IV thiamine. Naloxone blocks opioid receptors and is given for opioid overdose. Flumazenil is a benzodiazepine receptor antagonist and is given for benzodiazepine overdose. Vitamin K is given for warfarin overdose.

Objective: Communicable Diseases

Subobjective: Substance Abuse

168. A

Rationale: Herpes zoster, also known as shingles, is caused by the reactivation of dormant varicella virus. It can occur several times over the lifetime of a patient who has had an initial varicella infection. The varicella vaccine is not known to cause herpes zoster. Herpes zoster can be spread by contact with the rash; someone who has never had varicella may contract it from contact with a herpes zoster rash. The zoster vaccine may prevent a second or third outbreak in patients who have had active herpes zoster.

Objective: Communicable Diseases

Subobjective: Herpes Zoster

169. A

Rationale: A pseudomembrane, or thick gray membrane, covering the tonsils, the pharynx, and sometimes the larynx is characteristic of diphtheria infection. Patients with diphtheria may have a low-grade fever; they will not have a macular rash or headache.

Objective: Communicable Diseases

Subobjective: Childhood Diseases

170. C

Rationale: The nurse demonstrates personal insight that further help is needed via the Critical Incident Stress Management (CISM) system. CISM does not require or recommend that nurses needing debriefing or assistance meet with managers specifically about the event or experience. The nurse should not depart the debriefing before it is complete, and future debrief sessions may or may not occur. Scheduling appointments is a concrete action that demonstrates the nurse's effective participation.

Objective: Professional Issues

Subobjective: Nurse (Critical Incident Stress Management)

171. B

Rationale: Participation and engagement in Evidence-Based Practice (EBP) projects supports an environment of quality and safe care using up-to-date evidence and practices that have been thoroughly researched. Reading research articles is important, but the data must be synthesized through formal processes to implement evidence into practice.

Objective: Professional Issues

Subobjective: Nurse (Evidence-Based Practice)

172. D

Rationale: Patient income is not directly relevant to transitions of care and is not appropriate for ED nurses to ask about when managing care transitions. Safety, community partnerships, and accessibility of services are all appropriate considerations.

Objective: Professional Issues

Subobjective: Patient (Transitions of Care)

173. D

Rationale: The current (2015) AHA and NRP guidelines for newborn resuscitation is 3 compressions to 1 ventilation. A ratio of 30:2 is appropriate for all adults or a single rescuer infant/child; a ratio of 15:2 is appropriate for

2 rescuers with children and infants. A ratio of 15:1 is not recommended for anyone.

Objective: Obstetrical

Subobjective: Neonatal Resuscitation

174. D

Rationale: A Foley catheter is not necessary to decompress the bladder in this patient. Typically, these patients are eligible for eye donation, and the head should be at 20 degrees, with artificial tears or saline in the eyes to preserve the tissue. Tape should be used if eyes do not close after death.

Objective: Professional Issues

Subobjective: Patient (End-of-Life Issues)

175. B

Rationale: Annular lesions with raised borders and cleared central areas of the rash indicate ringworm. Scabies are characterized by red pruritic rashes, and cellulitis and impetigo do not present in this way.

Objective: Environmental

Subobjective: Parasite and Fungal Infestations

Follow the link below to take your SECOND CEN practice test:

www.ascenciatestprep.com/cen-online-resources

A SIGNS & SYMPTOMS GLOSSARY

abdominal guarding: involuntary contraction of the abdominal muscles to prevent pain caused by pressure

agonal respiration: breathing pattern characterized by labored breathing, gasping, and myoclonus

amenorrhea: abnormal absence of menstruation

anisocoria: unequal pupil size

anosmia: inability to smell

anuria (anuresis): inability to urinate or production of < 100 mL of urine a day

aphasia: impairment in ability to speak, write, and understand others

apnea: temporary cessation of breathing

ascites: abdominal swelling caused by fluid in the peritoneal cavity

asterixis: bilateral tremor or "flapping" of the wrist or fingers

ataxia: abnormal, uncoordinated movements

aura: unusual sensations (e.g., flashing lights, odors) that precede a migraine

blepharospasm: involuntary contractions of the eyelids

bradycardia: slow heart rate

bradypnea: slow respiration rate

chemosis: edema of the conjunctiva

clonus: rhythmic, involuntary muscular spasms

crepitus: abnormal cracking sounds heard in fractures, joints, or the lungs or in subcutaneous emphysema

cyanosis: blueish skin

decerebrate posturing: arms and legs extended and the head arched back

decorticate posturing: arms flexed onto chest, fists clenched, and legs extended

diaphoresis: excessive sweating

diplopia: double vision

dysarthria: slurred speech caused by muscle weakness

dysesthesia: uncomfortable or painful sensation caused by nerve damage

dyspareunia: painful sexual intercourse

dysphagia: difficulty swallowing

dyspnea: difficulty breathing

dysuria: difficult or painful urination

ecchymosis: bruising

edema: swelling caused by excess fluid

edentulous: without teeth

effusion: accumulation of fluid

emesis: the act of vomiting

enophthalmos: posterior displacement of the eyeball

epistaxis: bleeding from the nose

erythema: redness of the skin

exophthalmos: bulging of the eyeball out of the orbit

febrile: related to fever

halitosis: foul-smelling breath

hematemesis: blood in vomit

hematochezia: bright red blood in stool

hematuria: blood in urine

hemiplegia: unilateral paralysis

hemoptysis: blood in expectorate from respiratory tract

hemotympanum: blood in the middle ear

hepatomegaly: enlargement of liver

herniation: protrusion of tissue from a cavity

hydrophobia: fear of water

hypercapnia: high levels of CO_2 in blood

hyperpyrexia: body temperature > 106.7°F (41.5°C)

hyperreflexia: overreactive reflexes

hypertension: high blood pressure

hypertonia: tightness of muscles due to nerve damage

hypotension: low blood pressure

hypoxemia: low levels of oxygen in the blood

hypoxia: lack of oxygen supplied to tissues

ileus: lack of movement in the intestines

ischemia: restricted blood flow to tissue

jaundice: yellowing of the skin or sclera

Kussmaul respirations: deep, labored breathing

lacrimation: excessive secretion of tears

laryngospasm: spasm of the vocal cords

lymphadenopathy (adenopathy): swollen lymph nodes

lymphopenia: low levels of lymphocytes

malocclusion: misalignment of the upper and lower teeth

melena: dark, sticky digested blood in the stool

menorrhagia: heavy bleeding during menstruation

myoclonus: twitches or jerks of muscles

nocturia: excessive urination at night

nystagmus: repetitive, uncontrolled movement of the eyes

oliguria: low urine output

orthopnea: dyspnea that occurs while lying flat

orthostatic (postural) hypotension: decrease in blood pressure after standing

otalgia: ear pain

otorrhea: drainage from the ear

pallor: pale appearance

pancytopenia: low levels of RBCs, WBCs, and platelets

papilledema: swelling of the optic disk

paresthesia: abnormal dermal sensation such as burning or "pins and needles"

parotitis: inflammation of the parotid glands

periorbital ecchymosis: bruising under and around the eyes ("raccoon eyes")

petechiae: tiny red or brown spots on the skin caused by subcutaneous bleeding

photophobia: sensitivity to light

photopsia: perceived flashes of light

photosensitivity: immune system response to UV light

pleurisy: inflammation of the pleura

poikilothermia: inability to regulate body temperature

polydipsia: excessive thirst

polyphagia: excessive hunger

polyuria: abnormally high urine output

presyncope: feeling of weakness and light-headedness

pruritus: severely itchy skin

ptosis: drooping of upper eyelid

pulsus alternans: alternating strong and weak pulse

pulsus paradoxus: abnormally large drop in blood pressure during inspiration

rhinorrhea: drainage from the nose

scotoma: loss of vision restricted to part of the visual field ("blind spot")

steatorrhea: excretion of excess fat in the stool

stenosis: narrowing of a passage

strangury: blockage at the base of the bladder causing a painful need to urinate

stridor: high-pitched wheezing sound caused by a disruption in airflow

syncope: temporary loss of consciousness

tachycardia: fast heart rate

tachypnea: fast respiratory rate

tetany: muscle spasms and cramps usually caused by hypocalcemia

tinnitus: perception of sounds that are not present ("ringing in the ears")

trismus: restricted movement of mandible ("lockjaw")

urticaria: hives

vertigo: sensation of dizziness and loss of balance

B MEDICAL SIGNS

Babinski sign (reflex): dorsiflexion of big toe when bottom of foot is stroked (normal in infants; sign of disease in adults)

Battle's sign: ecchymosis over the mastoid process

Chvostek's sign: twitching of facial muscles caused by tapping the facial nerve (CN VII) near the tragus

Cullen's sign: a bluish discoloration to the umbilical area

Grey Turner's sign: ecchymosis in the flank area

Homan's sign: discomfort behind the knee or increased resistance in response to dorsiflexion of the foot

Kehr's sign: pain in the tip of the shoulder caused by blood in the peritoneal cavity

Kussmaul's sign: rise in jugular venous pressure during inspiration

Levine's sign: a clenched fist held over the chest in response to ischemic chest pain

Markle test (heel drop): pain caused when patient stands on tiptoes and drops heels down quickly or when patient hops on one leg

McBurney's point: RLQ pain at point halfway between umbilicus and iliac spine

Murphy's sign: cessation of inspiration when RUQ is palpated

Prehn's sign: lack of pain relief after scrotal elevation

Psoas sign: abdominal pain when right hip is hyper-extended

Rovsing's sign: pain in the RLQ with palpation of LLQ

Schafer's sign: presence of pigmented cells in the anterior vitreous

Trousseau sign: flexing of wrist and adduction of fingers when brachial artery is obstructed for > 3 minutes

C

DIAGNOSTIC TESTS & CRITICAL

TEST	DESCRIPTION	NORMAL Range
Basic Metabolic Panel		
Potassium (K⁺)	electrolyte that helps with muscle contraction and regulates water and acid-base balance	3.5 – 5.2 mEq/L
Sodium (Na⁺)	maintains fluid balance and plays a major role in muscle and nerve function	135 – 145 mEq/L
Calcium (Ca⁺)	plays an important role in skeletal function and structure, nerve function, muscle contraction, and cell communication	8.5 – 10.3 mg/dL
Chloride (Cl⁻)	electrolyte that plays a major role in muscle and nerve function	98 – 107 mEq/L
Blood urea nitrogen (BUN)	filtered by the kidneys; high levels can indicate insufficient kidney function	7 – 20 mg/dL
Creatinine	filtered by the kidneys; high levels can indicate insufficient kidney function	0.6 – 1.2 mg/dL
BUN to creatinine ratio	increased ratio indicates dehydration, AKI, or GI bleeding; decreased ratio indicates renal damage	10:1 – 20:1
Glucose	tests for hyper- and hypoglycemia	non-fasting: < 140 mg/dL fasting: 70 – 99 mg/dL
Bicarbonate (HCO₃ or CO₂)	measures amount of CO_2 in the blood; decreased levels indicate acidosis or kidney damage; increased levels indicate alkalosis or lung damage	23 – 29 mEq/L
Other Serum Tests		
Magnesium	electrolyte that regulates muscle, nerve, and cardiac function	1.8 – 2.5 mg/dL
Glomerular filtration rate (GFR)	volume of fluid filtered by the renal glomerular capillaries per unit of time; decreased GFR rate indicates decreased renal function	men: 100 – 130 mL/min/1.73m² women: 90 – 120 mL/min/1.73m² GFR < 60 mL/min/1.73m² is common in adults > 70 years

TEST	DESCRIPTION	NORMAL Range
Other Serum Tests (continued)		
Total cholesterol (LDL and HDL)	a steroid produced by the liver that is needed to build and maintain animal cell membranes and that has protective properties for the heart; goals for low-density lipoprotein (LDL) and high-density lipoprotein (HDL) levels are based on the patient's risk factors for cardiovascular disease	< 200 mg/dL LDL: < 100 mg/dL HDL (men): 40 – 50 mg/dL HDL (women): 50 – 59 mg/dL
Triglycerides	stores fat	< 150 mg/dL
B-type natriuretic peptide (BNP)	protein produced by the heart; high levels can indicate heart failure	< 100 pg/ml
Highly selective CRP test for C-reactive protein	marker for inflammation used to determine a patient's risk for heart disease	low risk: < 1.0 mg/L average risk: 1.0 – 3.0 mg/L high risk: > 3.0 mg/L
Homocysteine	an amino acid used as a marker for heart disease and vitamin deficiency (B_6, B_{12}, and folate)	4 – 14 µmol/L
Prostate-specific antigen (PSA)	enzyme produced by prostate gland; high levels can indicate prostate cancer, prostatitis, or BPH	< 4 ng/mL
Erythrocyte sedimentation rate (ESR or sed rate)	measures rate at which RBCs sediment (fall); increased ESR may indicate inflammation, anemia, or infection; decreased ESR may indicate heart failure or liver or kidney disease; ESR increases with age	men: 12 – 14 mm/h women: 18 – 21 mm/h
Ammonia	produced by bacteria in the intestines during the breakdown of proteins; increased levels may indicate liver or kidney damage; decreased levels are associated with hypertension	15 – 45 mcg/dL
Serum lipase (LPS)	protein secreted by the pancreas that helps break down fats; increased levels can indicate damage to the pancreas	0 – 160 U/L
Amylase	enzyme produced by pancreas and salivary glands; increased levels may indicate damage to the pancreas	23 – 85 U/L
Complete Blood Count (CBC)		
White blood cells (WBCs)	number of WBCs in blood; an increased number of WBCs can be an indication of inflammation or infection	4,500 – 10,000 cells/mcL
Red blood cells (RBCs)	carry oxygen throughout the body and filter carbon dioxide	men: 5 – 6 million cells/mcL women: 4 – 5 million cells/mcL
Hemoglobin (HgB)	protein that holds oxygen in the blood	men: 13.8 – 17.2 g/dL women: 12.1 – 15.1 g/dL
Hematocrit (Hct)	percentage of the blood composed of red blood cells	men: 41% – 50% women: 36% – 44%

Complete Blood Count (CBC) (continued)

Red blood cell indices	mean corpuscular volume (MCV): average size of the red blood cells mean corpuscular hemoglobin (MCH): average amount of hemoglobin per RBC mean corpuscular hemoglobin concentration (MCHC): average concentration of hemoglobin in RBCs	MCV: 80 – 95 fL MCH: 27.5 – 33.2 pg MCHC: 334 – 355 g/L
Platelets	play a role in the body's clotting process	150,000 – 450,000 cells/mcL

Coagulation Studies

Prothrombin time (PT)	tests how long it takes blood to clot	10 – 13 seconds
International normalized ratio (INR)	determines the effectiveness of an anticoagulant in thinning blood	healthy adults: < 1.1 patients receiving anticoagulants: 2.0 – 3.0
Partial thromboplastin time (PTT)	assess the body's ability to form blood clots	60 – 70 sec
Activated partial thromboplastin time (aPTT)	measures the body's ability to form blood clots using an activator to speed up the clotting process	20 – 35 sec

Cardiac Biomarkers

Troponin I (cTnI) and troponin T (cTnT)	proteins released when the heart muscle is damaged; high levels can indicate a myocardial infarction but may also be due to other conditions that stress the heart (e.g., renal failure, heart failure, PE); levels peak 24 hours post MI and can remain elevated for up to 2 weeks	cTnI: cutoff values for MI vary widely between assays cTnT: possible MI: > 0.01 ng/mL
Creatine kinase (CK)	responsible for muscle cell function; an increased amount indicates cardiac or skeletal muscle damage	22 – 198 U/L
Creatine kinase–muscle/brain (CK-MB or CPK-MB)	cardiac marker for damaged heart muscle; often used to diagnose a second MI or ongoing cardiovascular conditions; a high ratio of CK-MB to CK indicates damage to heart muscle (as opposed to skeletal muscle)	5 – 25 IU/L possible MI: ratio of CK-MB to CK is 2.5 – 3

Urinalysis

Leukocytes	presence of WBCs in urine indicates infection	negative
Nitrate	presence of nitrates in urine indicates infection by gram-negative bacteria	negative
Urobilinogen	produced during bilirubin reduction; presence in urine indicates liver disease, bilinear obstruction, or hepatitis	0.2 – 1 mg
Protein	presence of protein in the urine may indicate nephritis or eclampsia	negative

TEST	DESCRIPTION	NORMAL Range
Urinalysis (continued)		
pH	decreased (acidic) pH may indicate systemic acidosis or diabetes mellitus; increased (alkali) pH may indicate systemic alkalosis or UTI	4.5 – 8
Blood	blood in urine may indicate infection, renal calculi, neoplasm, or coagulation disorders	negative
Specific gravity	concentration of urine; decreased may indicate diabetes insipidus or pyelonephritis; increased may indicate dehydration or SIADH	1.010 – 1.025
Ketone	ketones are produced during fat metabolism; presence in urine may indicate diabetes, hyperglycemia, starvation, alcoholism, or eclampsia	negative
Bilirubin	produced during the breakdown of heme; presence in urine may indicate liver disease, biliary obstruction, or hepatitis	negative
Glucose	presence of glucose in urine indicates hyperglycemia	0 – 15 mg/dL
Urine hCG	determination of pregnancy	N/A
Urine culture and sensitivity	study of urine with growth on a culture medium to determine which pathogenic bacteria is present and which antibiotic the pathogen is sensitive to	N/A
Liver Function Tests		
Albumin	a protein made in the liver; low levels may indicate liver damage	3.5 – 5.0 g/dL
Alkaline phosphatase (ALP)	an enzyme found in the liver and bones; increased levels indicate liver damage	45 – 147 U/L
Alanine transaminase (ALT)	an enzyme in the liver that helps metabolize protein; increased levels indicate liver damage	7 – 55 U/L
Aspartate transaminase (AST)	an enzyme in the liver that helps metabolize alanine; increased levels indicate liver or muscle damage	8 – 48 U/L
Total protein	low levels of total protein may indicate liver damage	6.3 – 7.9 g/dL
Total bilirubin	produced during the breakdown of heme; increased levels indicate liver damage or anemia	0.1 – 1.2 mg/dL
Gamma-glutamyltransferase (GGT)	an enzyme that plays a role in antioxidant metabolism; increased levels indicate liver damage	9 – 48 U/L
L-lactate dehydrogenase (LD or LDH)	an enzyme found in most cells in the body; high levels may indicate liver damage, cancer, or tissue breakdown	adult: 122 – 222 U/L

Arterial Blood Gas (ABG)

pH	measure of blood pH	7.35 – 7.45
Partial pressure of oxygen (PaO$_2$)	amount of oxygen gas in the blood	75 – 100 mm Hg
Partial pressure of carbon dioxide (PaCO$_2$)	amount of carbon dioxide gas in the blood	35 – 45 mm Hg
Bicarbonate (HCO$_3$)	amount of bicarbonate in the blood	22 – 26 mEq/L
Oxygen (O$_2$) saturation	measurement of the amount of oxygen-saturated hemoglobin relative to unsaturated hemoglobin	94 – 100%
Lactate	molecule produced during anaerobic cellular respiration; high levels indicate lack of available oxygen in cells	4.5 – 14.4 mg/dL

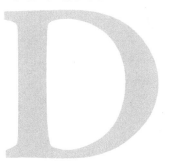

D ABBREVIATIONS

A

ABC: A1c (hemoglobin), blood pressure, and cholesterol

ABG: arterial blood gas

ACE inhibitors: angiotensin-converting enzyme inhibitors

ACLS: advanced cardiovascular life support

ACS: acute coronary syndrome

ACTH: adrenocorticotropic hormone stimulation test

A-fib: atrial fibrillation

ALL: acute lymphocytic leukemia

ALP: alkaline phosphatase

ALS: amyotrophic lateral sclerosis

ALT: alanine aminotransferase

AMA: against medical advice *or* American Medical Association

AML: acute myeloid leukemia

AND: allow natural death

AOM: acute otitis media

aPTT: activated partial thromboplastin time

ARBs: angiotensin II receptor blockers

ARDS: acute respiratory distress syndrome

ARF: acute renal failure

AST: aspartate aminotransferase

AUB: abnormal uterine bleeding

aVF: augmented vector foot (ECG lead)

aVL: augmented vector left (ECG lead)

AVM: arteriovenous malformation

aVR: augmented vector right (ECG lead)

B

BBB: bundle branch block

BNP: B-type natriuretic peptide

BPH: benign prostatic hyperplasia

bpm: beats per minute

BPM: breaths per minute

BRAT: banana, rice, applesauce, toast (e.g., BRAT diet)

BUN: blood urea nitrogen

BZK: benzalkonium chloride (e.g., BZK wipes)

C

CAD: coronary artery disease

CA-MRSA: community-acquired methicillin-resistant *Staphylococcus aureus*

CAP: community-acquired pneumonia

CBC: complete blood count

CDC: Centers for Disease Control and Prevention

CISD: critical incident stress debriefing

CISM: critical incident stress management

CIWA-Ar: Clinical Institute Withdrawal Assessment for Alcohol

CK-MB: creatine kinase–muscle/brain

CLL: chronic lymphocytic leukemia

CML: chronic myelogenous leukemia

CMP: comprehensive metabolic panel

CO: cardiac output

COBRA: Consolidated Omnibus Budget Reconciliation Act

COCA: color, odor, clarity, amount (urinary assessment)

COWS: Clinical Opiate Withdrawal Scale

CPG: clinical practice guideline

CPP: cerebral perfusion pressure

CPR: cardiopulmonary resuscitation

CRF: chronic renal failure

CRI: cutaneous radiation injury

CRP: C-reactive protein

CRT: capillary refill time

CS: culture and sensitivity

CSF: cerebrospinal fluid

CSM: circulation, sensation, and movement

CT scan: computed tomography scan

CTPA: computed tomography pulmonary angiography

CVA: cerebrovascular accident

CVP: central venous pressure

D

D&C: dilation and curettage

D50: dextrose 50% solution

D5W: dextrose 5% in water

DAI: diffuse axonal injury

DBP: diastolic blood pressure

DIC: disseminated intravascular coagulation

DKA: diabetic ketoacidosis

DMARDs: disease-modifying antirheumatic drugs

DNI: do not intubate

DNR: do not resuscitate

DT: diphtheria and tetanus (vaccine)

DTaP: diphtheria, tetanus, and pertussis (vaccine)

DTI: deep tissue injury

DTPA: diethylenetriamine pentaacetate

DTs: delirium tremens

DUBB: dangerous underwater breath-holding behaviors

DVT: deep vein thrombosis

E

EAPs: Employee Assistance Programs

EBP: evidence-based practice

ECF: extracellular fluid

ECG: electrocardiogram

ECR: extracorporeal core rewarming

EEG: electroencephalogram

EGD: esophagogastroduodenoscopy

EIA: enzyme immunoassay

ELISA: enzyme-linked immunosorbent assay

EMB: ethambutol

EMTALA: Emergency Medical Treatment and Active Labor Act

ESI: Emergency Severity Index

ESR: erythrocyte sedimentation rate

ESWL: extracorporeal shock wave lithotripsy

ET tube: endotracheal tube

F

FAST ultrasound: focused assessment with sonography for trauma

FFP: fresh frozen plasma

FLT3: fms-related tyrosine kinase 3

FSH: follicle-stimulating hormone

G

GCS: Glasgow Coma Scale

GFR: glomerular filtration rate

GSW: gunshot wound

GU: genitourinary

H

H/H: hemoglobin and hematocrit

HA-MRSA: hospital-acquired methicillin-resistant *Staphylococcus aureus*

HAP: hospital-acquired pneumonia

HBSS: Hanks' Balanced Salt Solution

HCAHPS: Hospital Consumer Assessment of Healthcare Providers and Systems

hCG: human chorionic gonadotropin

HCS: Hazard Communication Standard

HELLP syndrome: hemolysis, elevated liver enzymes, low platelet count

HgB: hemoglobin

HHS: hyperosmolar hyperglycemic state

HIPAA: Health Insurance Portability and Accountability Act

HIT: heparin-induced thrombocytopenia

HR: heart rate

HSV: herpes simplex virus

I

IBS: irritable bowel syndrome

ICD: implantable cardioverter defibrillator

ICF: intracellular fluid

ICP: intracranial pressure

ICS: incident command system

IgM: immunoglobulin M

INH: isoniazid

INR: international normalized ratio

IO: intraosseous (infusion)

ITP: idiopathic thrombocytopenic purpura

IUD: intrauterine device

IV: intravenous

IVIG: intravenous immunoglobulin

IVP: intravenous pyelography

J

JVD: jugular vein distention

K

KUB: kidney, ureter, bladder

L

LFT: liver function test

LLQ: left lower quadrant

LMA: laryngeal mask airway

LOC: level of consciousness

LPN: licensed practical nurse

LUQ: left upper quadrant

LVN: licensed vocational nurse

M

MAP: mean arterial pressure

MCI: mass casualty incident

MD: muscular dystrophy

mEq: milliequivalent

MG: myasthenia gravis

MI: myocardial infarction

MMI: maximum medical improvement

MODS: multiple organ dysfunction syndrome

MRI: magnetic resonance imaging

MRSA: methicillin-resistant *Staphylococcus aureus*

MS: multiple sclerosis

MSDS: material safety data sheets

MVA: motor vehicle accident/motorized vehicle accident

MVC: motor vehicle crash/motorized vehicle crash

N

NAAT: nucleic acid amplification test

NG tube: nasogastric tube

NIH: National Institutes of Health

NIHSS: National Institutes of Health Stroke Scale

NPE: noncardiac pulmonary edema

NSAID: nonsteroidal anti-inflammatory drug

NSTEMI: non-ST-elevation myocardial infarction

O

OME: otitis media with effusion

P

PALM-COEIN: polyp, adenomyosis, leiomyoma, malignancy, coagulopathy, ovulatory disorder, endometrial, iatrogenic, not otherwise classified (risk factors for abdominal uterine bleeding)

PCI: percutaneous coronary intervention

PCR: polymerase chain reaction

PE: pulmonary embolism

PEA: pulseless electrical activity

PHI: protected health information

PID: pelvic inflammatory disease

PO: *per os* (by mouth)

PPE: personal protective equipment

PRN: *pro re nata* (as needed)

PSP: primary spontaneous pneumothorax

PT: prothrombin time

PTH: post-traumatic headaches

PTT: partial thromboplastin time

PTU: propylthiouracil

PVD: peripheral vascular disease

PZA: pyrazinamide

R

RhoGAM: Rho(D) immune globulin

RIF: rifampin

RIG: rabies immune globulin

RLQ: right lower quadrant

ROM: range of motion

ROSC: return of spontaneous circulation

RPR: rapid plasma reagent

RR: respiration rate

RSI: rapid sequence intubation

RSV: respiratory syncytial virus

RT–PCR: real-time polymerase chain reaction

RUQ: right upper quadrant

S

SANE: sexual assault nurse examiner

SARS: severe acute respiratory syndrome

SBP: systolic blood pressure

SDS: safety data sheets

SSP: secondary spontaneous pneumothorax

START: simple triage and rapid treatment

STEMI: ST-segment elevation myocardial infarction

STI: sexually transmitted infection

SV: stroke volume

SVT: supraventricular tachycardia

T

TBSA: total body surface area

TCP: transcutaneous pacing

Td: tetanus and diphtheria (vaccine)

Tdap: tetanus, diphtheria, and pertussis (booster DTaP vaccine)

TEE: transesophageal echocardiogram

TIA: transient ischemic attack

TMJ: temporomandibular joint

tPA: tissue plasminogen activator

TPN: total parenteral nutrition

TSH: thyroid stimulating hormone

TTM: targeted temperature management

U

U/L: units per liter

ULQ: upper left quadrant

URQ: upper right quadrant

UTI: urinary tract infection

V

VDLR: venereal disease research laboratories

V-fib: ventricular fibrillation

VRE: vancomycin-resistant enterococci

V-tach: ventricular tachycardia

W

WBC: white blood cell

WHO: World Health Organization

COMMON ECG STRIPS

Sinus Rhythms

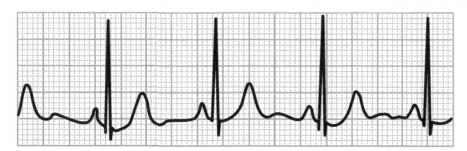

Normal sinus rhythm: Regular rhythm with a rate of 60-100 bpm. Every ORS is preceded by a P wave.

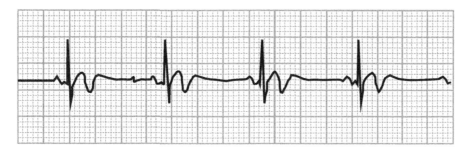

Sinus bradycardia: Regular rhythm with a slow rate <60. All other measurements are normal.

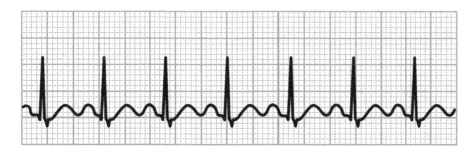

Sinus tachycardia: Regular rhythm with a fast rate >100 bpm. All other measurements are normal. Although P wave can merge with the T wave at very fast rates.

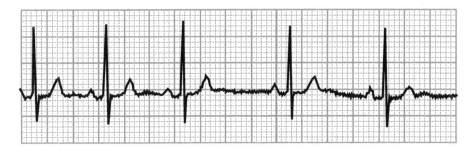

Sinus arrythmia: An irregular rhythm that can vary with respirations. All measurements are normal besides a varying R-R interval.

Atrial Rhythms

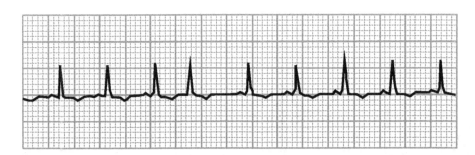

Premature atrial contractions: Irregular rhythm with premature, irregular P waves and QRS complexes.

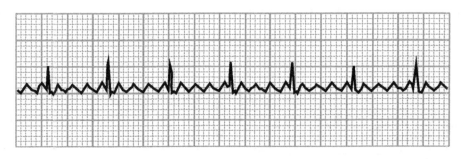

Atrial flutter: Rhythm can be regular or irregular with no observable P wave, but saw-toothed waves can be seen.

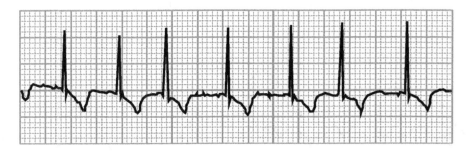

Atrial fibrillation: Irregular rhythm with absent P wave and PR interval.

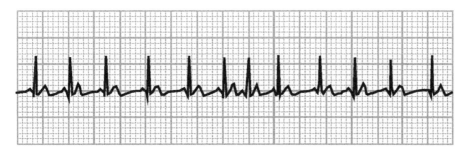

Atrial tachycardia: Irregular, fast rhythm (>100 bpm) with a variable PR interval and abnormal T wave.

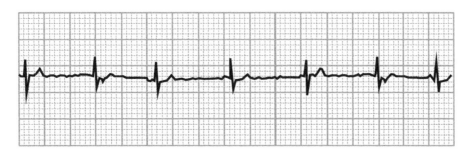

Wandering pacemaker: This rhythm can be regular or irregular and have a normal rate of 60-100 bpm. The P wave will change shape and size from one beat to another.

Junctional Rhythms

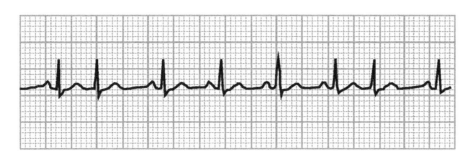

Premature junctional contractions: Regular rhythm with premature beats and a short or absent PR interval.

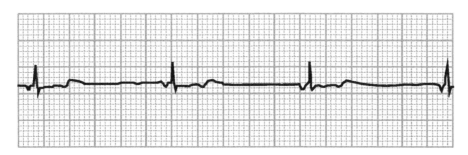

Junctional escape rhythm: A regular rhythm with a slow rate (40-60 bpm) and a PR interval that is unmeasurable. If a P wave can be seen it is inverted.

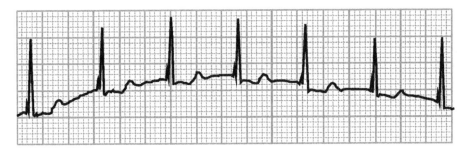

Accelerated junctional rhythm: A regular rhythm with a rate of 60-100 bpm and an unmeasurable PR interval.

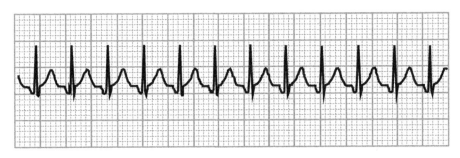

Junctional tachycardia: A regular rhythm with a rate of 100-180 bpm, with an absent or shorter PR interval. If a P wave is present it will be inverted.

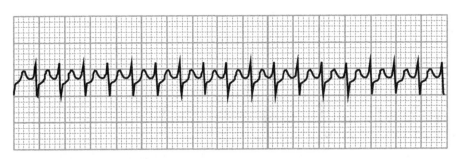

Supraventricular tachycardia: A regular rhythm with a rate of 150-250 bpm and T waves that are hidden in the QRS complex.

Heart Blocks

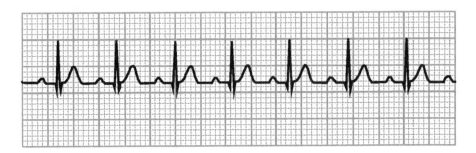

First degree block: A regular rhythm with a prolonged PR interval (>0.20 seconds).

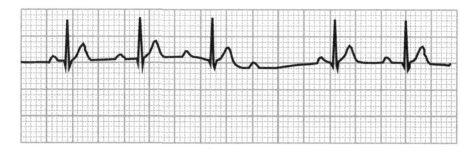

Second degree block type I Wenckebach: An irregular rhythm that has a PR interval that gets progressively longer until a QRS complex is dropped and then the cycle repeats itself.

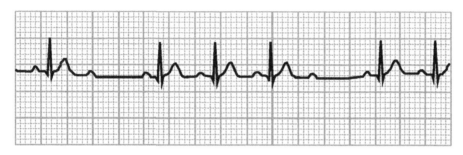

Second degree block type 2 Mobitz: An irregular rhythm with more P waves than QRS complexes.

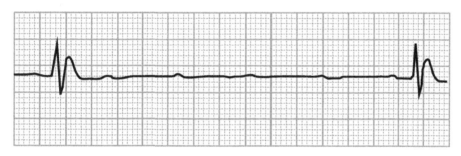

Third degree block/Complete heart block: An erratic rhythm that has no communication between the atria and ventricles.

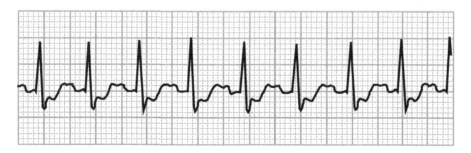

Bundle branch block: A regular rhythm with a wide QRS interval (>0.12 seconds).

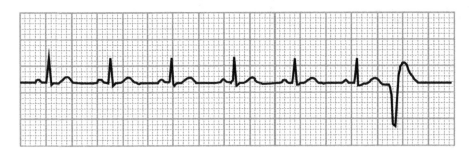

Premature ventricular contractions: A regular rhythm that possesses a wide and bizarre beat with a QRS interval greater than 0.10 seconds.

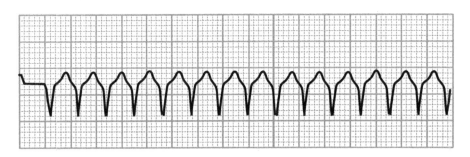

Ventricular tachycardia: A regular and fast rhythm (100-250 bpm) without P waves and wide bizarre QRS complexes.

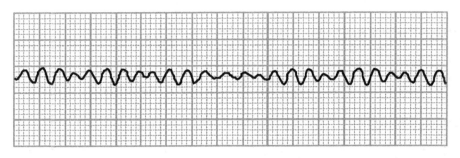

Ventricular fibrillation: An extremely irregular rhythm with an unmeasurable rate and no P waves. This rhythm does not have QRS complexes.

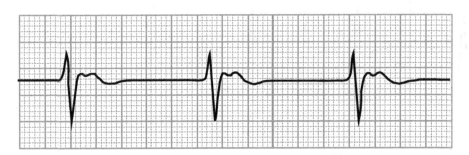

Idioventricular rhythm: A regular, but slow rhythm (20-40 bpm) without P waves and a wide bizarre QRS complex (>0.10 seconds).

Asystole

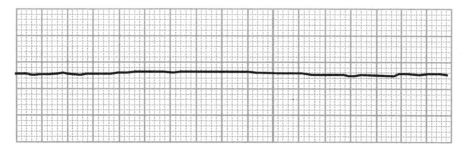

Asystole: This rhythm does not have a rate, P wave, or QRS complex.

APPENDIX

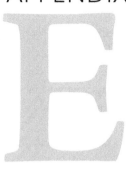

GENERIC Name	BRAND Name(s)	DOSAGE	CONTRAINDICATIONS and Nursing Considerations
ACE Inhibitors			
benazepril	Lotensin	5 – 10 mg/day	+ not indicated for patients with history of angioedema + may cause a dry, hacking cough + patients with ascites or cirrhosis should avoid
captopril	Capoten	+ Initial: 6.25 mg 3×/ day + Target: 50 mg 3×/ day	+ neutropenia a risk for patients with renal impairment + symptomatic hypotension may occur to include syncope, may occur in first few doses
enalapril	Vasotec	+ Initial: 5 mg/day + Target: titrate up to 40 mg/day + Max: 40 mg/day	+ in patients with severe aortic stenosis, may reduce coronary perfusion resulting in ischemia + possible exaggerated response in patients > 65 to this and other ACE inhibitors
lisinopril	Zestril	5 – 10 mg/day; max dose: 40 mg/day	+ may cause a dry, hacking cough + increased BUN and serum creatinine and/or deteriorated renal function have been associated with it, especially in patients with low renal blood flow

GENERIC Name	BRAND Name(s)	DOSAGE	CONTRAINDICATIONS and Nursing Considerations
Analgesics			
acetaminophen	Tylenol	+ Regular strength: 650 mg every 4 – 6 hours + Extra strength: 1,000 mg every 6 hours + Max dose: 4 g/day	+ associated with acute liver failure, liver transplant, and death + associated with serious/fatal skin reactions, including Stevens–Johnson syndrome and toxic epidermal necrolysis + use with caution in patients with alcoholic liver disease
acetaminophen/ butalbital/ caffeine	Fioricet	+ 1 – 2 tablets every 4 hours + Max: 6 tablets	use may not be advised in patients with renal, hepatic, or respiratory impairment
Anesthetics			
capsaicin	Zostrix	Topical via cream or patch; ≤ 4 applications/ day	+ patients with uncontrolled hypertension or a history of cardiovascular events may experience increased blood pressure + may impair physical or mental abilities; inform patients mental alertness may be diminished
lidocaine	Xylocaine	Dosage dependent on method of application and concentration	+ use with caution in patients with known drug sensitivities + application to broken or inflamed skin may lead to increased systemic absorption + reduce dose for acutely ill patients
Antacids			
aluminum hydroxide	Alternagel	1.9 – 4.8 mg up to 4×/ day	+ anti-ulcer agent, also used as adjunct for treatment of high serum phosphate in kidney failure + avoid taking other medications within 2 hours of use
magnesium hydroxide	Maalox	400 – 1,200 mg/day	+ used for constipation + used for indigestion + not indicated for patients in acute severe renal failure

Antibiotics

amoxicillin	Augmentin	250 – 500 mg 2 – 3×/day	+ dosage based on weight and clinical picture + patients should use alternate forms of birth control + indicated for use in otitis media, UTIs, skin infection
ampicillin	Principen	250 – 500 mg every 6 hours	+ used in respiratory infections, meningitis, UTIs, and GI infections + contraindicated in patients with PCN allergy
azithromycin	Zithromax	+ Dosing based on clinical picture + 250 – 600 mg 3x/day	+ used for chancroid type infections, respiratory infections, and some STIs + may result in elongated QT interval on ECG
ceftriaxone	Rocephin	1 – 2 g every 12 – 24 hours	+ used in endocarditis, bite wounds, cholecystitis + may increase INR + serious hypersensitivity may occur
ciprofloxacin	Cipro	500 – 750 mg 2×/day	+ used for infections resulting from bite wounds, cat scratches, chancroids + used for anthrax exposure/infection + may cause photosensitivity
clindamycin	Cleocin	600 – 1,800 mg/day in 2 – 4 divided doses	+ used for anthrax infection, bacterial vaginosis, bite wounds + use with caution in patients with GI disease or hepatic impairment + risk of colitis with use
doxycycline	Acticlate	100 – 200 mg/day in 1 – 2 divided doses	+ broad spectrum use, used for acne vulgaris, cellulitis, bite infections, Lyme disease + may cause abdominal pain and discomfort + used as malaria prophylaxis
gentamicin	Gentak	3 – 5 mg/kg/day in divided doses every 8 hours	+ used in endocarditis, brucellosis, gonococcal infection, plague + use with caution in patients with electrolyte imbalance + do not use in pregnancy
isoniazid	Nydrazid	5 mg/kg/doses 1×/day	+ treatment of nontuberculous mycobacterium + may result in fatal hepatitis

GENERIC Name	BRAND Name(s)	DOSAGE	CONTRAINDICATIONS and Nursing Considerations
Antibiotics (continued)			
meropenem	Merrem	1.5 – 6 g/day divided every 8 hours	+ confusion, seizures, and other adverse CNS effects + use with caution in patients with renal impairment
metronidazole	Flagyl	500 mg 2×/day for 7 days	+ most frequently used for bacterial vaginosis + *Clostridioides* may be treated with this medication + possibly carcinogenic
penicillin	N/A	Oral: 125 – 500 mg every 6 – 8 hours	+ used in bite wounds, pneumococcal prophylaxis, streptococcal infections + use caution in patients with renal impairment and seizure disorders
piperacillin-tazobactam	Zosyn	3.375 g every 6 hours	+ used in bite wounds, sepsis, cystic fibrosis + may cause serious skin reactions + may cause electrolyte abnormalities
rifampin	Rifadin	10 mg/kg/day 1×/day (max: 600 mg/day)	+ used for treatment of active tuberculosis + may cause vitamin K–dependent coagulopathy
streptomycin	N/A	1 g every 12 hours for 1 week	+ used for Ménière's disease and mycobacterium infections + may cause neuromuscular blockade and respiratory paralysis
sulfamethoxazole	Bactrim	1 – 2 double-strength tablets every 12 – 24 hours	+ used for bite wounds, brain abscess, infectious diarrhea + may cause blood dyscrasias + may cause hyperkalemia + may cause hepatic necrosis
vancomycin	Vancocin	15 – 20 mg/kg/dose	+ used in catheter-related infections, endocarditis, community-acquired pneumonia + may cause nephrotoxicity, neutropenia, and ototoxicity

Antiemetics

ondansetron	Zofran	4 – 8 mg every 8 hours	+ used for nausea + may cause prolonged QT interval + may cause serotonin syndrome
promethazine	Phenergan	12.5 – 25 mg/dose	+ used for persistent nausea + may cause respiratory depression + extravasation may cause severe tissue injury, including gangrene

Anti-Inflammatories

ibuprofen	Motrin	200 – 800 mg 3 – 4×/ day	+ used for analgesia and antipyretic properties + may have impact on liver enzymes and function + may cause skin reactions

Anticonvulsants

carbamazepine	Tegretol	400 mg/day in 2 divided doses or 4 divided doses	+ treatment for seizures, bipolar disorder + may cause blood dyscrasias + may cause hyponatremia + may cause psychiatric effects
fosphenytoin	Cerebyx	20 mg PE/kg as a single dose	+ used for status epilepticus + may cause cardiac events if infused too quickly + may cause hepatotoxicity
gabapentin	Neurontin	100 – 300 mg 1 – 3×/ day	+ used for neuropathic pain, psychiatric disorder adjunct, and alcohol withdrawal + can be used for intractable hiccups + may cause anaphylaxis + neuropsychiatric effects may occur
levetiracetam	Keppra	+ 500 mg 2×/day + Increase every 2 weeks by 500 mg/ dose based on response	+ used in status epilepticus, subarachnoid hemorrhage, and traumatic brain injury + may cause CNS depression + may cause hypertension + may cause increase in suicidal ideation
phenytoin	Dilantin	20 mg/kg at a max rate of 50 mg/minute	+ used in status epilepticus + can be used in seizures + chronic use may lead to decreased bone density

GENERIC Name	BRAND Name(s)	DOSAGE	CONTRAINDICATIONS and Nursing Considerations
Anticoagulants			
enoxaparin	Lovenox	40 – 60 mg every 12 hours	+ monitor patient closely for signs of bleeding + monitor for hyperkalemia; can cause hyperkalemia
heparin	N/A	+ 60 units/kg (max 4,000 units), then 12 units/kg/hour + Max: 1,000 units/ hour	+ adjunct to fibrinolysis in the presence of STEMI + bleeding may occur, causing fatal events + high-alert medication
warfarin	Coumadin	2 – 5 mg 1×/day (may be higher; varies by patient age and physical status)	+ used for prophylaxis and treatment of thromboembolic disorders + may cause hypersensitivity reactions, including anaphylaxis
Anticholinergics			
dicyclomine	Bentyl	20 mg 4×/day for 7 days	+ gastrointestinal motility disorders/ irritable bowel + use with caution in patients with coronary artery disease + use with caution in patients with autonomic neuropathy
Antidysrhythmics			
adenosine	Adenocard	Initial: 6 mg; if not effective within 1 – 2 minutes, another 6 mg may be given	+ used in the ED for supraventricular tachycardia for cardioversion + A-fib may occur + may cause conduction disturbances
amiodarone	Cordarone	150 mg over 10 minutes	+ used for A-fib + can cause life-threatening arrhythmias + pulmonary toxicity
digoxin/digitalis	Digox	+ 0.25 – 0.5 mg over several minutes + Maintenance dose: Oral: 0.125 – 0.25 mg 1×/day	used to control heart rate
lidocaine	Xylocaine	1 – 1.5 mg/kg bolus	+ can be used as an antidysrhythmic or in V-fib or V-tach + extreme caution in patients with severe hepatic dysfunction + risk of lidocaine toxicity

procainamide	Procan	10 – 17 mg/kg at a rate of 20 – 50 mg/minute or 100 mg every 5 minutes	+ used for hemodynamically stable ventricular arrhythmias + reduce dose if first-degree heart block occurs

Antidepressants

paroxetine	Paxil	20 mg 1×/day, preferably in the morning	+ may increase suicidal ideation or behavior + make cause extrapyramidal symptoms + may cause CNS depression
sertraline	Zoloft	50 mg 1×/day	+ may be used in a variety of depressive disorders, anxiety disorders, eating disorders + will not be initiated in ED + increased risk for suicidal ideation

Antihistamines

dimenhydrinate	Dramamine	50 – 100 mg every 4 – 6 hours	+ used for motion sickness and post-op vomiting + use with caution in patients with cardiovascular disease + some antibiotics can cause ototoxicity; if patient consumes, use dimenhydrinate with caution
diphenhydramine	Benadryl	25 – 50 mg every 4 – 8 hours	+ for use in allergic reactions, headaches, nausea + may cause CNS depression + use with caution in patients with asthma
meclizine	Antivert	Oral: 25 – 100 mg/day	+ used for symptoms caused by vertigo + use with caution in patients with narrow-angle glaucoma + use with caution in patients with hepatic disease

Antihypertensives

clonidine	Catapres	0.1 mg 2×/day; max dose: 2.4 mg/day	+ primary use for antihypertensive, secondary use for sedating side effects + may cause dose-dependent reductions in heart rate + symptomatic hypotension may occur with use
doxazosin	Cardura	Initial: 1 mg 1×/day	+ used for HTN and BPH + skin rash, urticaria, pruritus, angioedema, and respiratory symptoms may occur + use with caution in patients with heart failure, angina pectoris, or recent acute myocardial infarction

GENERIC Name	BRAND Name(s)	DOSAGE	CONTRAINDICATIONS and Nursing Considerations
Antihypertensives (continued)			
hydralazine	Apresoline	25 – 50 mg 3 or 4×/day	+ used for heart failure with reduced ejection fraction, hypertension emergency + may induce a lupus-like syndrome including glomerulonephritis + use with caution in patients with mitral valvular disease
nifedipine	Procardia	10 mg 3×/day; usual dose: 10 – 20 mg 3×/day	+ used for stable angina, hypertension, high-altitude pulmonary edema + possibility of increased angina and/or MI with initiation or dosage titration
Anthelmintic Agents			
albendazole	Albenza	800 mg/day in 2 divided doses for 8 – 30 days	+ used to treat infections with parasitic worms + in sensitized individuals, anaphylaxis may occur within minutes of exposure
Antifungals			
amphotericin B	Amphotec	3 – 4 mg/kg/day	+ used to treat invasive aspergillosis, candidiasis, and endocarditis + acute infusion reactions, sometimes severe, may occur 1 – 3 hours after starting infusion
fluconazole	Diflucan	Up to 1,600 mg/day	+ use in candidiasis infection + associated with QT prolongation and torsades de pointes + serious (sometimes fatal) hepatic toxicity
nystatin	Bio-Statin	400,000 – 600,000 units 4×/day	+ oral candidiasis and intestinal infections + in oral infections: patients who wear dentures must remove and clean them to prevent reinfection
terbinafine	Lamisil	250 mg 1×/day for 6 weeks	+ finger and toe infections and tinea capitis + use caution in patients sensitive to allylamine antifungals + patients should be alert to depressive symptoms/mood changes
Antiparasitics and Antimicrobials			
ivermectin	Stromectol, Soolantra	150 – 200 mcg/kg	+ parasitic infections + repeated treatment may be required in immunocompromised patients

| nitazoxanide | Alinia | 500 mg every 12 hours for 3 days | + used in *C. difficile* infection or in giardiasis
+ possible hypersensitivity to nitazoxanide or inactive ingredients |

Antiplatelets

| aspirin | Ecotrin, Bayer Aspirin | + Primary preventative: 81 mg/day
+ Medical therapy (post-MI): 162 – 325 mg | + increases risk of GI bleeding
+ should not be given to children or infants with viral infections (Reye syndrome) |
| clopidogrel | Plavix | Loading dose of 300 mg followed by 75 mg 1×/day | + increased bleeding risk
+ patients with renal impairment should be closely monitored |

Antipsychotics (Conventional and Atypical)

chlorpromazine	Thorazine	30 – 800 mg/day in 2 – 4 divided doses	+ may alter cardiac conduction + chlorpromazine can suppress the cough reflex; aspiration of vomit is possible
droperidol	Inapsine	5 – 10 mg	+ used for undifferentiated agitation + can also be used for postoperative nausea and vomiting + possible impaired physical or mental abilities from CNS depression + black box warning due to arrhythmias
haloperidol	Haldol	0.5 – 10 mg depending on degree of agitation	+ used for acute agitation + patients > 65 with dementia-related psychosis exhibit increased mortality + possible impaired physical or mental abilities from CNS depression
olanzapine	Zyprexa	+ 5 – 10 mg 1×/day + Max: 60 mg/day	+ patients > 65 with dementia-related psychosis exhibit increased mortality + risk of post-injection delirium/sedation syndrome
ziprasidone	Geodon	10 mg every 2 hours or 20 mg every 4 hours	+ in the ED used for acute agitation + risk for leukopenia, neutropenia, and agranulocytosis + possible esophageal dysmotility and aspiration

ARBs

| telmisartan | Micardis | 20 – 40 mg 1×/day | + management of hypertension
+ salt- or volume-depleted patients may experience symptomatic hypotension |

GENERIC Name	BRAND Name(s)	DOSAGE	CONTRAINDICATIONS and Nursing Considerations
ARBs (continued)			
valsartan	Diovan	80 mg or 160 mg 1×/day	+ used for management of hypertension or CHF + hyperkalemia possible in case of renal dysfunction, diabetes mellitus, use of potassium-sparing diuretics, potassium supplements
losartan	Cozaar	50 mg 1×/day; titrate as needed based on patient response up to 100 mg/day	+ unlikely to be newly prescribed in ED + management of hypertension + salt- or volume-depleted patients may experience symptomatic hypotension
Antitremors			
amantadine	Gocovri	137 mg 1×/day; after 1 week, increase to usual dose of 274 mg 1×/day	+ used for Parkinson's disease, extrapyramidal symptoms, and restless leg syndrome + risk of compulsive behaviors and/or loss of impulse control + suicidal ideation/attempt and depression in patients with and without a history of psychiatric illness
benztropine	Cogentin	1 – 2 mg 2 – 3×/day for reactions developing soon after initiation of antipsychotic medication	+ indicated for management of drug-induced extrapyramidal symptoms + used in parkinsonism + may be associated with confusion, visual hallucinations, or excitement + monitor patients with tachycardia
Antivirals			
acyclovir	Zovirax	400 mg 5×/day for 10 days	+ can be used for herpes simplex virus, cytomegalovirus, and new-onset Bell's palsy + neurotoxicity may be more common in patients with renal impairment + maintain adequate hydration during oral or IV therapy
valacyclovir	Valtrex	1 g 2×/day for 7 – 10 days	+ can be used for herpes simplex virus, cytomegalovirus, new-onset Bell's palsy, and shingles + risk for adverse CNS effects such as agitation, hallucinations, confusion, delirium, seizures, and encephalopathy

Benzodiazepines

alprazolam	Xanax	0.25 – 0.5 mg 3×/day	+ treatment of generalized anxiety disorder + associated with anterograde amnesia + possible impaired physical or mental abilities from CNS depression
diazepam	Valium	10 mg initially; may administer 5 – 10 mg 3 – 4 hours later	+ risks from concomitant use of opioids + used in anxiety and agitation or acute alcohol withdrawal
lorazepam	Ativan	2 – 3 mg/day	+ risks from concomitant use of opioids + used in anxiety and agitation or acute alcohol withdrawal
midazolam	Versed	2 – 3 mg	+ used for anxiety, sedation + used for status epilepticus + associated with anterograde amnesia + associated with respiratory depression and respiratory arrest

Beta-Blockers

atenolol	Tenormin	50 mg 1×/day	+ used for angina pectoris, A-fib, and ventricular arrhythmias + contraindicated in patients with bronchospastic disease + use caution in patients with conditions such as sick sinus syndrome
carvedilol	Coreg	6.25 mg 2×/day	+ used in heart failure and hypertension + measure apical heart rate before administering + hold for bradycardia
labetalol	Trandate	10 – 20 mg IV push over 2 minutes	+ indicated for hypertension or hypertensive urgency/emergency + monitor vitals (BP and pulse) throughout administration + symptomatic hypotension with or without syncope may occur
metoprolol	Lopressor	50 mg 2×/day	+ indicated for A-fib, atrial flutter, angina, and hypertension + monitor vitals (BP and pulse) throughout administration + symptomatic hypotension with or without syncope may occur

GENERIC Name	BRAND Name(s)	DOSAGE	CONTRAINDICATIONS and Nursing Considerations
Beta-Blockers (continued)			
propranolol	Hemangeol	10 – 30 mg/dose every 6 – 8 hours	+ used for A-fib, hypertension, migraine headache prophylaxis + contraindicated in patients with bronchospastic disease + monitor patients with myasthenia gravis closely
Bronchodilators			
albuterol	Proventil	2.5 mg 3 – 4×/day as needed	+ used for bronchospasm and asthma exacerbation + possibility of paradoxical bronchospasm
formoterol	Perforomist	12 mcg every 12 hours	+ used for treatment of asthma and COPD and exercise-induced bronchospasm + possibility of paradoxical, life-threatening bronchospasm
ipratropium	Atrovent HFA	2 inhalations (34 mcg) 4×/day	+ used in COPD and acute asthma exacerbations + often adjunct with albuterol + may cause dizziness and blurred vision
levalbuterol	Xopenex	1.25 – 2.5 mg every 20 minutes for 3 doses	+ indicated for bronchospasm or asthma exacerbation + use with caution in patients with cardiovascular disease + use with caution in hyperthyroidism; may stimulate thyroid activity
racemic epinephrine	Asthmanefrin	1 – 3 inhalations of 2.25%	+ for use in bronchospasm and croup as an upper airway instruction
Calcium Channel Blockers			
amlodipine	Norvasc	2.5 – 5 mg 1×/day	+ known to cause increased angina and/or MI with initiation + symptomatic hypotension can occur
diltiazem	Cardizem	120 mg 1×/day	+ transient dermatologic reactions have been observed + carefully consider use in patients with hepatic impairment
Diuretics			
bumetanide	Bumex	0.5 – 2 mg/dose 1 – 2×/day	+ in excess, can induce serious diuresis causing fluid and electrolyte loss + asymptomatic hyperuricemia has been reported with use

furosemide	Lasix	20 – 80 mg/dose	+ in excess, can induce serious diuresis causing fluid and electrolyte loss + fluid status renal function should be monitored to prevent oliguria
hydrochlorothi-azide	Microzide	25 – 100 mg/day	+ hypokalemia, hypochloremic alkalosis, hypomagnesemia, and hyponatremia may occur + hypersensitivity reactions may occur with hydrochlorothiazide
mannitol	Osmitrol	0.25 – 1 g/kg/dose	+ indicated for use in management of intracranial pressure + avoid extravasation of IV infusions of mannitol: vesicant

H₂ Blockers

ranitidine	Zantac	150 mg 2×/day	+ rare cases of reversible confusion have been associated with ranitidine + elevation in ALT levels has occurred with higher doses

Inotropes

milrinone	Primacor	50 mcg/kg administered over 10 minutes	+ indicated for use in inotropic support in heart failure + some cases of ventricular dysrhythmias (non-sustained V-tach and supraventricular dysrhythmias)

Immunosuppressants

methotrexate	Otrexup; Rasuvo; Rheumatrex	100 – 500 mg/m²	+ indicated for use in the ED for ectopic pregnancy + black box warning for fetal toxicity, chemotherapeutic agent

Mood Stabilizers

lithium	Lithobid	600 – 900 mg/day	+ lithium toxicity is possible at doses close to therapeutic levels and is closely related to serum concentrations + may cause CNS depression + may cause behavior changes

Muscle Relaxants/Paralytics

rocuronium	Zemuron	8 – 12 mcg/kg/minute	+ resistance may occur in burn patients + carefully consider use in patients with cardiovascular disease
succinylcholine	Anectine	0.6 mg/kg	+ risk of bradycardia may be increased with second dose + may cause a transient increase in intracranial pressure

GENERIC Name	BRAND Name(s)	DOSAGE	CONTRAINDICATIONS and Nursing Considerations
Muscle Relaxants/Paralytics (continued)			
vecuronium bromide	Norcuron	0.08 – 0.1 mg/kg	+ severe anaphylactic reactions possible + carefully consider use in patients with hepatic impairment
Nitrates			
nitroglycerin	Nitro-Bid; Nitro-Dur	2.5 – 6.5 mg 3 – 4×/day	+ indicated for use in angina, myocardial infarction + may cause headache + may lead to syncope or near syncope
Nonsteroidal Anti-Inflammatory Drugs (NSAIDs)			
naproxen	Aleve	500 – 1,000 mg/day	+ increased risk of serious (sometimes fatal) cardiovascular thrombotic events + increased risk of GI inflammation, ulceration, bleeding
Opioids			
codeine	N/A	15 – 60 mg every 4 hours as needed	+ may cause CNS depression + may cause or aggravate constipation
fentanyl	Duragesic; Fentora	0.35 – 0.5 mcg/kg every 30 – 60 minutes as needed	+ may cause severe hypotension + life-threatening or fatal respiratory depression possible
hydrocodone	Vicodin	10 – 20 mg/dose	+ possible impaired physical or mental abilities from CNS depression + life-threatening or fatal respiratory depression possible
hydromorphone	Dilaudid	2 – 4 mg every 4 – 6 hours	+ black box warning for high risk for addiction + possibility of severe hypotension (including orthostatic hypotension and syncope); patients with hypovolemia should be monitored
morphine sulfate	Duramorph	2.5 – 5 mg every 3 – 4 hours	+ possible impaired physical or mental abilities from CNS depression + life-threatening or fatal respiratory depression possible
oxycodone	OxyContin	5 – 15 mg every 4 – 6 hours as needed	+ high risk for addiction, should be used carefully + life-threatening respiratory depression possible

Potassium-Removing Agents

sodium polystyrene sulfonate	Kayexalate	15 g 1 – 4×/day	+ use for hyperkalemia + severe hypokalemia may occur + intestinal necrosis and other serious gastrointestinal events may occur

Proton-Pump Inhibitors

lansoprazole	Prevacid	15 mg 1×/day for up to 8 weeks	+ symptomatic GERD, erosive esophagitis, peptic ulcer disease + risk of fundic gland polyps; long-term use increases risk
pantoprazole	Protonix	20 – 40 mg 1×/day for 4 weeks	+ used for GERD and for erosive esophagitis + long-term use may result in *C. difficile* infection + increased risk of GI infection

Sedatives/Hypnotics

etomidate	Amidate	0.2 – 0.6 mg/kg	+ used in the ED for induction of anesthesia for rapid sequence intubation + may induce cardiac depression in elderly patients
ketamine	Ketalar	0.5 – 2 mg/kg (IV)	+ used for moderate sedation and for pain in the ED + ketamine increases the risk of laryngospasm in the presence of upper respiratory disease + may cause dependence
propofol	Diprivan	100 – 150 mcg/kg/minute	+ used for sedation in procedures or for sedation of patients with ET tubes + use with caution in patients with severe cardiac disease + use with caution in patients with increased intracranial pressure

Steroids

dexamethasone	Decadron	0.75 – 9 mg/day	+ has many indications + generally used to reduce inflammation + contraindicated in systemic fungal infections
fluticasone	Flovent Diskus	44 mg/actuation	+ indicated for use in prevention of asthma attacks + avoid use with concurrent infections + contraindicated in immunosuppressed patients

GENERIC Name	BRAND Name(s)	DOSAGE	CONTRAINDICATIONS and Nursing Considerations
Steroids (continued)			
methylpredniso-lone	Medrol	4 – 48 mg orally, gradual taper off	+ has many uses, such as dermatologic concerns and endocrine disorders + may result in mild allergic reaction
prednisolone	Millipred	5 – 60 mg/day	+ acute myopathy has been reported with high-dose corticosteroids + psychiatric disturbances associated with corticosteroid use
prednisone	Deltasone	5 – 60 mg/day	+ may cause hypercortisolism + Kaposi's sarcoma associated with prolonged use of corticosteroids
Tricyclic Antidepressants			
amitriptyline	Elavil	75 – 100 mg/day	+ patients newly prescribed may have increased suicidal ideation + should not be given with MAOIs + may take up to 3 weeks to be effective
Triptans			
sumatriptan	Imitrex	+ 25 – 100 mg + Max dose: 200 mg/day	+ indicated for migraine headache + treats cluster headaches
Thrombolytics			
streptokinase	Streptase	+ MI: 1.5 million intl units + PE/DVT: 250,000 intl units	+ indicated in MI, DVT, and pulmonary embolism + may cause bleeding + may cause syncope
tenecteplase	TNKase	+ Dosage based on weight chart + Max dose: 50 mg	+ indicated for use in patients experiencing heart attack who cannot get to a cath lab in a reasonable period of time + increases risk of bleeding or hemorrhage + contraindicated in trauma patients
tPA (tissue plasminogen activator)	n/a	+ Dose is based on weight and time of infusion + 100 mg max dose	+ for use in patients with ischemic stroke + must be administered in specific window of time + window is measured from onset of symptoms + inclusion criteria is strict

Vasodilators

sildenafil	Viagra, Revatio	10 mg injected 3×/day	+ used in pulmonary hypertension + also used for erectile dysfunction + may cause persistent hypotension
sodium nitroprus-side	Nipride, Nitro-press	+ HTN dose: 0.3 mcg/kg/minute + CHF dose: 1,015 mcg/minute	+ used in congestive heart failure and hypertension + not suitable for IV push or direct injection, must be diluted + can cause severe hypotension and cyanide toxicity

Vasopressors

dobutamine	Dobutrex	2.5 – 15 mcg/kg/minute	+ inotropic medication in cardiac muscle failure + may cause severe changes in blood pressure, high or low
dopamine	Intropin	0.5 – 20 mcg/kg/minute	+ used for hypotension in the presence of shock + do not use in patients with uncorrected tachyarrhythmias or V-fib
epinephrine	Adrenalin, EpiPen	+ 1 mg (cardiac arrest) + 0.3 – 0.5 mg (anaphylaxis)	+ used in anaphylaxis + used in cardiac arrest + be cautious in the presence of hypertension

Other Drugs

acetylcysteine	Mucomyst	+ Initial: 140 mg/kg + Follow on: 70 mg/kg every 4 hours	+ used in acetaminophen overdose (antidote) + pay special care to dosing and administration schedule + do not wait for plasma results in overdose to administer antidote
atropine	AtroPen	+ 0.5 – 1 mg every 5 minutes + Max dose: 2 mg	+ used in symptomatic bradycardia + contraindicated with acute hemorrhage + use cautiously with patients with renal or hepatic disease
calcium gluconate	Kalcinate	1 – 2 g/day	+ given for hypocalcemia + should be considered with multiple transfusions of blood products + risk for toxicity, monitor serum levels
filgrastim	Neupogen	6 mcg/kg 2×/day	+ bone marrow stimulant + treats radiation exposure + used in severe neutropenia + monitor for signs of allergic reaction

GENERIC Name	BRAND Name(s)	DOSAGE	CONTRAINDICATIONS and Nursing Considerations
Other Drugs (continued)			
flumazenil	Romazicon	+ 0.2 mg/dose + Max dose: 1 mg	+ GABA receptor antagonist + treats benzodiazepine overdose + institute seizure precautions
hydroxocobal-amin	Cyanokit	5 g/dose; max dose 10 g	+ cyanide treatment + use cautiously in concurrent infection
levothyroxine	Synthroid	75 – 125 mcg/day	+ given for thyroid supplementation + assess apical pulse before administration + monitor for toxicity
magnesium sulfate	N/A	1 g every 6 hours, max 4 doses	+ prevents seizures + high-alert medication + assess deep tendon reflexes frequently
methylene blue	ProvayBlue	0.1 – 0.2 mL/kg	+ used to treat methemoglobinemia + contraindicated in G6PD deficiency
naloxone	Narcan	Initial: 0.4 – 2 mg; may need to repeat doses every 2 – 3 minutes	+ for the complete or partial reversal of opioid depression + use with caution in patients with cardiovascular disease
naltrexone	Vivitrol	50 mg/day	+ treatment of alcohol-use disorder + naltrexone may cause a patient to respond to lower opioid doses than previously used
physostigmine salicylate	N/A	Initial: 0.5 – 2 mg	+ reversal of central nervous system anti-cholinergic syndrome + patient must have a normal QRS interval, as measured by ECG, in order to receive
pralidoxime	Protopam Chloride	+ Loading: 30 mg/kg + Maintenance: 8 – 10 mg/kg/hour	+ treatment for organophosphate poisoning + pralidoxime is NOT indicated for the treatment of carbamate poisoning + patients with renal impairment should be closely monitored
rasagiline mesylate	Azilect	1 mg 1×/day	+ antiparkinson + contraindicated in concomitant use of an MAO inhibitor + may cause psychiatric and behavioral disturbances

scopolamine	Transderm Scop	0.6 – 1 mg	+ antiemetic + lower doses (0.1 mg) may have vagal mimetic effects
sodium nitrate	N/A	300 mg; 10 mL of a 3% solution	+ used for cyanide poisoning, given in conjunction with sodium nitrate + administer sodium nitrite first, followed immediately by the administration of sodium thiosulfate
sodium thiosulfate	N/A	12.5 g; 50 mL of a 25% solution	+ used for cyanide poisoning + use with caution with patients for whom the diagnosis of cyanide poisoning is uncertain
tamsulosin	Flomax	0.4 mg/day	+ used for urinary retention + if angina occurs or worsens, discontinue + may exacerbate heart failure symptoms + priapism has been associated with use

Made in the USA
Monee, IL
27 May 2022

97121528R00254